Pandemics and Health Care:
Principles, Processes and Practice

Pandemics and Health Care: Principles, Processes and Practice

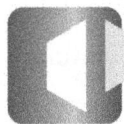

juta

Pandemics and Health Care: Principles, Processes and Practice

First published 2021

© Juta and Company (Pty) Ltd
First Floor, Sunclare Building, 21 Dreyer Street,
Claremont, 7708, Cape Town
www.juta.co.za

ISBN: 978 1 48513 174 8 (print)
ISBN: 978 1 48513 175 5 (webpdf)
ISBN: 978 1 48513 176 2 (ipub)

Production Specialist: Zainub Gamieldien
Editor: The Black Letter
Proofreader: Deidre du Preez
Cover Designer: Simplicitas Design
Indexer: Lexinfo
Typeset in 11 on 13 pt Minion Pro Regular
Typesetting by Elinye Ithuba DTP Solutions

CONTENTS

CHAPTER 1
INTRODUCTION TO PANDEMICS AND HEALTHCARE: PRINCIPLES, PROCESSES AND PRACTICE

CHAPTER 2
PANDEMICS: GLOBAL HEALTH SECURITY

DEDICATIONS

This book is dedicated to our South African healthcare practitioners and healthcare practitioners around the globe who have been treating patients infected by COVID-19, often under difficult circumstances. Many succumbed during this outbreak.

Several colleagues have helped in managing this pandemic on a policy and implementation level. Some of these actions have been seminal in the South African and global response while others have done so by speaking truth to power. We thank them for their contributions.

We also acknowledge the many colleagues who have assisted with disseminating honest and objective information during this time.

IN ADDITION:

Daynia Ballot dedicates this book to her late husband, Charles, and their wonderful children – Nina, James, Lisa and George.

Ames Dhai dedicates this book to her husband, Faruk, her granddaughter, Nura, and all the children who have lost a significant part of their childhood due to the pandemic.

PREFACE

Public health experts regularly warn that pandemics are not rare events. While the highly publicised more recent pandemics, H1N1 Influenza, the original SARS corona virus and the tick-borne Zika virus epidemics are top of mind, current international experience suggests that the world will experience one new, deadly infectious organism each year. Fortunately, most of these outbreaks are geographically localised and/or only cause minimal morbidity and mortality. The consequence of this is that the world continues to be complacent, resulting in the global lack of preparedness for the occasional seismic outbreak such as the COVID-19 outbreak we are currently experiencing.

That all countries and regions were underprepared for the current pandemic is patently clear. Given that the SARS-Cov-2 virus initially evaded detection – with some evidence suggesting that it was already well established prior to the first reported cases in Wuhan – and was then able to spread across the world, overcoming all supposed barriers put in place to limit its spread, is overwhelming testament to this.

What is also clear is that no country or region had adequate public health structures in place to manage the current pandemic. Even in the best-resourced countries and regions, the virus spread with ease. Once the pandemic had taken hold, it rapidly became clear that the treatment facilities required were inadequate, not only in the poor regions but also in Milan, New York and Madrid. Even the most basic of medical interventions such as oxygen supplementation was and continues to be short in supply. Most poignant in this regard is the experience in India, where many are reported to have died from hypoxia alone. How can this be?

The fact that the origin of this new variant of the beta-corona virus is still disputed, despite the currently available gene sequencing and bioinformatics technologies, suggests that even in such a crisis, the resources needed to understand the most recent and severe pandemic, are still not being made available. Similarly, while the rapid pace of vaccine development using new biotechnologies is impressive, the fact that virus mutations seem to be outstripping the efficiency of the vaccines is concerning. Undoubtedly, earlier investment in identifying a more stable immunological target on the virus would have probably been of value.

Perhaps most concerning has been the political and social response to the COVID-19 pandemic. On the political front, the lack of consistent messaging and, at times, illogical decision-making has been widespread. Unfortunately, the pandemic has also been used to drive political agendas with devastating consequences in many parts of the world. Corruption at all levels has been rife: from the procurement of urgent PPE and medical supplies to the sanitising of public facilities are small examples of what has happened in our country and several others globally. On the social front, without clear guidance, it is not surprising that the simple preventive measures of mask-wearing, social distancing and self-imposed quarantining and isolation have not been effective. The jumping of queues to gain early access to vaccines outside of national priority guidelines has also been evident worldwide.

Failure to effectively manage such a pandemic occurs because we are human and fallible. What is however clear is that we cannot just leave it at this. That there will be another outbreak is inevitable, and that such an outbreak may have the possibility of being more dangerous is an unavoidable reality. We must be prepared for such an eventuality. It is clear that all countries must improve their systems of preparedness and the quality of their response. This is important to save lives, protect livelihoods and to alter the trajectories of pandemics. The requirements for this are well-established. Amongst others, they include the need for:

- Tracking systems to know if and where new infectious organisms are developing.
- Trained disease detectives that identify such events as they develop.
- Well-funded country-based public health institutions which are able to coordinate and manage all epidemics, both of a communicable and of a non-communicable nature. These country-based institutions must cooperate with regional and international bodies and must be able to do so without restriction.
- Support from national, regional and international laboratory networks.

It is essential that when 'fires' start, that they are put out before there is a conflagration. The continued mantra must be to find, stop and prevent! When a crisis develops, public health interests must trump (pun intended) all vested political interests. To do so requires that public health experts are trusted and that their advice is used in managing these complex, emotive and treacherous times. It also requires strict adherence to evidence-based policy implementation and clinical decision-making. Those who are prepared to set these basic tenets of modern health care aside must be scorned. Anything less than adhering to these principles will be paid for in lives.

Pandemics and Health Care has been compiled to bring together some of the many lessons learnt over the last 18 months in South Africa, since the first South African patient with the SARS-Cov-2 virus was detected in March 2020. Since then, globally, there have been more than 219 million recorded cases of people infected with the virus and 4.55 million deaths (as of 21 September 2021). The book draws from global experiences as well and will be relevant to readership both locally and abroad. It has been written to assist readers in navigating the new landscape and provides information on the appropriate management of pandemics and emergencies in the healthcare context not only from the medical perspective, but also from economic, social, ethical, legal and human rights considerations. The book comprises two sections. The first section, made up of the first 14 chapters, straddles disciplines related to health care. It has generic application. The second section, comprising the next 10 chapters, are specific to relevant health science disciplines, with its focus being on technical and clinical management. It is hoped that individuals at various levels, including academics, educators, researchers, students and civil society, will benefit from engaging with the book.

CONTRIBUTORS

Ames Dhai (MASSAf, PhD, MBChB, FCOG, LLM, PGDip-IntResEthics) is the founder and past director of the Steve Biko Centre for Bioethics at the Wits Faculty of Health Sciences (2007–2019), visiting professor of bioethics and health law at the Wits School of Clinical Medicine, specialist ethicist at the Office of the President and CEO of the South African Medical Research Council (SAMRC) and member of the Academy of Science South Africa. She is a leading authority in bioethics both internationally and locally, and can be credited with entrenching bioethics and human rights as an integral aspect of health sciences in South Africa. She serves on a number of ethico-regulatory bodies in the country and internationally, including being chairperson of the SAMRC Bioethics Advisory Panel, vice-chairperson of the Ministerial Advisory Committee on COVID-19 Vaccinations and vice-chairperson of the International Bioethics Committee of UNESCO.

Daynia Ballot (MBBCh (Wits – 1982), PhD (Wits – 1989), Fellow of the College of Paediatrics of South Africa – 1990, (registered subspecialist in Neonatology with Health Professions Council of SA – 1993) is a neonatologist and is currently head of the School of Clinical Medicine at Wits University. She worked with Prof Bothwell in his Iron and Red Cell Metabolic Unit and obtained her PhD in Iron Nutrition and Metabolism in 1989. Professor Ballot qualified as a paediatrician in 1990 and registered as a neonatologist in 1992. She has a strong interest in neonatal research in South Africa, particularly in neonatal sepsis, determinants of survival in very low birth weight infants and the neurodevelopmental outcome of high-risk newborns. She is an NRF-rated researcher and has more than 120 peer-reviewed publications. She was promoted to associate professor in 2002 and personal professor in 2019.

Martin Veller (MBBCh, FCS (SA), MMed (Surg)), a vascular surgeon, is the past dean of the Faculty of Health Sciences of the University of the Witwatersrand (June 2014 to December 2020). Prior to this, he was the professor and head of the Department of Surgery, (November 2001 to February 2013) and the head of the Division of Vascular Surgery (January 1992 to June 2014). His pre- and post-graduate training also occurred at the University of the Witwatersrand, where he qualified in general surgery in 1987. He subsequently undertook a vascular surgical research fellowship at St. Mary's Hospital, Imperial College, London (1990 to 1991). In April 2002, he was awarded an *ad hominem* professorship and became professor emeritus in January 2021. He previously has been the chairman of the Association of Surgeons, president of the World Federation of Vascular Societies, president of the Vascular Society of Southern Africa and president of the College of Surgeons of the Colleges of Medicine of South Africa.

Paula Barnard-Ashton (BSc OT, MSc OT, PhD, PGDip HPEL) established and manages eFundanathi – Learn with Us in the School of Therapeutic Sciences, Faculty of Health Sciences at the University of the Witwatersrand. eFundanathi supports the online and blended learning initiatives across the School through professional learning engagement with lecturers and students, supporting the redesign of curricula and establishing an active learning environment – the eZone. Her PhD investigated the integration of blended learning into the undergraduate occupational therapy curriculum. She is recognised as a leader in health professions education and is chair of the Northern Chapter of the Sub-Saharan African Association of Health Educationalists.

Lucille Blumberg (DSc (Med) *Honoris Causa* (Wits) MB BCH MMed (Clin Micro) ID (SA) FFTM (RCPS, Glasgow) DTM&H DOH DCH) is a deputy director at the National Institute for Communicable Diseases (NICD) of the National Health Laboratory Service, and founding head of the Division of Public Health Surveillance and Response. She is currently a medical consultant to this division and the Centre for Emerging, Zoonotic and Parasitic Diseases, and an infectious diseases consultant to 'Right to Care' as of October 2021. Her major interests are in outbreak response, malaria, rabies, the viral haemorrhagic fevers and zoonotic diseases, travel–related infections and mass gatherings. Professor Blumberg has worked on a large number of outbreaks including COVID-19, the 2009 A H1N1 influenza pandemic, polio, avian influenza A H5N2, rabies, cholera, typhoid, and the new arenavirus – the Lujo virus. During the COVID-19 pandemic she established the DATCOV surveillance system for hospitalised patients, and was vice-chair of the WHO IHR COVID-19 review committee. She is a medical graduate of the University of the Witwatersrand, an associate professor at the University of Stellenbosch, and lecturer in the Faculty of Veterinary Medicine, University of Pretoria, South Africa. She is a member of a number of national and international advisory bodies.

Lawrence Chauke (MBCHB (UCT), BTh (ATS), Dip HIV Man (SA), Mmed (O&G) (Pret), FCOG (SA), Cert Maternal and Fetal Medicine (SA), MSc (Clinical Research) (Liverpool), PhD) is an adjunct professor, Maternal and Fetal Medicine Specialist, an assistant head of the School of Clinical Medicine responsible for Cluster C at the University of the Witwatersrand, and the clinical head of the Department of Obstetrics and Gynaecology at Charlotte Maxeke Johannesburg Academic Hospital. He is also the head of Charlotte Maxeke Cluster, former Gauteng Provincial Chair of Maternal Clinical Governance Committee and former member of Gauteng Provincial Clinical Advisory Committee, an advisory committee to the MEC of Gauteng Department of Health. His interest is in perinatal and maternal health. He has received a number of local and international awards in recognition of his work in the field. He is a member of local and international organisations.

Indhrin Chetty (MBChB, FCPsych, LLB, Certificate in Forensic Psychiatry) is academic head of the Division of Forensic Psychiatry, Department of Psychiatry, Faculty of Health Sciences, University of the Witwatersrand, Johannesburg. Dr Chetty practices as a forensic psychiatrist in the Forensic Neuroscience Unit at Sterkfontein Hospital, Krugersdorp. This allows him to indulge his interest in psychiatry and the law. He has a keen interest in ethics and its practical application in the area of animal rights in his endeavour towards a cruelty-free lifestyle.

Shren Chetty (MBChB, DMH, MMED, FC Psych) is a psychiatrist working at Weskoppies hospital in general adult psychiatry, and previously at Sterkfontein hospital in forensic psychiatry. She completed her MBChB at UKZN in 2011. Her interest developed while working in psychiatry during her community service at Addington Hospital. Thereafter, she was a medical officer in psychiatry at Dora Nginza Hospital and obtained her DMH (SA) in 2015. Her MMED topic was HIV and mental illness, which was published. Both MMED(Psych) and FC Psych (SA) training was completed in Weskoppies Hospital through UP in 2019. At her leisure, she enjoys travelling and adventuring outdoors with her two dogs.

David Chiriboga (MD, MPH) is a physician focused on sustainability, health equity and human rights advocacy. He established a healthcare system to serve indigenous peoples living in conditions of extreme poverty in Ecuador. He is former Minister of Health of Ecuador, president of the Council of Health Ministers of South America and member of the Executive Board of the World Health Organization. He supported strengthening the healthcare system in Liberia, post-Ebola. He is also associate professor of medicine at the University of Massachusetts Medical School and co-founder of the Global Movement for Sustainable Health Equity (SHEM), with over 200 institutions united in the fight for equity in the response to the pandemic.

Tobias Chirwa (PhD, PGDip, MSc, BSc) is an Associate Professor and Head of the Wits School of Public Health. He is the Director for the Wellcome Trust funded Sub-Saharan Africa Consortium for Advanced Biostatistics (SSACAB) Training and Principal Investigator (PI) for Fogarty grant on Expanding Capacity in HIV Implementation Science in South Africa, together with the Phase I WHO/TDR Implementation Research. He has contributed towards research projects on Disease Surveillance, STI Care and Maternal and Newborn Health. He continues to work on tuberculosis diagnosis, treatment adherence and post-treatment survival, and child health. His methodological interest is in longitudinal data analysis.

Yahya E. Choonara (BPharm, MPharm, PhD) is chair and head of the department of Pharmacy and Pharmacology at the University of the Witwatersrand (Wits), Johannesburg, South Africa (SA). He is a professor of pharmaceutics, Head of Pharmaceutics and director of the Wits Advanced Drug Delivery Platform (WADDP) research unit and National Research Foundation (NRF) Chair in Pharmaceutical Biomaterials and Polymer-Engineered Drug Delivery Technologies. He features in Stanford University's Top 2% of pharmaceutical scientists globally and holds a strong research position globally in targeted drug delivery, nanomedicines, regenerative medicine and functional biomaterials. For 21 years, he has been at the forefront of producing targeted medicines to treat infectious, hereditary and lifestyle diseases and continues to make a major impact centred on intellectual property generation and translational research in the pharmaceutical sciences. He is an inventor of 12 patent families across infectious diseases, neurotrauma, oral peptide delivery, targeted cancer therapy and complex therapeutic devices for the most challenging illnesses. He has published >300 research articles in ISI-accredited journals, 42 book chapters, 10 editorials, and was the editor of two books. His work is highly cited, with more than 8 000 citations.

Cheryl Cohen (MD, PhD) is professor in epidemiology at the University of the Witwatersrand and heads the Centre for Respiratory Disease and Meningitis at the National Institute for Communicable Diseases in South Africa. Through her work she aims to generate evidence to guide policy for the control of respiratory diseases and meningitis. She heads up a team responsible for the national surveillance of respiratory diseases and meningitis for South Africa. Her main research focus is infectious respiratory diseases including burden of disease, disease transmission and risk groups for severe illness. This includes assessment of the impact and effectiveness of interventions, such as vaccination, aiming to reduce disease burden. She is a member of several national and international advisory committees and working groups mainly related to influenza, SARS-CoV-2 and other respiratory diseases.

Richard Cooke (B. Business Science, MBBCh, MMed Family Medicine) is department head of Family Medicine and Primary Care, Faculty of Health Sciences, University of the Witwatersrand. He is director of the Faculty Centre for Rural Health. After an early finance career, he switched to medicine, specialising as a family physician. Joining Wits in 2011, he chairs the Graduate Entry Medical Programme Curriculum Committee. He is director of the Wits Nelson Mandela Fidel Castro (NMFC) Collaboration, serving on the NMFC Ministerial Task Team. He is a Fellowship of the College of Family Physicians (FCFP) examiner. A keen advocate of partnerships, Adj Prof Cooke shares responsibility for various COVID-19-related responses in the Johannesburg Metro Health District during the pandemic.

David Francis (MDev, BSocSci) is deputy director of the Southern Centre for Inequality Studies, University of the Witwatersrand, Johannesburg. His research interests focus on labour market economics, the informal economy, and inequality. He is a PhD candidate in economics at Wits University. He was the researcher for the Advisory Panel on the minimum wage in South Africa. He has previously worked as a development consultant, and a policy and budget analyst at South Africa's National Treasury, where he worked in health and social policy.

Mallorie Govender (MBChB, FC Psych (SA), MMED Psych) is a psychiatrist at Waitemata District Health Board currently based in He Puna Waiora in Auckland, New Zealand. She is a former associate lecturer at the University of Witwatersrand Faculty of Health Sciences and is currently an honorary academic for the University of Auckland.

Glenda E. Gray (MBBCh (Wits), FCPaeds (SA), DSc (*honoris causa* Simon Fraser University), DSc (*honoris causa* Stellenbosch University), and LLD (*honoris causa* Rhodes University)) is the first female president of South African Medical Research Council, has received the country's highest honour, the Order of Mapungubwe, granted by the president of SA for achievements in the international area which have served South Africa's interest. She was listed by *Forbes* as one of Africa's 50 most powerful women. She is co-principal investigator of the Sisonke study an open-label, single-arm phase 3B COVID-19 vaccine implementation study for healthcare workers and spearheads the SAMRC funding for COVID-19.

Marc D. Grodman (MD) is a physician-entrepreneur-innovator, founder of two companies in diagnostics and genomics, a board member and chair of Patient Safety and Quality Task Force of the Health Care Leadership Council, a trustee of the New York Academy of Medicine and a member of the CUIMC (Columbia) Board of Advisors. Dr Grodman has been on staff at Columbia University Vagelos College of Physicians and Surgeons since 1983 where he made teaching rounds for over 25 years.

S. Zane Grodman (MD, MS) is currently a third-year pediatrics resident at the Texas Tech-Amarillo programme. He received a BA from the University of Pennsylvania with a double major in History and Anthropology and graduated from the Vagelos College of Physicians and Surgeons at Columbia University, where he also received a Master in Science (Global Health) while working on issues in global health security and research in Zika.

Wilmot James (PhD) is a senior research scholar at Columbia University's Institute for Social and Economic Research and Policy (ISERP) and an honorary professor of public health at the University of the Witwatersrand. He is the author and/or editor of 17 books which include the policy-oriented *Vital Signs: Health Security in South Africa* (2020). He leads the Center for Pandemic Research at ISERP and is an associate director in the programme in vaccine education at the Vagelos College of Physicians and Surgeons. Wilmot serves as a senior consultant in biosecurity to the Nuclear Threat Initiative, is a member of the Accessible Medicines Advisory Board to Chimeron Bio as well as to Resolve to Save Lives. He co-chairs the National Frameworks Focal Group of the G7-led Global Partnership (Against the Spread of Weapons and Materials of Mass Destruction) Africa Signature Initiative.

Waasila Jassat (MBBCh, MMed, FCPHM) works at the National Institute for Communicable Diseases (NICD), where she leads the DATCOV hospital surveillance for COVID-19. She is currently registered towards a PhD at the School of Public Health, University of Western Cape, focused on understanding the gap between health policy and its implementation. Waasila has experience in clinical practice, research and management in the South African public health sector for the past 20 years. Dr Jassat has a strong interest in health systems, particularly in using information for health planning and effective implementation of health programmes.

Preethi Jayrajh (FCPsych, MMed, MBBCh) is currently a consultant psychiatrist at the Auckland District Health Board as well as an honorary academic in the School of Medicine at the University of Auckland, New Zealand. In 2011 she obtained her MBBCh from the University of Witwatersrand (Wits) in Johannesburg and in 2019 went on to qualify with her FCPsych (SA) and MMed (Psychiatry). She held the post of associate lecturer at Wits and was involved in research focusing on post-traumatic stress and depression among refugees and asylum seekers. In her spare time, she enjoys sport, reading and cooking.

Andrew Wooyoung Kim (PhD) is a biological and medical anthropologist whose research integrates biological, epidemiological, and anthropological approaches to understand how social oppression becomes embodied and produces health inequities in historically marginalised communities. His current work traces the biosocial mechanisms underlining the life course and intergenerational mental health effects of violence from apartheid in Soweto, South Africa. Through a collaboration with the Department of Psychiatry at the University of the Witwatersrand, he is also leading a study on the perceptions, experiences, and mental health impacts of COVID-19 in tertiary psychiatric hospitals in Johannesburg. He is a postdoctoral fellow at the Center for Global Heath at the

Massachusetts General Hospital in Boston, USA and an Honorary Researcher at the SAMRC Developmental Pathways for Health Research Unit in the Faculty of Health Sciences at the University of the Witwatersrand.

Lazarus Kuonza (MPH, MBChB) a medical doctor with over 18 years' experience in clinical medicine, public health practice and research, is currently working as senior medical epidemiologist in the Division of Public Health Surveillance and Response of the National Institute for Communicable Diseases (NICD) for South Africa. He heads the South African Field Epidemiology Training Programme (SAFETP), and is jointly appointed as senior lecturer of epidemiology at the School of Public Health of the University of the Witwatersrand and the School of Health Systems and Public Health of the University of Pretoria. Dr Kuonza has keen interests in infectious disease surveillance and outbreak investigations, particularly the use of epidemiological methods to understand their transmission dynamics and inform public health interventions.

Melodie Labuschaigne (MA, DLitt, LLB, LLD) is professor in medical law and ethics in the Department of Jurisprudence in the School of Law, University of South Africa. She has published extensively on legal issues relating to stem cell research, human tissue regulation, genomic and genetic research and assisted reproduction. She is the recipient of a number of research awards and has been involved with the revision and drafting of health legislation and development of policy for the past two decades. She serves on the South African Medical Research Bioethics Advisory Panel and is currently the legal member of the South African National Health Research Ethics Council.

Pralene Maharaj (MBChB, FCPsych, Cert Child and Adolescent Psychiatry, Cert Forensic Psychiatry) is a forensic psychiatrist currently working at Sterkfontein Hospital in Krugersdorp. In addition to establishing a standardised assessment process for the forensic evaluation of children in conflict with the law, Dr Maharaj has also implemented a psychotherapy programme for adult male state patients at Sterkfontein Hospital. She has also contributed to undergraduate and postgraduate teaching. Her professional endeavours highlight her passion for education, advocacy, and the provision of quality clinical and academic services.

Mia Malan (MPhil) founded the Bhekisisa Centre for Health Journalism in 2013. She is the Editor-in-Chief of the Centre and has 25 years of journalism and institution-building experience in legacy media and digital native publications, working in newsrooms and at media development organisations in Johannesburg, Nairobi and Washington, DC. Malan has won over 20 African and international journalism awards. Most recently she received the Excellence in Public Health

Award from the Charlotte Mannya-Maxeke Institute. Mia is a former Knight International Journalism fellow of the International Centre for Journalists and a Reuters Institute for the Study of Journalism fellow at Oxford University. Malan serves on the council of the South African National Editors' Forum.

Maurice Mars (MBChB, MD) is an emeritus professor of teleHealth at the University of KwaZulu-Natal, a department he started in 2002, adjunct professor at Flinders University in Adelaide, and formerly professor of physiology at the University of Natal. He chaired the eHealth sub-committee of the Ministerial Advisory Committee on Health Technology in South Africa and served as an advisor on eHealth in Rwanda. Mars is editor of the *Journal of the International Society for Telemedicine and eHealth*, and has served on committees of the American Telemedicine Association, the International Society for Telemedicine and eHealth and the American Medical Informatics Association.

Maureen Masha (MPH, MBChB, AMP) is a medical advisor at Right to Care, seconded to the National Institute for Communicable Diseases (NICD) Public Health Surveillance and Response Department. She was part of the team that established DATCOV digital platform at NICD in 2020 to report on COVID-19 hospital admissions in both the private and the public sector in all nine provinces in South Africa. She also participated in the Ministerial Advisory Committee (MAC) COVID-19 Pregnancy and Lactating Women Technical Working Group. Her work and dedication to women and children's health, has led to her focus of attention on the impact of COVID-19 pandemic on these two groups of the population. Her greatest philosophy is that a healthy nation starts with excellent mother–child healthcare.

David J. McQuoid-Mason (B Comm (Natal) LLB (Natal) LLM (London) PhD (Natal)), is a professor of law based at the Centre for Socio-Legal Studies at the University of KwaZulu-Natal, Durban and president of the Commonwealth Legal Education Association. He has published more than 300 articles in law and medical journals, contributed more than 60 chapters to books, and co-authored 21 books and manuals in the medical and nursing field. He has visited over 132 countries, and has delivered over 180 papers at national and over 250 at international law and medical conferences.

Bruce Mellado (PhD) is a professor at the University of the Witwatersrand, a senior researcher of iThemba LABS and serves as the Director of the Institute for Collider Particle Physics. He is the National Contact Physicist of South Africa at the ATLAS experiment at CERN, the Chairman of the Institutional Board of the Tile Calorimeter and the co-Chair of the Nuclear Particle and Radiation Division of South African Institute of Physics. He is the recipient of several awards and fellowships. He is an Internationally acclaimed, B1 rated researcher of the NRF. He is a member of the Gauteng Premier's COVID-19 Advisory Committee, where he leads work on predictions. He is also the Co-President of the Africa-Canada Artificial Intelligence Data Modelling Consortium.

Mongezi Mdhluli (PhD, MBA) is the chief research operation officer at the office of the South African Medical Research Council's (SAMRC) President and CEO and is a member of the SAMRC Executive Management Committee. He has been involved in research ethics for over 10 years, is a member of the South African National Bioethics Committee and served on several ethics committees. He was instrumental in revitalising the SAMRC's ethics committee, establishing the Bioethics Advisory Panel and continues to promote a culture of responsible conduct of research in the SAMRC. He serves on many national and international bodies. With the emergence of COVID-19, he contributed in the development of the Framework for Fair, Equitable and Timely Allocation of COVID-19 Vaccines in Africa, which has been endorsed by the Africa Centres for Disease Control and Prevention.

Colin Nigel Menezes (MD, MMed (Int Med), Dip HIV Mang (SA), DTM&H, FCP (SA), Cert ID (SA), MSc Med (Bioethics and Health Law), PhD)) is an associate professor at the University of the Witwatersrand. He is the academic head of the Department of Internal Medicine, and the clinical head of the Division of Infectious Diseases at Chris Hani Baragwanath Academic Hospital. His research interests are in the field of infectious diseases and other conditions in general medicine. He also has an interest in health law and medical ethics.

Mervyn Mer (MBBCh, Dip PEC (SA), FCP (SA), Pulmonology subspecialty, Cert Critical Care (SA), M Med (Int Med,) FRCP (London), FCCP, PhD)) is professor, specialist physician, pulmonologist and intensivist based at Charlotte Maxeke Johannesburg Academic Hospital (CMJAH) and Faculty of Health Sciences, University of the Witwatersrand. He is the clinical head of the Adult Multidisciplinary Intensive Care Unit at CMJAH and academic head of Critical Care at the University of the Witwatersrand. He is the current chairperson of the Global Intensive Care Working Group of the European Society of Intensive Care Medicine and is extensively involved in multiple local, regional and global bodies, societies, panels and organisations. He is the recipient of numerous awards.

Mantoa Mokhachane (MBBCh, FCPaeds, MMed Paeds, PGDip-Health Science Education) is currently the director of the Unit of Undergraduate Medical Education at the University of Witwatersrand, Johannesburg, which she joined in 2015. She worked as a neonatologist at the Chris Hani Baragwanath Hospital Neonatal Unit for 18 years prior to branching into Medical Education. Dr Mokhachane has been a member of the Human Research Ethics Committee at the University of Witwatersrand for over 18 years and is also a member of the SAMRC Bioethics Advisory Panel. She has been a member of several ethics' committees, including SAMRC and South African Human Sciences Research Council.

Oluseyi Ajayi Mojisola (MSc Epidemiology and Biostatistics (Wits), MBChB (OAUTHC)) is an epidemiologist, researcher, and general practitioner. She is a lecturer and serves as the course coordinator for the year-five medical students at the Department of Family Medicine and Primary Care (Wits University). She is currently pursuing a doctoral degree in paediatrics at the Clinical School of Medicine, Wits University. Dr Mojisola is a full member of the International AIDS Society. She possesses solid research abilities and her areas of interest include maternal and child health, communicable and non-communicable diseases.

Rachel Moore (MBBCH, FCS (SA)) established the Acute Care Surgery Unit at Chris Hani Baragwanath Academic Hospital in September 2018, and is the head of the unit. She chairs the committee that is responsible for the staffing of the interdepartmental COVID response at CHBAH, as well as assisting in overseeing the COVID response of the Department of Surgery. Dr Moore is actively involved in Global Surgery with a focus on improving access to quality surgical care in South Africa; and heads a research hub, which is part of an international network across low- and middle-income countries.

Hellen Myezwa (DHT, MSc, PhD) is professor and head of the School of Therapeutic Sciences, Faculty of Health Sciences at the University of the Witwatersrand. She has held several leadership positions in both the clinical, practice and the academic setting and is a trained executive coach. She has been involved in several education-related projects throughout her career and is an active researcher in Health science education. Hellen Myezwa is an expert in HIV and disability, and the study of service delivery systems and has research involving service delivery management, models, their structure and monitoring and evaluation systems. Professor Myezwa has published 80 articles and co-authored a book in special education with input on community approaches and a book chapter.

Galenda Jeniffer Nagudi (MSc, BPharm) is an independent contractor at the Aurum Institute, South Africa, working on research in the fields of HIV and TB. She holds a BSc degree in pharmacy (Anadolu University, Turkey) and an MSc in epidemiology and biostatistics (University of the Witwatersrand, South Africa). Nagudi has gained experience in health service delivery in both the public and private health sectors. She has previously worked as a research assistant at the National Institute of Communicable disease (NICD) on a long-COVID study. She has collaborated with fellow researchers on diverse fields such as hypertension, Intimate Partner Violence, and COVID.

Stavros Nicolaou (BPharm (Wits), MPS (SA), FPS (SA) PhD (Medicine) Wits) is a member of Aspen Pharmacare's Group Executive team and its senior executive responsible for Strategic Trade Development. Nicolaou has over 30 years' experience in the South African and International pharmaceutical industry working across a number of geographies and therapeutic areas. He was instrumental in introducing the first generic ARV's on the African Continent developed by Aspen, which has gone on to save hundreds of thousands of lives in South Africa and on the African Continent. He has been the recipient of a number of awards, including the Monte Rubenstein Award for proficiency in pharmaceutics at an undergraduate level from the Wits University Pharmacy School, the SA Institute of Marketing Management (IMM) Health Marketer of the Year Award, induction as a fellow of the Pharmaceutical Society of South Africa (PSSA) and the Order of the Lion of St Mark by the Greek Orthodox Pope and Patriarch, Theodoros II for his work in HIV. He was recently awarded an Honorary Doctorate of Science in Medicine from Wits University.

Nathan D. Nielsen (MD, MSc, FCCM) is an Intensivist and Transfusion Medicine specialist presently based in Albuquerque, New Mexico in the United States. He is the International Representative for North America on the Council of the European Society of Intensive Care Medicine (ESICM), and also serves on the Editorial Board of the ESICM Academy. He has been the Scientific Content Editor of the Global Sepsis Alliance since 2018, and has lectured on sepsis and other critical care topics on four continents. Dr Nielsen is an active educator locally and internationally, and has been a major contributor to several innovative global intensive care training initiatives.

Peter Suwirakwenda Nyasulu (PhD, MScMed, PgDip Epi, Adv Dip Derv, Dip Clin Med, MACE) is a professor of epidemiology at the Faculty of Medicine and Health Sciences, Stellenbosch University. He is a C2-Rated Scientist with extensive experience in epidemiological and clinical research in infectious diseases, including HIV/AIDS, tuberculosis, pneumococcal diseases, among others. He is also actively involved in the COVID-19 research response initiative of the Stellenbosch University, Faculty of Medicine and Health Sciences.

He has an extensive network of research collaboration both locally and internationally. He is a member of the American College of Epidemiology and serves on the Editorial Board of the *BMC Infectious Diseases Journal* and the *Malawi Medical Journal*.

Warren Parker (PhD, MA, BA hons, B Journ, Dip Adult Ed) is an international public health specialist. His work on HIV in South Africa has informed diverse aspects of the epidemic including prevention, epidemiology and communication since the early 1990s. He has developed and guided research approaches for understanding community perspectives on preventive health in more than 20 countries and contributes to intervention design and health policy at country and global levels. In support of the response to the COVID-19 pandemic, Dr Parker has guided prevention initiatives and contributed to research and strategic policy development.

Laetitia Rispel (PhD) is professor of public health, National Research Foundation-rated researcher, and a chair holder of the South African Research Chairs Initiative (SARChI) at the University of the Witwatersrand (Wits) in Johannesburg, South Africa. Her research focuses on human resources for health and its intersection with the performance of the health system and other social determinants of health. She has published extensively, and has won several national and international awards. She is a former president of the World Federation of Public Health Associations (2018–2020), the first woman from Africa to achieve this honour.

Lewis Rubin-Thompson has worked as a research assistant for the Columbia University Institute for Social and Economic Research and Policy and for the Programs for Vaccine Education at the Vagelos College of Physicians and Surgeons. He has helped support research related to global health security and global vaccine infrastructure and safety monitoring. Lewis completed his premedical studies at Columbia University and is currently an MD candidate at the University of Rochester School of Medicine and Dentistry.

Robin Saggers (MBBCh, DCH, DipHIVMan, FCPaed, MMed Paed) is a paediatrician employed at Charlotte Maxeke Johannesburg Academic Hospital. Having previously gained experience in neonatology, he is currently sub-specialising in critical care medicine. He completed his MMed under the supervision of Professor Ballot, going on to co-supervise paediatric registrars with her and participate in her research project PRINCE (Project to Improve Neonatal Care). Additionally, he is an Advanced Paediatric Life Support instructor playing to his interests in paediatric ventilation. Other interests include sports medicine, where he acts as academic director of Wits of Sports and Health.

Richard E. Scott (PhD), a Global e-Health expert, is an honorary professor (University of KwaZulu Natal, Durban, South Africa), and adjunct professor (Department of Community Health Sciences, University of Calgary, Alberta, Canada). Richard is also a Fulbright New Century Scholar (2001–2002; Healthcare in a Borderless World), a Canadian Harkness Associate (2004–2005; Health Policy – International Comparisons), and a Mary Weston Scholar (2008; eHealth in the Developing World). For over 20 years, Richard has focused on examining the role of eHealth in the globalisation of healthcare, including aspects impacting the implementation, integration, and sustainability of eHealth globally and locally (*'glocal' eHealth*).

Hayley Anne Severance (MPH) serves as the senior director for NTI's Global Biological Policy and Programs team. Ms Severance previously served as senior policy advisor in the Office of the Deputy Assistant Secretary of Defense for Countering WMD, where she developed strategic policy guidance for the Cooperative Threat Reduction's Biological Engagement Program and led efforts to advance the U.S. commitment under the Global Health Security Agenda. Severance holds an M.P.H. in Infectious Disease Epidemiology from George Washington University and a BS in Public Health from Rutgers University. Severance is an alumna of the Emerging Leaders in Biosecurity Initiative Fellowship.

Scott Smalley (MSPAS, PGDHSE, BSc, PA-C) is the head of division of Clinical Associates, University of Witwatersrand, Johannesburg, South Africa. He has developed and implemented an integrated curriculum for the Bachelor of Clinical Medical Practice degree, leading to registration as a clinical associate in South Africa. During COVID-19, he implemented a policy for academic continuation in the Faculty of Health Sciences. He serves on national policy boards for clinical associate training and practice. He is the president of the International Academy of Physician Associate Educators (IAPAE), a non-profit to promote global teaching and learning of clinical associates, physician associates/assistants.

Martin D. Smith (MBBCh (Wits), FCS (SA) UEMS (HPB surgery), FRCS (Edin)) is currently clinical head of surgery at Chris Hani Baragwanath Academic Hospital (CHBAH) and the professor and academic head of the Surgery Department at the University. He has been the president of a number of International Professional Associations, including the PAAS, E-AHPBA and the IHPBA. His research interests include chronic pancreatitis and pancreatic cancer. He is actively involved in Global Surgery initiatives and research that serve to improve access to quality surgical care especially in low- and middle-income countries. He chairs the task team to establish a National Surgical, Obstetrics and Anesthesia Plan for South Africa.

Eddie Eung Sok Pak (MBBCh (Wits), FCPsych (SA)) qualified as a psychiatrist at Wits University in Johannesburg. Thereafter, he worked at Sterkfontein Hospital in Krugersdorp, where he served as head of the Forensic Unit during the period 2007–2020. When the COVID-19 pandemic hit South Africa in early 2020, he was appointed chairperson of the hospital's COVID-19 management committee. From 2013 till 2020, he also served on the Aeromedical Committee of the South African Civil Aviation Authority. In late 2020, Dr Pak relocated to Auckland, New Zealand, where he currently works as a consultant psychiatrist in community mental health.

Lawrence Stanberry (MD, PhD) is professor of paediatrics, associate dean for International Programs and director of the programmes in Global Health at the Vagelos College of Physicians and Surgeons, Columbia University. Dr Stanberry is an authority on viral diseases and vaccine development. He has served on numerous advisory and review panels including serving as the chair of the Vaccine Study Section and the Pediatrics Review Panel at the National Institutes of Health. He has received research funding from the National Institutes of Health, the Centers for Disease Control and Prevention, numerous vaccine, pharmaceutical and biotech companies, and the Bill and Melinda Gates Foundation. He is the co-editor of several textbooks, including *Vaccines for Biodefense and Emerging and Neglected Diseases, Understanding Modern Vaccines*, and *Viral Infections of Humans: Epidemiology and Control*.

Garth Stevens (BA, BA (Hons) Psychology, MPsych, DLitt et Phil) is a clinical psychologist at the University of the Witwatersrand, Johannesburg, South Africa. His enduring research interests include foci on race, racism and related social asymmetries; critical violence studies; applied psychoanalytic theorising of contemporary socio-political issues; and historical/collective trauma and memory. Professor Stevens is a member of the Academy of Science of South Africa (ASSAf), serves as the dean of the Faculty of Humanities at the University of the Witwatersrand, and president of the Psychological Society of South Africa (PsySSA).

Ugasvaree (Ugash) Subramaney (PhD, BSc(honours) (Psychology), MMED, FCPsych (SA), MBBCh) is the academic head of department of psychiatry at Wits as well as clinical HOD at Sterkfontein hospital. She works as a forensic psychiatrist and has an interest in female murderers and trauma amongst other things. Following her internship at Chris Hani Baragwanath Academic Hospital she started training in psychiatry at Wits, after a brief stint in paediatrics. Her PhD is in the area of traumatic stress disorders. When not dealing with staff and administration issues as HOD, she enjoys dabbling in art and writing.

Imraan Valodia (DEcon, MSc, BCom) is professor of economics, dean of the Faculty of Commerce, Law and Management, and director of the Southern Centre for Inequality Studies, University of the Witwatersrand. He has published extensively in leading academic journals and the popular press on issues related to his research interests. He is a part-time member of the Competition Tribunal, a member of the National Minimum Wage Commission and a member of the Academy of Science of South Africa Standing Committee on Science for the Reduction of Poverty and Inequality. He is a member of President Ramaphosa's Presidential Economic Advisory Council.

Alex van den Heever (MA Economics) holds the chair of Social Security Systems Administration and Management Studies at the Wits School of Governance. He has worked in the areas of health economics, public finance and social security since 1989. Adjunt Professor van den Heever has worked for the Department of Finance, Industrial Development Corporation, Centre for Health Policy (WITS), the Gauteng Department of Health, and the Council for Medical Schemes. He also formed part of the Melamet Commission on Medical Schemes, the Taylor Committee of Inquiry, the Medicines Pricing Committee, the Ministerial Task Team on Social Health Insurance and the Health Market Inquiry.

Charles Shey Wiysonge (MPhil, MD, PhD, MASSAf) is the director of Cochrane South Africa at the South African Medical Research Council, an extraordinary professor of global health at Stellenbosch University, and an honorary professor of epidemiology and biostatistics at the University of Cape Town in South Africa. He is a physician with expertise in epidemiology, evidence-based health care, and vaccinology. Professor Wiysonge's research interests include vaccine hesitancy, acceptance, and uptake in Africa. He is a member of numerous national, continental, and global scientific and policy advisory committees.

ACKNOWLEGEMENTS

Figure 8.1: Covid graphic from https://www.avert.org/coronavirus/infographics. www.avert.org is a website operated by the international HIV and AIDS charity, Avert

Figure 8.1: Covid graphic: PPE is key to protect healthworkers from COVID-19. Copyright World Health Organization (WHO). Sourced at: https://www.weforum.org/agenda/2020/04/10-april-who-briefing-health-workers-covid-19-ppe-training/

Figure 9.1: Figure adapted from *Social Dererminants of Health*. https://www.paho.org/en/topics/social-determinants-health. © Pan American Health Organization, 2020. Some rights reserved. This work is available under license CC BY-NC-SA 3.0 IGO

Figure 9.2: © Angus Maguire Ltd.2021 from Peter Levine: A Blog for Civic Renewal "defining equity and equality". Interaction Institute for Social Change. Artist Angus Maguire. interactioninstitute.org and madewithangus.com. Used with permission

Table 9.2: University of Massachusetts Medical School. Open Access Articles Open Access Publications by UMMS Authors 2017-08-01. *A paradigm shift for socioeconomic justice and health: from focusing on inequalities to aiming at sustainable equity.* Juan E. Garay, University of California Berkeley, Et al

Table 9.3: Based on the Report: *Overcoming Poverty and Inequality in South Africa: An Assessment of Drivers, Constraints and Opportunities* March 2018. https://documents1.worldbank.org/curated/en/530481521735906534/pdf/124521-REV-OUO-South-Africa-Poverty-and-Inequality-Assessment-Report-2018-FINAL-WEB.pdf

Figure 12.3: Barnard-Ashton Paula, Adams Fasloen, Rothberg Alan, & McInerney Patricia. (2018). Digital apartheid and the effect of mobile technology during rural fieldwork. South African Journal of Occupational Therapy, 48(2), 20-25. https://dx.doi.org/10.17159/23103833/2018/vol48n2a4

Table 16.1: National Institute for Communicable Diseases. Copyright © NHLS 2010. This report summarises data of COVID-19 cases admitted to DATCOV hospital surveillance sites in all provinces. Copyright © NHLS 2010.

Figure 16.2: National Institute for Communicable Diseases. Copyright © NHLS 2010. This report summarises data of COVID-19 cases admitted to DATCOV hospital surveillance sites in all provinces. Copyright © NHLS 2010.

Table 16.3: Ruth, G. and Susan J, C. (2016) 'Public Health Surveillance', *Nature Public Health Emergency Collection*, 19(10). Copyright © Springer International Publishing Switzerland 2016

Table 16.4: National Institute for Communicable Diseases. Copyright © NHLS 2010. This report summarises data of COVID-19 cases admitted to DATCOV hospital surveillance sites in all provinces. Copyright © NHLS 2010.

Table 16.5: National Institute for Communicable Diseases. Copyright © NHLS 2010. This report summarises data of COVID-19 cases admitted to DATCOV hospital surveillance sites in all provinces. Copyright © NHLS 2010.

Figure 16.3: Reddy Tarylee, Shkedy Ziv, Janse van Rensburg Charl, Mwambi Henry, Debba Pravesh, Zuma, Khangelani & Manda Samuel. (2021). *Short-term real-time prediction of total number of reported COVID-19 cases and deaths in South Africa: a data driven approach.* BMC Medical Research Methodology. 21.10.1186/ s12874-020-01165-x. Springer, January 2021

Figure 16.4: Reddy Tarylee, Shkedy Ziv, Janse van Rensburg Charl, Mwambi Henry, Debba Pravesh, Zuma, Khangelani & Manda Samuel. (2021). *Short-term real-time prediction of total number of reported COVID-19 cases and deaths in South Africa: a data driven approach.* BMC Medical Research Methodology. 21. 10.1186/s12874-020-01165-x. Springer, January 2021

Figure 16.5: Reddy Tarylee, Shkedy Ziv, Janse van Rensburg Charl, Mwambi Henry, Debba Pravesh, Zuma, Khangelani & Manda Samuel. (2021). *Short-term real-time prediction of total number of reported COVID-19 cases and deaths in South Africa: a data driven approach.* BMC Medical Research Methodology. 21. 10.1186/s12874-020-01165-x. Springer, January 2021

Figure 16.6: Reddy Tarylee, Shkedy Ziv, Janse van Rensburg Charl, Mwambi Henry, Debba Pravesh, Zuma, Khangelani & Manda Samuel. (2021). *Short-term real-time prediction of total number of reported COVID-19 cases and deaths in South Africa: a data driven approach.* BMC Medical Research Methodology. 21. 10.1186/s12874-020-01165-x. Springer, January 2021

Table 16.6: Amawi, H. et al. (2020). Amawi, H. et al. (2020) 'COVID-19 pandemic: An overview of epidemiology, pathogenesis, diagnostics and potential vaccines and therapeutics', *Therapeutic Delivery*, 11(4), pp. 245–268. Copyright © 2020 Newlands Press. This work is licensed under the Creative Commons Attribution 4.0 License

Figure 16.7: Reddy Tarylee, Shkedy Ziv, Janse van Rensburg Charl, Mwambi Henry, Debba Pravesh, Zuma, Khangelani & Manda Samuel. (2021). *Short-term real-time prediction of total number of reported COVID-19 cases and deaths in South Africa: a data driven approach.* BMC Medical Research Methodology. 21. 10.1186/s12874-020-01165-x. Springer, January 2021

Figure 18.1: Lewis-O'Connor A, Warren A, Lee JV, Levy-Carrick N, Grossman S, Chadwick M, Stoklosa H, Rittenberg E. The state of the science on trauma inquiry. *Womens Health* (Lond). 2019 Jan-Dec;15:17

Table 19.1: Adapted from/Based on: Penchansky R. and Thomas J. W. (1981) 'The concept of access: definition and relationship to consumer satisfaction', *Medical Care*, 19(2), pp. 127–140

Table 19.2: Adapted from Wilkinson L. S. et al. (2020) 'Preparing healthcare facilities to operate safely and effectively during the COVID-19 pandemic: The missing piece in the puzzle', *South African Medical Journal* 110(9), pp. 835–836

Figure 23.1: Based on the *Framework for the Response of Integrated Health Service Delivery Networks to COVID-19.* https://iris.paho.org/bitstream/handle/10665.2/52269/ PAHOIMSHSSHSCOVID19200021_eng.pdf?sequence=1&isAllowed=y © Pan American Health Organization, 2020. Some rights reserved. This work is available under license CC BY-NC-SA 3.0 IGO

ACRONYMS AND ABBREVIATIONS

3D:	Three-dimensional
4IR:	Fourth Industrial Revolution
AAS:	African Academy of Sciences
ACOG:	American College of Obstetricians and Gynaecologists
ACS:	Acute Care Surgery
ACSU:	ACS Unit
ACT:	Access to COVID-19 Tools
Africa CDC:	Africa Centre for Disease Control and Prevention
AGSA:	Auditor-General of South Africa
AI:	Artificial Intelligence
AIDS:	Acquired immunodeficiency syndrome
ALOS:	Average Length of Stay
ALT:	Alanine transaminase
AMR:	Antimicrobial resistance
ANC:	African National Congress
ARVs:	Antiretroviral therapy
ASSA:	Association of Surgeons of South Africa
AU:	African Union
B4SA:	Business for South Africa
B-BBEE:	Broad-Based Black Economic Empowerment
BBC:	Black Business Council
BMI:	Body Mass Index
BMJ:	British Medical Journal
BUR:	Bed Utilisation Rate
BUSA:	Business Unity South Africa
BWC:	Biological Weapons Convention
CCMDD:	Central Chronic Medicine Dispensing and Distribution
CCTV:	Closed-Circuit Television
CDC:	Center for Disease Control

CEPI:	Coalition for Epidemic Preparedness
CHBAH:	Chris Hani Baragwanath Academic Hospital
COMEST:	World Commission on the Ethics of Scientific Knowledge and Technology
CONCVACT:	COVID-19 Vaccine Clinical Trial
COVID-19:	Coronavirus disease 2019 (this novel coronavirus was identified in 2019; it is linked to the same family of viruses as Severe Acute Respiratory Syndrome and some types of common cold), also SARS-CoV-2
CPD:	Continuing Professional Development
CRAM:	Coronavirus Rapid Mobile Survey
CRP:	C-Reactive protein
CSDH:	Commission on Social Determinants of Health
DNN:	Deep Neural Network
DoS:	Department of Surgery
Ebola:	Haemorrhagic fever that is caused by a virus. Ebola is named for the river in Africa where the disease was first recognised in 1976
ECDC:	European Centre for Disease Prevention and Control
ECG:	Electrocardiography
ELT:	Experiential Learning Theory
EMR:	Electronic Medical Record
ESR:	Erythrocyte Sedimentation Rate
EUA:	Emergency Use Authorisation
FDA:	Food and Drug Administration
FFP2:	Filtering Facepiece 2
FFP3:	Filtering Facepiece 3
Gavi:	Global Vaccine Alliance
GDOH:	Gauteng Department of Health
GHSA:	Global Health Security Agenda
GHSI:	Global Health Security Index
GLASS:	Global Antimicrobial Resistance and Use Surveillance System.

GPMB:	Global Preparedness Monitoring Board
GPS:	Global Positioning System
GSK:	GlaxoSmithKline
HCPs:	Healthcare Professionals
HCU:	High Care Unit
HICs:	High-income countries
HIV:	Human immunodeficiency virus
HPCSA:	Health Professions Council of South Africa
IBC:	International Bioethics Committee
ICARES:	Information, Clinical, Administration, Research, Education, and Surveillance
ICESCR:	International Covenant on Economic, Social and Cultural Rights
ICFJ:	International Centre for Journalists
ICT:	Information and Communication Technology/ies
ICU:	Intensive Care Unit
IDVI:	Infectious Disease Vulnerability Index
IHR:	International Health Regulations (2005)
IHS:	Imperial Health Sciences
IL-1RA:	Interleukin-1 Receptor Antagonist
IL-6:	Interleukin 6
INR:	International Normalised Ratio
IP:	Intellectual Property
IQR:	Interquartile range
ISID:	International Society for Infectious Diseases
ISO:	International Organization for Standardization
IUCD:	Intrauterine Contraceptive Device
IVIG:	Intravenous Immunoglobulin
IV-Ig:	Intravenous immunoglobulins
JEE:	Joint External Evaluations

KD:	Kawasaki disease
LCOGS:	Lancet Commission on Global Surgery
LLP:	Lead Logistics Provider
LMICs:	Lower- and middle-income countries
LSTM:	Long Short-Term Memory
MAC:	Ministerial Advisory Committee
MCWH:	Maternal, Child and Women's Health
MERS:	Middle East respiratory syndrome
MERS-CoV:	Middle East Respiratory Syndrome-Coronavirus
MERV:	Minimum Efficiency Reporting Value
MIC:	Middle-income country
MIS-C:	Multisystem Inflammatory Syndrome in Children
MMR:	Maternal Mortality Ratio
MSNBC:	Microsoft National Broadcasting Company
N95:	Non-Oil respirator rating letter class with 95% efficiency
NASREC:	National Recreation Centre
NCCEMD:	National Confidential Enquiry Committee into Maternal Deaths
NCDs:	Non-communicable diseases
NCEMD:	National Confidential Enquiry into Maternal Deaths
NDoH:	National Department of Health
NEDLAC:	National Economic Development and Labour Council
NHLS:	National Health Laboratory Services
NICD:	National Institute of Communicable Diseases
NIDS:	National Income Dynamics Study
NIDS-CRAM:	National Income Dynamics Study – Coronavirus Rapid Mobile Survey
NIOH:	National Institute for Occupational Health
NIOSH:	National Institute for Occupational Safety and Health
NMC:	Notifiable Medical Condition
NPI:	Non-pharmaceutical Interventions

NPIs:	Non-Pharmacological Interventions
NRSC:	National Regulator for Compulsory Specifications
NSOAP:	National Surgical, Obstetric and Anaesthesia Plans
OEMs:	Original Equipment Manufacturers
OHS:	Occupational Health and Safety
OHSC:	Office of Health Standards Compliance
OxCGRT:	The Oxford COVID-19 Government Response Tracker
PC:	Personal Computer
PCR:	Polymerase chain reaction
PEAC:	Presidential Economic Advisory Council
PEPFAR:	President's Emergency Plan For AIDS Relief
PHC:	Primary health care
PHE:	Public Health England
PHEIC:	Public Health Emergency of International Concern
PIMS-TS:	Paediatric Multisystem Inflammatory Syndrome Temporally associated with SAR-CoV-2
PPE:	Personal protective equipment
ProMED:	Program for Monitoring Emerging Diseases
PUI:	Patient-Under-Investigation
Q&I:	Quarantine & Isolation
QR codes:	Quick Response codes
RCOG:	Royal College of Obstetricians and Gynaecologists
REC:	Research Ethics Committee
RNA:	Ribonucleic acid
RNN:	Recurrent Neural Network
RT-PCR:	Reverse Transcriptase Polymerase Chain Reaction
SA:	South Africa
SABS:	South African Bureau of Standards
SAHPRA:	South African Health Products Regulatory Authority
SAMED:	South African Medical Technology Industry Association

SAMRC:	South African Medica Research Council
SANC:	South African Nursing Council
SARS:	Severe acute respiratory syndrome
SARS:	South African Revenue Services
SARS-CoV-2:	Severe Acute Respiratory Syndrome Coronavirus 2 (a novel severe acute respiratory syndrome coronavirus)
SDGs:	Sustainable Development Goals
SDH:	Social determinants of health
SIRD:	Susceptible–Infected–Recovered–Dead
SIU:	Special Investigative Unit
SMEs:	Small and medium-sized enterprises
SOGC:	Society of Obstetricians and Gynaecologists of Canada
SPAR:	State Party Self-Assessment Annual Reporting
SRD:	COVID-19 Social Relief of Distress Grant
SSA:	Sub-Saharan Africa
TB:	Tuberculosis
TERS:	Temporary Employer/Employee Relief Scheme
TOP:	Termination of Pregnancy
TRIPS:	Agreement on Trade-Related Aspects of Intellectual Property Rights
UHC:	Universal Health Coverage
UN:	United Nations
UNICEF:	United Nations Children's Emergency Fund
UNODA	United Nations Office of Disarmament Affairs
UNSC 1540:	United Nations Security Council Resolutions 1540 (2004)
US:	United States
VIDA	Vaccines and Infectious Disease Analytics
WHO:	World Health Organization
WMA:	World Medical Association
WTO:	World Trade Organization

CHAPTER 1

INTRODUCTION TO PANDEMICS AND HEALTH CARE: PRINCIPLES, PROCESSES AND PRACTICE

Ames Dhai

Daynia Ballot

Martin Veller

1.1 INTRODUCTION

It became clear soon after the World Health Organization (WHO) declared COVID-19 a pandemic that not much was known about the management of pandemics in the healthcare context. This topic had received little to no attention in health sciences and other training curricula. Accordingly, there was much uncertainty as to the management of infected patients, their families and communities at large. There had been a flurry of academic and non-academic publications, social media reports and fake information resulting in an 'infodemic' of alarmingly confusing proportions. This unfortunately did not assist with processes and practice at macro-, meso- and micro-levels of healthcare delivery with many critical issues arising at the coalface.

Infectious disease outbreaks, such as Ebola and influenza, have featured prominently at an international level over the last few decades, with data suggesting that these catastrophes are increasing in frequency. Since the sixteenth century, at least three pandemics per century have occurred at between 10- to 50-year intervals with varying levels of morbidity and mortality. It has not been possible to predict the impact of future pandemics. This was also evident early in the COVID-19 pandemic, which has resulted in an unprecedented burden on human health, major disruptions in healthcare systems, and grave social and economic consequences. The pandemic has affected a large part of the population and it will last for several years. Changes in the twenty-first century due to *inter alia* travel, trade, urbanisation and environmental degradation increase the risk of disease outbreaks and their spread, which rapidly amplify into epidemics and pandemics. There is much uncertainty as to the management of infected patients, their families and communities at large.

As the COVID-19 pandemic evolves, many critical issues arise impacting on teaching, learning, and healthcare delivery through the spectrum of primary to quaternary care, public health and the social determinants of health. A peer-reviewed book with pertinent theoretical and practical information has therefore become necessary.

1.2   A BRIEF HISTORY OF PANDEMICS

Throughout history, very few phenomena have shaped societies the way infectious disease outbreaks have done. Entire populations have been wiped out, societies decimated and the outcomes of wars determined by pandemic outbreaks (Huremović, 2019). The spread of infectious diseases was facilitated by the shift from hunter-gatherers to agrarian societies. As trade between communities expanded, interactions between humans and animals increased, and so did the transmission of zoonotic pathogens. Cities expanded, trade territories were extended and travels increased. The human population increased, resulting in ecosystems being effected, fuelling the emergence and spread of infectious diseases leading to higher risks for outbreaks, epidemics and pandemics. The transmission of pathogens has also been influenced by climate changes (Piret and Boivin, 2021; Dasgupta and Crunkhorn, 2020).

1.2.1   The Plagues

The earliest recorded pandemic in history is the plague. Originating from the Greek word *plaga* (strike, blow), the word plague was used as a general term for any epidemic disease causing a high rate of mortality or to denote the flea-borne Yersinia pestis virulent contagious febrile disease. More generally, it was used as a metaphor for any sudden outbreak of a disastrous evil or affliction (Piret and Boivin, 2021). Plagues have also been recorded in several religious scriptures and even today continue to be commemorated in religious practices throughout the world (Huremović, 2019).

The Athenian plague occurred in 430–26 BC during the Peloponnesian War between Athens and Sparta. Originating in Ethiopia, the Athenian plague spread throughout Egypt and Greece. Initially, the symptoms included headaches, conjunctivitis, a rash covering the body, and fever. This was followed by coughing up blood and severe gastrointestinal symptoms with cramping and vomiting and ultimately death by day seven or eight. Those who survived remained partially paralysed, with amnesia, or blind for the remainder of their days. Many doctors and other caregivers succumbed to the illness during the course and scope of their work. Because of wartime overcrowding in Athens, there was a rapid spread of the plague, with more than 25% of the population being killed. While the cause of the Athenian plague of 430 BC has not been clearly determined and typhoid fever remains the most popular possibility, more recently it has been postulated that the cause of the Athenian plague could have been Ebola virus hemorrhagic fever (Huremović, 2019).

The next plague, the Antonine plague of 165–180 AD, recorded a few centuries later, was documented by the physician Galen. It is also known as the Plague of Galen. It occurred in the Roman Empire and was possibly caused by smallpox. It reached the Roman Empire by soldiers returning from Seleucia. It had also affected Asia Minor, Egypt, Greece, and Italy. While the Athenian plague affected a geographically limited region, the Antonine plague spread widely across the entire Roman Empire, which was an economically and politically integrated, cohesive society occupying vast territory. In some areas it destroyed a third of the population. It decimated the Roman army resulting in the weakening of the Roman Empire's military and economic supremacy, possibly resulting in its decline and later its fall in the West in the fifth century AD (Huremović, 2019; Piret and Boivin, 2021; Dasgupta and Crunkhorn, 2020).

The Justinian plague during the Byzantine Empire was the first documented bubonic plague caused by Yersinia pestis. It originated in the mid-sixth century AD, possibly in Ethiopia and then spread through Egypt or Central Asia, where it travelled along the caravan trading routes. It then spread widely throughout and beyond the Roman world. It generally followed trading routes and was therefore particularly ferocious in coastal cities. The spread from Asia Minor to Africa, Italy and other parts of Western Europe is attributed to military movement at that time. Many victims succumbed within days of contracting the disease, and gravesites were full beyond capacity. Where patients survived, they were left with physical deformities and had to live with the stigmata of survivors. Streets became deserted, all trade was abandoned, economic output decreased, the tax base shrank, staple foods became scarce and people died of starvation as well as of the disease itself. Following the initial outbreak in 541, several cycles of infection followed and by 600, it is possible that the population of the Empire had been reduced by 40% with this figure exceeding 50% in the city of Constantinople itself (Huremović, 2019; Piret and Boivin, 2021).

A global outbreak of bubonic plague originating in China in 1334, followed the Silk Road, spread through Central Asia and North India and arrived in Sicily, Europe in 1347. It was called 'The Plague' (also the Black Death), and by 1400 (within 50 years), it had killed over 150 million, reducing the global population from 450 million to possibly less than 300 million. Up to 60% of people in Europe succumbed. Within five years of arriving in Europe, it had spread throughout the continent, into Russia and in its first wave, claimed 25 million lives. The Black Death relentlessly wiped out entire neighbourhoods and even entire towns. It broke down the established divisions between the upper and lower classes and led to the emergence of a new middle class. Many professions, particularly that of medical doctors, were severely affected and lost to the plague.

Several municipalities contracted young doctors and established dedicated practitioners to deal with the duty of the plague doctor (*medico della pes*). Learning from the experiences of ancient cultures that dealt with contagious diseases, medieval societies started instituting mandatory isolation with the first quarantine enacted in Ragusa in 1377. Anyone arriving at this city had to spend 30 days (later extended to 40 days) on a nearby island of Lokrum before entering the city (Huremović, 2019). As the notion of quarantines took hold, armed guards were placed along transit routes and at access points to cities to create a sanitary cordon. Infected individuals were separated from healthy people and placed into camps or permanent plague hospitals. Ships arriving from areas with The Plague were not allowed into port cities and suspicious vessels were thoroughly fumigated and retained in isolation for 40 days. The Black Death decimated Medieval Europe with major impacts on its socioeconomic development, culture, art, religion and politics (Piret and Boivin, 2021). The use of quarantine quickly spread throughout Europe and currently remains in effect as an effective and regulated public health measure to combat contagions globally. Since the 1990s, plague is classified as a re-emerging infectious disease by the World Health Organization (WHO) (Piret and Boivin, 2021).

1.2.2   The Spanish Flu

The Spanish flu pandemic (1918–1920) is recorded as the first true global pandemic and the first one occurring in the era of modern medicine. The nature and course of the pandemic and its illness as it evolved was studied by specialities such as infectious diseases and epidemiology. Caused by the H1N1 strain of the Influenza virus, it was the last true global pandemic with devastating consequences for societies across the globe before the COVID-19 pandemic. Its true origin, despite its name, remains unknown. Possible sources are postulated to be the USA, China, Spain, France, or Austria. Of note, it took place in the middle of World War I when fairly advanced modes of transportation, including intercontinental travel, had already been established, and within months, its deadly strain had spread around the world. Over 25% had contracted the virus globally, with a mortality rate between 10% and 20%. It has been suggested that between 50 million to 100 million died. More individuals died in one year than the Black Death had killed in a century, and by August 1918, the virus had mutated to a much more virulent and lethal form, killing many who had avoided it during the first wave (Huremović, 2019). Health authorities in large cities of the Western world implemented a number of containment strategies to prevent its spread. These included the suspension of public gatherings and the closure of schools, churches and theatres. Respiratory hygiene and social distancing were encouraged. Because of the war, these measures were uncoordinated and implemented too late, and travel restrictions and border controls were impossible to institute (Piret and Boivin, 2021). Despite the magnitude of its impact, the Spanish flu rapidly evaporated from public and scientific attention, with some historians calling it the forgotten pandemic. Unfortunately, this seems to have been the trend with pandemics that followed; societies would initially display immense interest, followed by horror and panic, and then dispassionate disinterest once the pandemic subsided (Huremović, 2019).

1.2.3   Swine Flu

The 2009 H1N1 pandemic, colloquially known as the swine flu, was a harsh reminder of the 1918 Spanish flu but fortunately with far less devastating consequences. Its origins trace back to Mexico in April 2009. It reached pandemic proportions within weeks, began to taper off toward the end of the year and by May 2010, it was declared over. Ten per cent of the global population were infected and the numbers that succumbed are estimated to vary from 20,000 to 500,000. It was very threatening because it disproportionately and severely affected previously healthy young adults, possibly because older adults had developed immunity due to a similar H1N1 outbreak in the 1970s (Huremović, 2019). The average age of people who died was 37 years. Hand washing, use of face masks and cough etiquette were among the non-pharmaceutical preventative measures implemented. This was the first pandemic where vaccines and antiviral use were combined (Piret and Boivin, 2021). It is interesting to note the dissonance between public sentiment about the outbreak and the public health steps recommended and undertaken by the WHO and national health institutions. Because of WHO releases and warnings, public alarm rapidly transitioned to discontent and mistrust as the initial bleak outlook failed to materialise with health agencies being accused of creating 'panicdemics' and pushing unproven vaccines so the pharmaceutical industry could be promoted. A lesson to be learnt from this pandemic is how difficult it is to understand and manage public expectations and public sentiments when attempting to mobilise a response (Huremović, 2019). This can be compared to the anti-vaccine sentiment and lack of confidence in state players during the current COVID-19 pandemic.

1.2.4   The Corona Viruses

SARS-CoV originated in Guangdong province (China) in 2003, with bats being the likely natural reservoir. During the 2002–2003 outbreak, SARS-CoV infection was reported in 29 countries in North America, South America, Europe and Asia. About 8,437 were infected, with 813 fatalities. Respiratory failure was the most common cause of death among patients infected with SARS-CoV. MERS-CoV was reported in Jeddah in Saudi Arabia in 2012, ten years after the first emergence of SARS-CoV, with the potential animal reservoirs being bats and dromedary camels. Between 2012 and 2020, there have been 2,519 cases of MERS-CoV, with at least 866 deaths in 27 countries. In all cases, there has been a link to persons in the Arabian Peninsula or persons who had returned from travelling in MERS-CoV endemic areas.

Given that MERS-CoV is still circulating currently and its outbreak in South Korea, its potential to spread around the world and pose a threat for global health must be kept in mind (Piret and Boivin, 2021).

1.3 AN APPRAISAL OF EVENTS EARLY ON IN THE COVID-19 PANDEMIC

Understanding the COVID-19 pandemic and responses both nationally and globally requires an appraisal of the early events. December 2019 witnessed the first cohort of patients with COVID-19 when patients with pneumonia of unknown origin were admitted to hospitals in Wuhan, China. When clinicians became concerned about a patient with pneumonia not responding to treatment, they sent a sample to a private laboratory for testing on 24 December. By 2 January 2020, there were already 41 patients with COVID-19 in the city. There appeared to be an association with visiting the Huanan Seafood Market in Wuhan and the pneumonia between several of these patients. However, not all the patients had attended the seafood market and it was noted that contacts and family members of some of the first patients also presented with similar patterns of pneumonia. Studies confirmed that only 55–66% of cases were linked to exposures at the market. This suggested that the market may have been a site of amplification of the virus rather than its origin. Initial evidence of human-to-human transmission of a new pathogen was not definitive. However, there were signs of this being likely by the end of December when the Wuhan Municipal Health Commission issued two urgent notices on 30 December to hospital networks in the city about cases of pneumonia of unknown origin linked to the Huanan Seafood Market. These notifications were subsequently reported in the Chinese media and detected by disease surveillance systems, including the Centers for Disease Control (CDC), Taiwan, which then informed the WHO. By 2 January 2020, almost the entire genome of the virus had been sequenced by the Wuhan Institute of Virology, and on 5 January, the complete genetic sequence was submitted to the open-access website GenBank from a sample sequenced by the Shanghai Public Health Center. This was made public on 11 January. China CDC successfully isolated the virus by 7 January, and Chinese scientists developed a polymerase chain reaction (PCR) testing reagent for the virus by 10 January (The Independent Panel for Pandemic Preparedness & Response, 2021).

The first confirmed case of an infected person outside of China was in Thailand on 13 January; a woman travelled to Thailand from Wuhan on the 8 January. On 16 January, Japan reported its first infection. The WHO undertook its initial fact-finding mission to Wuhan on 20–21 January. Chinese health experts confirmed human-to-human transmission in a public announcement on 20 January, where they also confirmed that health workers had been infected. Wuhan instituted a drastic population lockdown on 23 January in an attempt to contain the virus, as 830 cases and 25 deaths had already been reported (The Independent Panel for Pandemic Preparedness & Response, 2021).

Meanwhile, on 5 January, the WHO officially alerted all national governments about the cluster and published its first Disease Outbreak News notice on the issue. On 30 January, the WHO declared that the infectious disease outbreak constituted a public health emergency of international concern (PHEIC). At that time, 18 countries outside China had recorded 98 cases. There are four criteria, two of which must be met for an event to be categorised as a PHEIC: there must be potential for serious public health impact; it needs to be unusual or unexpected; there must be significant risk of international spread; and it must carry significant risk of travel or trade restrictions. The view of the Independent Panel for Pandemic Preparedness and Response, in its report 'COVID-19: Make it the last pandemic', is that the outbreak in Wuhan would have met the criteria to be declared a PHEIC as early as 22 January 2020.

The events evolving in Wuhan in the final two weeks of December 2019 and into January 2020, demonstrate the diligence of clinicians who acted on their concerns. However, it also illustrates the slowness of the WHO to act promptly and decisively when it became aware of the impending global threat. Not only has the current pandemic affected health and mortality catastrophically, but it has also had disastrous consequences on the socioeconomic fabric of life, forcing painstaking decisions when balancing saving lives with saving livelihoods. Almost 90% of schoolchildren were unable to attend school at the peak of the pandemic in 2020. The workload of women increased substantially as they tried to maintain the family income and well-being, care for the elderly and sick, and home-school their children (The Independent Panel for Pandemic Preparedness & Response, 2021). It is well known that the vulnerable become more vulnerable and those previously not vulnerable may become so for the first time during pandemics (UNESCO, 2020).

Current economic data indicates that the world's gross domestic product shrank by 6.5% in 2020 and while growth is expected in the years to come this will likely be flatter than previously expected (Statista, 2021). The COVID-19 pandemic is the most unsettling event to the global economy since World War II and the biggest reduction of national economies since the Great Depression of 1930–1932 (The Independent Panel for Pandemic Preparedness & Response, 2021). The COVID-19 pandemic, its lockdowns and other containment efforts has, without doubt, struck a brutal blow to the global economy and is predicted to drive between 40 to 60 million people into extreme poverty, 27 million of them in Sub-Saharan Africa (SSA). While the COVID-19 crisis may be perceived as primarily a health crisis, the spread of the disease in SSA is also being influenced by economic and labour conditions, especially within the informal sector. The informal sector in SSA accounts for more than 80% of the workforce. Given the high informal sector with almost no social protection, this pandemic has taught us in SSA that both saving lives and protecting livelihoods are extremely challenging. Similar to healthcare workers, informal workers and their families are most vulnerable to the disease, as they labour in overcrowded streets and bazaars. In addition, more often than not, these workers are generally indigent, do not have financial reserves and cannot afford to stockpile basic commodities required to weather such times of adversity (Nguimkeu and Okou, 2020).

1.4 CONTINUING COMPLEXITIES

The situation is compounded by the fact that national pandemic preparedness has been quite low on the priority list of most countries, albeit unambiguous evidence that the cost of responses and losses incurred when an epidemic occurs far outweighs the cost of being prepared to manage one (Global Health Security Index, 2019). In addition, failures of political leadership have led to the inability of countries to respond adequately, appropriately and in a timely manner. Distrust in government institutions is particularly high in countries like South Africa, where pandemic plundering and looting have been rife, and the pandemic has provided fertile ground for corruption at the highest levels (World Justice Project, 2020).

Of concern is the development of virus variants, which have also continued to devastate societies and economies. The emergence of these new variants continually exposes the global population to danger. While non-pharmaceutical preventative measures coupled with public health interventions are essential, we need additional measures to contain the spread of the virus. Vaccinations alone will not end this pandemic, but they are critical for the containment of the virus. Therefore, there is an urgent need to scale up vaccine rollout in all countries globally. Eradicating vaccine nationalism and reforming intellectual property law at the level of the World Trade Organization (WTO) coupled with technology transfer and upscaling manufacturing capabilities across the globe is imperative. Currently (June 2021), less than two years after the WHO declared COVID-19 to be a pandemic, 174 822 669 people have been infected and 3 764 513 have died (Worldometers, 2021). By April 2021, 16 months after the virus was first discovered and four months after the WHO authorised the first vaccine for emergency use, more than a billion people were administered the first dose. Given the significance of this achievement, it has been disheartening to see that 75% of these doses were administered in just 10 countries (Kreier, 2021). It is critical that wealthier countries realise that everyone benefits if the vaccines are distributed equitably worldwide. The situation is dire in SSA where, at the time of writing this book, the continent was importing 99% of all its vaccines because it lacks manufacturing capacity. Furthermore, countries in SSA lack the pre-order purchasing capacity of wealthier nations (Nature, 2021). Moreover, nine in 10 countries in Africa are likely to miss achieving their urgent COVID-19 vaccination goals (UN News, 2021).

It has become clear that pandemic preparedness programmes in SSA, while focusing on improvements of health systems and the social determinants of health, should also target the informal sector if lives and livelihoods are to be saved. It is imperative that social protection programmes are expanded. The lesson that Africa needs to learn from the COVID-19 pandemic is that health systems in all countries must be strengthened, access to health services ensured, and efforts towards achieving universal health coverage must be accelerated. It is essential that we get back on track towards realising the 2030 Agenda for Sustainable Development. We have entered the last decade to achieve the sustainable development goals, facing not only the challenge of COVID-19, but also pre-existing problems interfering with people living healthy lives and preventing them from reaching their full potential. This is particularly true for SSA, which has lagged far behind to meet the targets for health and well-being (African Academy of Sciences, 2021).

1.5   CONCLUSION

The pandemic needs to end as soon as possible. We should remember that COVID-19 is not the first pandemic, and neither will it be the last one. Zoonotic outbreaks are becoming more frequent. The huge increase in air travel over the last three decades makes it very easy for a virus to reach any place in the world in just a few hours. A new infectious disease outbreak could occur at any time, even before the COVID-19 pandemic ends. The urgency for better detection and vigorous preparedness is dire. We have been exposed to increasing vulnerability within our countries and the world at large, with inequalities deepening excessively. Therefore, it is imperative that we consider the lessons learnt from a global perspective and prepare to avert the pandemics that could follow. This peer-reviewed book serves as one of the initiatives towards preparedness for future pandemics.

1.6   SELF-ASSESSMENT QUESTIONS

1. What are some of the twenty-first century risks for epidemics and pandemics?
2. Discuss some considerations for pandemic preparedness programmes for Africa.

1.7   REFERENCES

Global Health Security Index. 2019. Building Collective Action and Accountability. Available at: https://www.ghsindex.org/wp-content/uploads/2019/10/2019-Global-Health-Security-Index.pdf.

Kreier, F. 2021. 'Unprecedented achievement': Who Received the First Billion COVID Vaccinations? *Nature News*. 29 April. Available at: https://www.nature.com/articles/d41586-021-01136-2.

Nguimkeu, Y.P. and Okou, C. 2020. A Tale of Africa Today: Balancing the Lives and Livelihoods of Informal Workers During the COVID-19 Pandemic. Africa Knowledge in Time Policy Brief Office of the Chief Economist, Africa Region. World Bank. October, 2020 Issue 1, No 3. Available at: https://openknowledge.worldbank.org/bitstream/handle/10986/34582/A-Tale-of-Africa-Today-Balancing-the-Lives-and-Livelihoods-of-Informal-Workers-During-the-COVID-19-Pandemic.pdf?sequence=1&isAllowed=y.

Nature. 2021. Editorial. A Patent Waiver on COVID Vaccines is Right and Fair. Available at: https://media.nature.com/original/magazine-assets/d41586-021-01242-1/d41586-021-01242-1.pdf.

Statista. 2021. Global gross domestic product (GDP) at current prices from 1985 to 2026 *(in billion U.S. dollars)*. Available at: https://www.statista.com/statistics/268750/global-gross-domestic-product-gdp/.

The African Academy of Sciences. 2021. Africa's Scientific Priorities. Available at: https://www.aasciences.africa/african-scientific-priorities.

The Independent Panel for Pandemic Preparedness & Response. 2021. Available at: https://theindependentpanel.org/wp-content/uploads/2021/05/COVID-19-Make-it-the-Last-Pandemic_final.pdf.

United Nations Educational, Scientific and Cultural Organisation. 2020. Statement On COVID-19: Ethical Considerations From A Global Perspective Statement of the UNESCO International Bioethics Committee (IBC) and the UNESCO World Commission on the Ethics of Scientific Knowledge and Technology (COMEST). Available at: https://en.unesco.org/inclusivepolicylab/e-teams/ethical-considerations-covid-19-responses-and-recovery/documents/unesco-ibc-comest-statement.

UN News. 2021. Nine in 10 African Nations Set to Miss Urgent COVID Vaccination Goal. Available at: https://news.un.org/en/story/2021/06/1093712.

World Justice Project. 2020. Corruption and the COVID-19 Pandemic. Available at: https://worldjusticeproject.org/sites/default/files/documents/2020-07-01%20Corruption%20and%20the%20COVID-19%20Pandemic_1.pdf.

Worldometers. 2021. Available at: https://www.worldometers.info/coronavirus/.

CHAPTER 2

PANDEMICS:
GLOBAL HEALTH SECURITY

Wilmot James

Lawrence R Stanberry

Hayley Severance

Marc Grodman

Schyler Grodman

Lewis Rubin-Thompson

2.1   INTRODUCTION

Although some national responses to COVID-19 have been more successful than others, no country has emerged unscathed by the pandemic. The containment, mitigation and suppression of any pandemic, especially one fuelled by a swiftly spreading novel respiratory virus is only possible with a proportionately bold level of international cooperation using multilateral institutions. Some have characterised the global response to COVID-19 as 'dismal', 'weak', and 'uncoordinated' (*Financial Times,* Jul/Aug 2020 pp. 8–42) but this tepid global response might have been preventable if not for key leaders of the world's most powerful countries failing to mobilise and, in some cases thwarting, the world's multilateral global health security ecosystem.

Present shortcomings aside, the world has not been idle in combating global health emergencies. The WHO managed – however imperfectly – to mount global responses to the SARS epidemic in 2003, the H1N1 flu pandemic in 2009, the Ebola epidemic in 2014–16, and the ZIKA epidemic in 2015–16. Lessons were learnt and adjustments were made at every step along the way. Poor member state compliance with the WHO's International Health Regulations of 2005 prompted the launch of the multi-country Global Health Security Agenda in 2014 and the resulting Joint External Evaluation (JEE) process in 2016. These efforts are part of an impressive multilateral ecosystem which includes the Global Fund to Fight Aids, TB and malaria, the Global Alliance for Vaccines and Immunization (Gavi), the Coalition for Epidemic Preparedness (CEPI), and, though more of an evaluator rather than an actor in this space, the Global Preparedness Monitoring Board (GPMB).

The COVID-19 pandemic has stressed this emerging ecosystem to levels never before anticipated and has brought profound awareness not only to the ecosystem's shortcomings, but has also highlighted areas and opportunities for improvement.

Since 2014 epidemic risks in over 100 countries have been independently assessed through the JEE process with the goal of identifying gaps in health security. Built on the JEE assessments, the Global Health Security Index (a project of the Nuclear Threat Initiative and Johns Hopkins Center for Health Security and developed with The Economist Intelligence Unit) was released in October 2019 and further examined the strengths and weaknesses in health systems, country compliance with international norms, and the political and security environments of 195 countries. The Index's results indicated that limited progress had been made in filling financing gaps in preparedness. Similarly, the GPMB reported in September 2019 that urgent actions are required to prepare the world for health emergencies, calling on heads of government to commit to obligations under the International Health Regulations (IHR) (2005) and highlighting the need for financing institutions to link preparedness with financial risk planning. Despite high-level calls for increased financing to bolster health security, there are still no concrete incentives for countries or donors to prioritise outbreak preparedness in national budgets (Cameron et al, 2019).

The COVID-19 pandemic revealed the human cost of our global failure to lead and act on the aforementioned evidence-based health security risk assessments. Across the globe, poor preparedness has unnecessarily exposed frontline healthcare professionals and essential workers to life-threatening hazards. Many countries – even those with ample resources – struggled to develop, procure, and deploy appropriate SARS-CoV-2 diagnostic and surveillance technologies. Perhaps more alarming was the manner in which nations were unable to adequately stock essential medical equipment and supplies. As clinicians learnt about the nature of the disease, there was a global real-time educational practicum in reporting and adopting successful treatment measures and guidelines while aggressively searching for effective therapies. Monumental investments were made in an accelerated effort to research and develop vaccines that promised delivery at an unprecedented speed. Despite these noble efforts, the absence of strategic coordination and collaboration, often driven by self-interested nationalist tendencies, often took precedence.

This chapter reviews the global health security ecosystem and serves as the context for the chapters that follow. It will make a case for the world to revitalise the multilateral health security system with stronger leadership from the United Nations (UN). We call on the UN Security Council and the G7 and G20 country processes to adopt pandemic prevention and response as high-priority issues in geopolitics.

2.2 OBJECTIVES

- Establish a permanent unit in the Office of the UN Secretary-General to monitor and coordinate multilateral responses to all high consequence infectious disease and biological events, whether they are natural, accidental or deliberate.

- Strengthen the Global Preparedness Monitoring Board to improve accountability for epidemic and pandemic preparedness significantly.

- Strengthen and invest more substantially in UNICEF to care for the welfare of children, especially during catastrophes.

- Develop a robust financing mechanism for a reformed World Health Organization which better shields it from nationalistic, opportunistic, and political disruptions.

- Introduce a catalytic global health security challenge fund to drive sustainable, measurable investments in pandemic preparedness specifically.

2.3 THE GLOBAL HEALTH SECURITY ECOSYSTEM AND COVID-19

The global health security ecosystem comprises numerous organisations, and while many may share some level of collaboration and governance, these organisations generally maintain independent functionality. Initiatives undertaken by any single organisation are often inextricably entwined with the others. With overlapping missions and priorities, this intricate network of actors will continue to work jointly towards the global response to not only the COVID-19 pandemic, but to future pandemics.

2.3.1 The World Health Organization (WHO)

As a specialised agency of the UN, the WHO provides international leadership for matters related to public health and global health security while serving as the main governance structure of global health security organisations. As a technical support organisation, it distributes resources – such as medical supplies and personnel – to help support developing healthcare systems and respond to public health crises worldwide. The WHO is also responsible for monitoring public health threats as they arise and providing ethical and evidenced-based international policy recommendations in the event of an outbreak of global concern.

Attending to conflicting member state interests has become an increasing source of controversy for the WHO. As an example, during the 2016 Zika epidemic, the WHO was criticised for not making timely recommendations for women to delay pregnancy and use contraception in order to help prevent the complications the virus can produce for developing foetuses; this was primarily designed to appease Catholic member states (McNeil, 2016). In response to COVID-19, the WHO has again been criticised for catering to member state interests. The WHO has on many occasions praised China's transparency and handling of the initial outbreak in Wuhan, while China had for several weeks actively suppressed information pertaining to SARS-CoV-2 during the early stages of the pandemic (Siji, 2020). This has led to significant diplomatic conflicts for the WHO, particularly with the United States (US), culminating with former President Donald Trump's directive to withdraw critical US funding from the WHO (Shear and Jr, 2020). Fortunately, with the inauguration of Joseph Biden as president in January 2021, the US has rejoined the WHO and has committed to help fund the international effort to combat COVID-19.

At present, the efficacy of the WHO is largely dependent on member state compliance with its constitution and International Health Regulations (IHR) (2005). However, consequences such as loss of voting rights and international sanctions for non-compliance with WHO regulations are usually not employed because the WHO is primarily funded by voluntary member state contributions – action against a member state for non-compliance could result in decreased funding for an already woefully underfunded organisation (Gostin, 2020).

Contributions to the WHO's budget can be categorised in one of two ways: flexible or specified. Flexible contributions, also known as Assessed Contributions, are often from member nations, and may be allocated as the WHO sees fit. In contrast, specified contributions are granted to the WHO with a clear directive determined largely by the donor. Since the 1980s, Assessed Contributions have fallen from approximately 80% to 20% of the WHO's budget. As recently as 25 May 2020, the Director-General of the WHO, Dr Tedros Gebreyesus, has renewed a call for increased Assessed Contributions from donors (WHO, 2019). In 2002, at the end of her tenure as Director-General, Dr Gro Harlem Brundtland gave an interview with the *British Medical Journal* in which she argued that increasing voluntary funding, and diversifying the sources of this funding, will decrease the influence of any one contributor and allow the WHO to carry out its mission more effectively (Yamey, 2002).

Top 10 contributors to WHO for 2018/19 biennium
Based on WHO revenue data (in US$ millions)

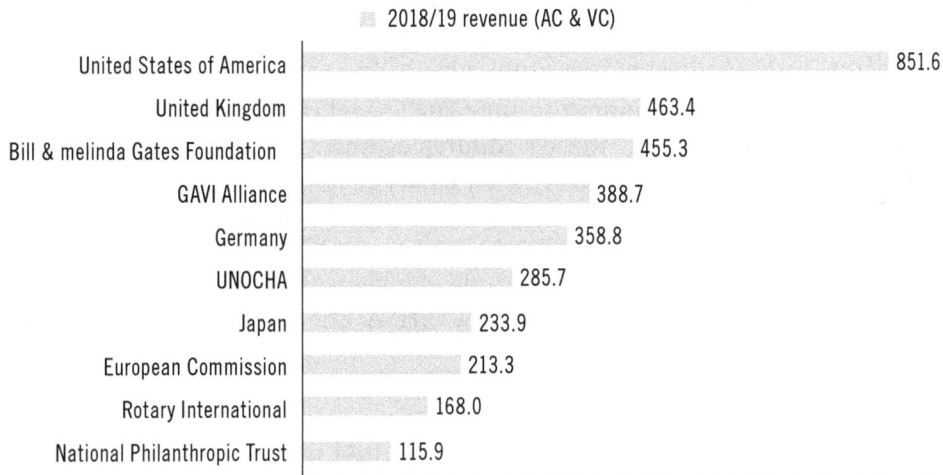

2018/19 revenue (AC & VC)

United States of America	851.6
United Kingdom	463.4
Bill & melinda Gates Foundation	455.3
GAVI Alliance	388.7
Germany	358.8
UNOCHA	285.7
Japan	233.9
European Commission	213.3
Rotary International	168.0
National Philanthropic Trust	115.9

Figure 2.1 Sources of Voluntary and Assessed Contributions to the WHO (WHO, 2019)

There have also been many calls for the restructuring of WHO governance and policies. During the 72nd World Health Assembly (WHA) in 2019, a transformation agenda for the organisation was proposed to increase the efficiency and efficacy of the WHO. The reforms to be implemented include increased collaboration with the UN; streamlining management and legislative practices so as to allow aid to reach member states faster; and increased partnerships with organisations outside the UN so as to allow more flexibility in implementing missions at the country level (World Health Assembly, 2019).

2.3.2   Global Alliance for Vaccines and Immunisation (Gavi)

In response to declining childhood vaccination efforts worldwide, Gavi was founded in 2000 as a partnership of the Bill and Melinda Gates Foundation, the WHO, UNICEF, and the World Bank. Its primary objective is to make vaccination accessible to children worldwide; Gavi also works with its partners to strengthen primary care facilities in developing countries. Together with the WHO and CEPI, Gavi co-leads the COVAX initiative to ensure equitable global access to a COVID-19 vaccine when one becomes available. The COVAX initiative is the vaccine pillar of the WHO's Access to COVID Tools accelerator (ACT) programme sponsored by a myriad of international philanthropic organisations such as the Bill and Melinda Gates Foundation and the Wellcome Trust (Gavi, 2020) (WHO, 2020a).

Gavi has faced criticisms regarding its allocation of resources and pricing of vaccines. Gavi primarily partners with and subsidises firms such as Pfizer, Johnson & Johnson, and GlaxoSmithKline (GSK). These firms have been known to charge premiums of up to 180% for their vaccines (Médecins Sans Frontières, 2011); (Médecins Sans Frontières, 2019).

At the global vaccine summit in June 2020, Gavi raised USD $8.8 billion to fund efforts to vaccinate the world's children against COVID-19 once a vaccine is made available (Gavi – the Vaccine Alliance, 2020). The United States is also making efforts to subsidise Gavi with the Global Health Security and Diplomacy Act of 2020, proposed in May by Senator Steve Risch (Republican–Idaho). The bill seeks to establish a trust fund which would help finance several international organisations, including the GHSA, the Global Fund, CEPI, and Gavi (Risch, 2020).

2.3.3   Coalition for Epidemic Preparedness (CEPI)

Originally founded in 2017, CEPI is a global vaccine research and development partnership founded by the Bill and Melinda Gates Foundation, the Wellcome Trust, the World Economic Forum, and the Indian and Norwegian governments. Worldwide contributions to CEPI have recently increased to support the rapid development and production of COVID-19 vaccines (Bernasconi et al, 2020).

CEPI's primary focus is on the research and development of vaccine technologies to increase global preparedness for emerging disease outbreaks. Research is split between developing new and safer vaccines for already known diseases and developing new vaccine technology platforms that can readily adapt to new pathogens and provide rapid immunisation in the event of a novel epidemic (Gouglas et al, 2018).

2.3.4   Global Preparedness Monitoring Board (GPMB)

Headed by former WHO Director-General Dr Gro Harlem Brundtland, the GPMB was first convened in 2018 at the behest of the UN, the WHO, and the World Bank Group. Its purpose is to monitor global threats and make recommendations for leaders of nations and multilateral institutions to increase preparedness for global health security emergencies.

The GPMB's first annual report was released in September 2019. Seven action items were given to global leaders to strengthen preparedness for threats to global health security. They include (1) Commitment to invest, as per compliance with the 2005 IHR; (2) G7, G20 and G77 Member States must lead by example by following through with their political and funding commitments for preparedness; (3) a commitment from all countries to build strong systems; (4) countries, donors, and multilateral institutions must be prepared for the worst (somewhat prophetically, a rapidly-spreading, lethal respiratory pathogen is listed among the worst-case scenarios); (5) financing institutions must account for the economic impact of disasters in their preparedness planning; (6) there must be incentive from donor organisations to increase funding for preparedness; (7) it is the responsibility of the United Nations to strengthen coordination mechanisms (Global Preparedness Monitoring Board, 2019).

2.3.5   United Nations Children's Emergency Fund (UNICEF)

A special agency of the United Nations, UNICEF provides humanitarian and developmental aid to children worldwide. Its primary activities include immunisation and disease prevention, providing treatment for children and mothers with HIV, enhancing childhood and maternal nutrition, improving sanitation conditions, promoting education, and providing emergency relief in the event of a disaster.

In response to COVID-19, UNICEF strategy is divided into two categories. The first strategic category is to advance public health measures to reduce SARS-CoV-2 transmission and mortality. The second focuses on continuity of health care; HIV care; water, sanitation and hygiene (WASH); child protection; gender-based violence; social protection and other social services. Both strategies rely heavily on up-to-date data collection, analysis and social science research (UNICEF, 2020).

UNICEF is the primary implementing instrument of childhood vaccination in low- and middle-income countries (LMICs), with Gavi as UNICEF's primary supplier. This has created a monopsony for many childhood vaccines, including those for polio, rotavirus, and pentavalent diphtheria, tetanus, pertussis, hepatitis B and Hemophilus influenza type B. The resulting market is inflated, and the cost of vaccination remains high, leading to diminished efforts to increase childhood vaccination rates (Clinton and Sridhar, 2017, pp. 86-87).

2.3.6   The Global Fund to Fight AIDS, Tuberculosis and Malaria (Global Fund)

Founded in 2000, the Global Fund collects donations and directs strategic investments to fight epidemics of AIDS, TB and malaria. The Global Fund has diverted up to USD$1 billion to fight COVID-19, strengthen healthcare systems, and mitigate the effects of the pandemic on lifesaving HIV, TB and malaria programmes. The Global Fund is also a founding partner of ACT, working with the WHO and philanthropic organisations to ensure that vulnerable populations receive equitable health care during the crisis.

In 2019, the Global Fund announced a partnership with the World Bank to increase financing for the Global Fund's mission. This partnership will allow the Global Fund to make the best use of its resources by facilitating loan buy-down programmes, establishing multi-donor trust funds, and implementing programmes with performance-based financing schemes in target countries (World Bank, 2019).

2.4   GLOBAL HEALTH SECURITY – LEGISLATION AND POLICY

The human and economic cost of the world's collective failure to respond multilaterally to the COVID-19 pandemic emphasises the importance of international coordination in response to the spread of a sinister pathogen in the future. The pandemic also exposed crippling weaknesses in a majority of international, national, and local public health strategies. Failed international cooperation is largely due to poor compliance with international laws and regulations regarding response to disease outbreaks.

The WHO's International Health Regulations (2005) (IHR), the Biological Weapons Convention (BWC), and United Nations Security Council Resolution 1540 (UNSC 1540) serve as international law for responding to emerging disease threats and the prevention of the deliberate misuse and weaponisation of pathogens and biological toxins. The Global Health Security Agenda (GHSA) (2014), the Joint External Evaluations (JEE) (2016), and the Global Health Security Index (GHSI) (2019) are multilateral efforts to assess and improve global health security capacities.

2.4.1   International Health Regulations (2005) (IHR)

The WHO's IHR (2005) currently serve as international law for the reporting of and response to disease outbreaks. A primary function of the IHR is to determine whether a disease outbreak in any member state is to be considered a Public Health Emergency of International Concern (PHEIC). Since the most recent IHR went into effect in June 2007, several diseases have received such a label. They include the H1N1 Swine Flu pandemic (2009), the West African Ebolavirus epidemic (2013–2016), Zika virus (2016), Kivu Ebola epidemic (2018–2019), and now COVID-19, first identified in late 2019. The IHR also provide guidelines to mitigate the impact of disease-related travel restrictions. The mounting economic toll resulting from COVID-19 has been fueled by widespread international travel bans that went beyond the scope of what is recommended by the IHR (Von Tigerstrom and Wilson, 2020).

Despite global efforts to increase member state compliance with the IHR, revisions are still necessary in order to make the regulations more effective; even after global efforts such as the GHSA and JEE, member state compliance with the IHR remains frightfully low. Furthermore, many member states have violated key provisions of the document, particularly those surrounding the reporting of outbreaks and implementing response mechanisms. In addition to further ensuring member state compliance, the IHR would benefit from revisions that allow its policies to be more enforceable (Tonti, 2020).

2.4.2   Biological Weapons Convention (BWC)

The BWC provides international regulations on the development, production and stockpiling of biological and toxin weapons. The regulations first went into effect on 10 April 1972; since then, the convention has been revised several times, most recently in 2017 (Nuclear Threat Initiative, 2011).

While there are currently 183 state parties to the convention, there is no formal verification regime for oversight to monitor compliance. Any country with a biodefense programme or pharmaceutical/biotech industry has the capability to produce biological weapons. There are concerns with instituting a verification regime because it is difficult to differentiate between agents that are being used for scientific and therapeutic reasons such as vaccines versus those that are being used for military purposes (Nuclear Threat Initiative, 2001). The COVID-19 pandemic has raised questions as to whether the virus SARS-CoV-2 was manufactured in a lab, was part of a weapons programme, or originated in an open-air market (European Leadership Network, 2020).

The BWC lacks the authority, workforce, and mandate to investigate and attribute an alleged use of biological weapons. Concerns surrounding the origin of COVID-19 and experiments such as the 2005 laboratory reconstruction of the 1918 Spanish influenza virus point to a need to strengthen the BWC. One recommendation is that the UN Secretary-General should provide the United Nations Office of Disarmament Affairs (UNODA) with the resources to conduct fact-finding missions which investigate the alleged use of biological weapons and determine whether the attack was carried out by a terrorist or was state-backed (Cameron et al, 2019).

2.4.3   United Nations Security Council Resolution 1540 (2004) (UNSC 1540)

Expanding upon the BWC, UNSC 1540 affirms that member states must not provide support to any non-state actors to develop, acquire, manufacture or transport chemical or biological weapons. The resolution is largely directed toward preventing terrorist organisations from acquiring, manufacturing, or using chemical and biological weapons.

The UNSC 1540 has been viewed internationally as an 'unfunded mandate', as concrete provisions to assist states directly in implementing the resolution's requirements do not exist. Even though a number of the major supporters of the resolution (including the United States, the European Union, and Japan) have actively offered assistance, many developing states fear that implementing the export controls required by UNSC 1540 will smother their nascent industries. Supporters of the resolution, however, counter that well-designed export controls laws do not hinder trade and investment (NTI, 2019).

2.4.4 Global Health Security Agenda (2014) (GHSA)

As of 2014, only 20% of countries were in compliance with IHR (2005). Recognising the global health and security risks of continued non-compliance with IHR, GHSA was launched in February 2014 by over 30 countries and non-governmental organisations with the goal of achieving a world safe and secure from infectious disease threats, whether naturally occurring or as a result of accidental or intentional release. GHSA is meant to serve as a catalyst for achieving compliance with IHR, as well as with the World Organization for Animal Health international standards and guidelines, UNSC 1540 measures, and States Parties obligations under the Biological Weapons Convention. GHSA centres around strengthening three pillars of global health security – prevent, detect, and respond. These three categories are further broken down into eleven action packages, forming a useful framework which includes capacity-related targets for each (CDC, 2019c). The 'prevent' action packages include antimicrobial resistance, zoonotic diseases, biosafety and biosecurity, and immunisation. The 'detect' action packages include national laboratory systems, real-time surveillance, reporting, and workforce development. And the 'respond' action packages include emergency operations centres, linking public health with law and multisectoral rapid response, and medical countermeasures and personnel deployment. GHSA members, in developing this clear framework for setting targets and measuring progress, have provided a useful tool for collaboration across sectors and among partner nations.

Since 2014, GHSA members have raised awareness of the importance of building national, regional, and global health security capacity, mainly through their regular ministerial meetings. Additionally, GHSA members have contributed to increased transparency within the global health security community through the creation of the GHSA assessment process, the precursor to and the model for the Joint External Evaluation (JEE) process which is discussed in the next session. Through these new processes, countries, many for the first time, began publicly publishing the results of these comprehensive assessments of their health security capacities in a demonstration of transparency and willingness to improve.

GHSA touts many accomplishments and its members, recognising its value, chose to extend it beyond the original five-year timeframe to 2024; however, GHSA also has its share of challenges. While GHSA led to the development of concrete targets across the prevent, detect, respond spectrum, it has not traditionally been successful at measuring progress globally and holding members accountable to their commitments to advance specific areas of health security. As GHSA entered its second five-year phase, members developed an overarching target as part of the GHSA 2024 Framework that reads:

> By 2024, more than 100 countries that have completed an evaluation of health security capacity will have undergone planning and resource mobilization to address gaps, and will be in the process of implementing activities to achieve impact. These countries will strengthen their capacities and demonstrate improvements in at least five technical areas to a level of "Demonstrated Capacity" or comparable level, as measured by relevant health security assessments, such as those conducted within the WHO IHR Monitoring and Evaluation Framework. (GHSA, 2018)

If GHSA as a collective can show that members are contributing toward achieving this target by advancing health security capacities globally, this will be a successful outcome of the second phase of GHSA and will effectively reduce existing health security risks highlighted by the COVID-19 pandemic.

The COVID-19 pandemic has revealed a disconnect between public health experts and political leadership, with the US being a prime example. While the US certainly possesses the resources and capacity, it is not clear if its capabilities were able to meet the extraordinary challenge of the pandemic. In addition, the ineffectiveness of leadership has led to disastrous consequences for the US. In spite of the US CDC's reputation as one of the top disease control and prevention agencies in the world, the lack of an immediate action plan, guidance, and testing at the outset of the first domestic cases demonstrated serious deficiencies in the organisation's capacity to react on a timely basis. Complicating matters further, the Trump administration frequently undermined CDC recommendations, sowing further public distrust in leadership and public institutions.

Finally, GHSA does not have funding associated with it, making it difficult for some countries to dedicate necessary time and effort to the initiative. National leadership from GHSA member states must fully buy into the value of GHSA in order to provide the dedicated resources necessary to advance progress toward prevent, detect, and respond targets. To increase the likelihood of investment, GHSA has recently formed a 'sustainable financing' action package which has the following mandate: '...develop a strategic approach for mobilizing resources to achieve sustainable financing for preparedness at the country, regional, and global levels' (GHSA, 2020). The current health crisis will certainly draw attention to and, hopefully, resources toward health security capacity building, but the challenge of securing sustainable funding remains. GHSA will have a role in ensuring the global community avoids the panic-neglect financing cycle that contributed to the struggle of many countries in bringing the COVID-19 crisis under control.

2.4.5   Joint External Evaluations (2016) (JEE)

First launched by the WHO in 2016, the JEE is designed to support the efforts of the GHSA to assess and increase member state compliance with the WHO's IHR. A JEE involves a voluntary collaboration between a country and a group of international experts to assess the country's capacities to prevent, detect and rapidly respond to public health risks, whether occurring naturally or due to deliberate or accidental events. In doing so, critical gaps in human and animal health systems may be identified in order to prioritise efforts to increase the country's preparedness and ability to respond (WHO, 2020c).

As of 2019, the JEE had been completed for 91 countries, with 19 future evaluations planned (Figure 2.1). An analysis of 55 countries' reports revealed that most countries were underprepared to prevent, detect and respond to an infectious disease outbreak (Gupta et al, 2018). The JEE are voluntary assessments, thus explaining the low rates of international participation. Concern over low rates of participation led to the formation of the Global Health Security Index, which evaluated the public health security capacities of 195 countries.

Completion of Joint External Evaluations Globally: End of 2018

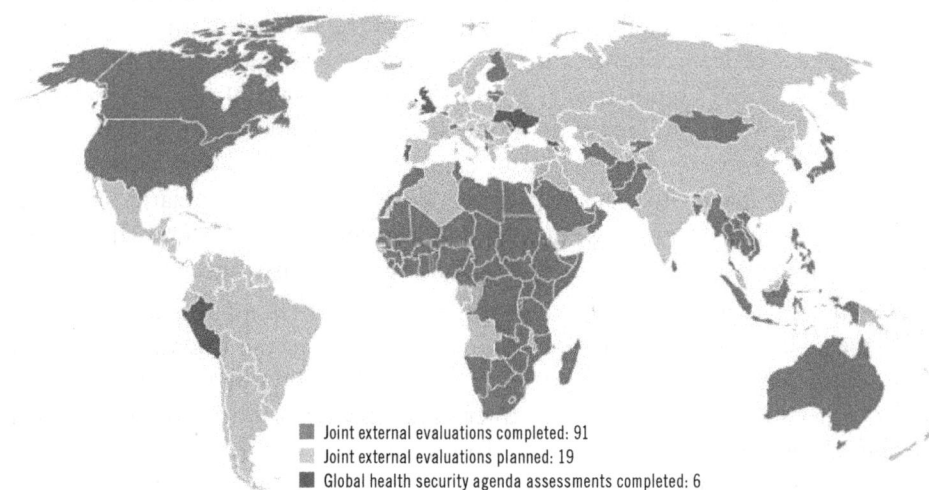

■ Joint external evaluations completed: 91
▨ Joint external evaluations planned: 19
■ Global health security agenda assessments completed: 6

Figure 2.2 Completion of Joint External Evaluations Globally: End of 2018 (CDC, 2019)

2.4.6   Global Health Security Index (2019) (GHSI)

As a partnership between the Nuclear Threat Initiative, Johns Hopkins University, and the Economist Intelligence Unit, the GHSI was designed and utilised to evaluate the global health security capacities of 195 countries. Participants were evaluated across six domains: (1) prevention of emergence or release of pathogens; (2) early detection and reporting of epidemics of potential international concern; (3) rapid response to and mitigation of outbreaks; (4) health system capabilities; (5) compliance with international norms; and (6) overall risk environments.

The GHSI concluded overall that health security was weak around the world. No country scored perfectly, and the global average score was 40.2 points out of a possible 100. Among high-income countries, the average was only 51.9. The findings of the GHSI are the most recent evidence that points to a need for all countries to strengthen health security practices.

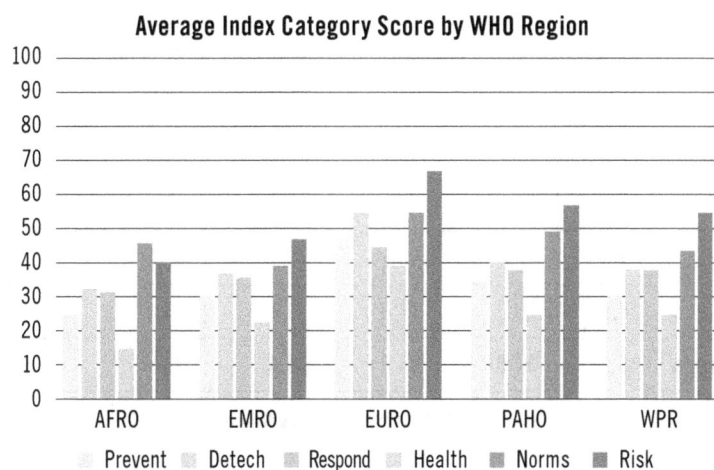

Average Index Category Score by WHO Region

WHO Region	Overall	Prevent	Detect	Respond	Health	Norms	Risk
AFRO	31.3	24.8	31.9	31.3	14.8	46.7	40.9
EMRO	35.3	30.4	37.0	35.9	23.2	40.3	47.7
EURO	51.3	48.5	55.8	45.4	39.6	54.7	68.0
PAHO	40.5	34.6	40.8	38.1	25.4	50.8	58.1
WPR	38.4	30.5	38.7	39.2	25.2	44.8	55.9
WORLD	40.2	34.8	41.9	38.4	26.4	48.5	55.0

Average Index Category Score by UN Region

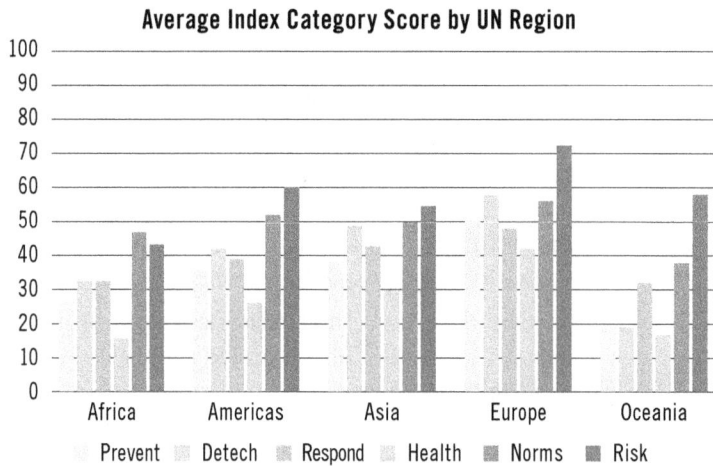

Prevent   Detech   Respond   Health   Norms   Risk

UN Region	Overall	Prevent	Detect	Respond	Health	Norms	Risk
Africa	31.0	24.9	31.3	31.6	14.9	45.1	40.9
Americas	40.5	34.6	40.8	38.1	25.4	50.8	58.1
Asia	42.3	37.2	47.5	41.1	29.1	48.1	53.2
Europe	53.0	49.3	58.1	46.9	42.1	55.1	71.1
Oceania	28.5	20.2	18.3	30.8	16.0	37.5	56.6
Grand Average	40.2	34.8	41.9	38.4	26.4	48.5	55.0

Figure 2.3 GHSI Scores by Region

2.5   STATE OF AFFAIRS: THERAPEUTICS, VACCINES, SURVEILLANCE, AND DIAGNOSTICS

Supply chain deficiencies and technological limitations of international surveillance and diagnostics contributed to the rapid global spread of COVID-19. When the disease first garnered international attention in late 2019, many countries lacked the capacity to identify local outbreaks and prevent wider spread. Compounding the lack of infrastructure were many instances of inconsistent or negligent government leadership, which hindered many countries' ability to scale up testing and prepare for increased demands on the healthcare system. New Zealand, Taiwan, and South Korea set examples by quickly developing their capacity to conduct widespread testing, screen international travellers and enact travel bans, and establish strong contact tracing networks. As a result of these efforts, the aforementioned nations saw relatively limited outbreaks, and were thus better able to mitigate the economic and social impacts of the pandemic than many other countries.

2.5.1 Therapeutics

Nearly two years into the pandemic, there remain few known effective options for the treatment of SARS-CoV-2 infections. High-flow nasal cannula oxygen therapy has proved to reduce mortality (Frat et al, 2015). Shortage of supplemental oxygen is a major problem in many LMICs, with an estimated cumulative need of 1.6 million oxygen cylinders per day (Market Dynamics, 2021). Dexamethasone, an inexpensive and widely available corticosteroid, has been shown to reduce mortality in patients hospitalised with COVID-19 requiring oxygen therapy (The RECOVERY Collaborative Group, 2020). While the drug has been recommended for use in LMICs (Islam et al, 2020), there have been concerns that international demand for the drug could result in a global shortage due to hoarding (Cahan, 2020). Other treatments such as convalescent plasma and the antiviral Remdesivir have shown mixed or detrimental results in clinical trials. While Remdesivir is being used in some countries for the treatment of patients hospitalised with COVID-19, the WHO has recommended against its use in hospitalised patients as there is currently no evidence of improved survival rates (NIH, 2021) (WHO, 2020e). Potential benefits of Remdesivir in treating paediatric cases are currently uncertain, though it is recommended over other antiviral agents (Chiotos et al, 2020). As of October 2021, the experimental drug molnupiravir, an antiviral agent designed by Merck, was shown in clinical trials to halve the chances of death and/or hospitalisation among individuals infected with SARS-CoV-2, with strong efficacy against variants (Beasley and O'Donnell, 2021).

Due to the presence of increased inflammatory markers in patients with COVID-19, il-6 receptor blockers, such as tocilizumab and sarilumab, have been administered to symptomatic patients; to apparently beneficial effect (REMAP-CAP Investigators, 2021). Monoclonal antibodies (e.g., bamlanivimab and estesevimab from Lily and casirivimab and imdevimab from Regeneron) also demonstrate promise in the treatment of mild to moderate cases, though their effectiveness in treating emerging variants of SARS-CoV-2 is currently unknown.

While progress with therapeutics has been slow, the underlying approach to treating COVID-19 patients in terms of medical management has contributed significantly to the ability of the global medical and scientific communities to share research and conduct reliable clinical studies within abbreviated timeframes. Basic treatment guidelines, such as early implementation of high-flow supplemental oxygen, prophylactic anti-coagulants, awareness of cardiac and renal complications, and prone positioning of patients on ventilators have led to improved outcomes in COVID-19 patients.

2.5.2   Vaccines

SARS-CoV-2 vaccines are currently the most effective tool for combatting the spread of COVID-19 and preventing death and hospitalisation. There are currently 194 SARS-CoV-2 vaccines in development, with many having already reached the third phase of clinical trials, which evaluates efficacy and safety (WHO, 2021). As of 3 October 2021, 22 vaccines have received approval in at least one country (RAPS, 2021).

With the approval of the vaccines, there remain issues of financing, mass production, and equitable distribution. History has shown that national interests will take priority in the distribution of a vaccine (Bollyky and Bown, 2020). Many rich countries have already secured vaccine doses for over 100% of their population, contributing to the shortage of doses allotted to LMICs. Organisations that support the COVAX initiative, such as Gavi and CEPI, will be critical in ensuring adequate funding for and equitable access to COVID-19 vaccines when they become available. It is estimated that widespread COVID-19 vaccination will prevent the loss of US$375 billion to the global economy per month; however, this will only be possible if a vaccine is made available globally, and to high-risk groups such as health care workers and the elderly (WHO, 2020c).

The US government commissioned millions of doses of vaccines from Pfizer and Moderna in anticipation of the results of Phase III clinical trials of their mRNA vaccines. The University of Oxford has partnered with the Serum Institute in India to mass-produce its vaccine ahead of results from its Phase III clinical trials. Countries in Africa and South America face a serious disadvantage when accessing vaccines, as there are no major manufacturers of vaccines on either continent. While programmes run by the WHO, Gavi, and CEPI exist to ensure vaccines are distributed to developing countries, it is unlikely that they will be sufficient to meet the demand presented by COVID-19. The COVAX facility projects delivery of 2 billion vaccine doses to African Union countries by the first quarter of 2022, 25% lower than was predicted in June 2021. The downgraded forecast is largely due to a prolonged pause of exports from the Serum Institute of India, production capacity constraints for Johnson & Johnson and AstraZeneca, and uncertainty surrounding the approval of additional vaccine candidates (Gavi, 2021). In order to combat inequitable distribution of vaccines in the long run, it will be necessary to bolster vaccine manufacturing capacity in regions of the world with high demand for vaccines and a lack of vaccine infrastructure such as on the African continent and in South America.

Another hurdle faced by vaccine efforts is vaccine hesitancy, which, as of 2019, was listed by the WHO as being among the top 10 threats to global health. A survey administered by Northeastern University, Harvard University, Rutgers University and Northwestern University, prior to any vaccine being approved in the USA, found that only two-thirds (66%) of Americans were likely to take a COVID-19 vaccine if it were available. Among African Americans, a demographic dispropor-tionately affected by SARS-CoV-2, only 50% of respondents reported that they would likely receive a vaccine if given the option (Lazer et al, 2020). Resistance to vaccine uptake will undermine the herd-immunity effects of vaccination campaigns and prolong the duration of the pandemic, as we have no antivirals that will be useful in bringing the pandemic to an end. This emphasises the need for the continued development of effective COVID-19 treatment strategies alongside ensuring equitable access to vaccines as they become available.

2.5.3 Surveillance

Surveillance, which has taken on a new meaning in the age of COVID-19, is a critical component to Global Health Security; it helps to ensure early detection of outbreaks, monitor the number of cases and hospitalisations, assess the severity of those cases, and monitor supply levels of the resources that admitted patients require (ICU status, ventilators, therapeutics, etc.). Comprehensive surveillance is also necessary to understand community infection rates so that appropriate public health measures can be evaluated and implemented. With the advent of new COVID-19 variants, which may possess different degrees of infectivity or trigger more severe disease in infected patients, appropriate global surveillance may be seen as more critical to achieving the endpoints of global health security than any one component alone; these new variants of COVID-19 may appear not only in large population centres, but also in smaller areas where the implementation of large-scale vaccination programmes may be problematic.

The principles of surveillance may face equal challenges on a global scale as well as within sovereign borders. On a local level, screening for COVID-19 currently comes in many forms, such as temperature checks, questions of the existence of symptoms and in many cases, required evidence of negative testing. Routine testing in the workplace, in schools, and for travel purposes have been increasingly adopted but often subject to local and private sector guidelines, even with consistent access to appropriate diagnostics tools. We have seen contact tracing become problematic in the face of such high community spread, as the numbers become too overwhelming to manage. At some point, environmental and wastewater testing to evaluate community spread will become essential. However, in order to slow the spread of infectious disease at any level – international, national, or local – routine functional surveillance mechanisms and infrastructure need to be in place to detect and respond to outbreaks promptly.

It is important to note that there is currently not enough data to determine whether a positive COVID-19 antibody test is indicative of immunity to reinfection (Metcalf et al, 2020).

Early detection and reporting are of critical importance to mitigate the spread of infectious diseases. The Program for Monitoring Emerging Diseases (ProMED) platform, founded in 1994 by the International Society for Infectious Diseases (ISID), relies on a global network of operators and moderators which scans for and reviews reports of infectious disease outbreaks. ProMED has been the first to report several outbreaks of note, including SARS, MERS, Ebola, and Zika. ProMED also offered one of the earliest reports of COVID-19 to the WHO – the report contributed significantly to early efforts by the WHO to mount an international response to the virus (WHO, 2020). Strengthening ProMED's surveillance and reporting capabilities is an effort that could greatly reduce the risk posed by emerging infectious diseases in the future.

2.5.4   Diagnostics

COVID-19 presented unanticipated challenges to the entire continuum of diagnostic testing. Initial SARS-CoV-2 diagnostic tests relied primarily on polymerase chain reaction (PCR) technology. Early shortcomings in testing stemmed from issues with the global supply chain of reagents and testing equipment. The global system was largely unprepared, and many countries failed to mount effective testing strategies in a timely manner, leading outbreaks to go unnoticed until infections had become widespread. WHO guidelines state that in order to control the spread of SARS-CoV-2 successfully, testing capacity must be such that less than 10% of test results are returned positive. Testing levels below this threshold allow many outbreaks to go undetected. In June, Nobel Laureate economist Paul Romer estimated that the US would need to conduct 30 million daily tests to generate less than 10% positive results (Nature Biotechnology, 2020).

The United States is a perfect illustration of the disconnect between possessing outstanding expertise and lacking the infrastructure to respond to the testing requirements necessitated by the pandemic successfully. In the United States, the prevailing system of testing is largely diagnostic. Laboratories, both commercial and those affiliated with public health systems, hospitals, and clinics, obtain an order for a test from a health care provider who thereby 'owns' and acts on the result. At the outset of the pandemic, where the goal was rapid identification and containment, efforts fell short. While the CDC was able to validate a test relatively quickly, despite not adopting the WHO testing kit that was used globally, they decided to create their own testing kit with the responsibility for containment delegated to 97 public health laboratories which lacked the capacity and infrastructure to accomplish this goal (CDC, 2020a). In order to meet the national demand of testing, commercial laboratories were required to obtain emergency certification and shift their operations to accommodate clinical test samples (CDC, 2020b). As if ramping up testing capacity was not challenging enough, there was up to a three-week delay for the public health laboratories to validate the assay due to a defect in one of the components sent by the CDC which was required to set up the assay.

Even if regulatory challenges were not in place, the pandemic evolved, the priority of containment shifted to mitigation, and whatever testing capacity existed needed to be diverted toward diagnostic purposes. By March 2020, in vitro diagnostic companies, those companies that build equipment aimed at automating the testing process, were given regulatory clearance to enable SARS-CoV-2 testing to be incorporated in their workflow so as to increase throughput. Once access to those testing systems was possible, commercial laboratories, hospitals, and related health facilities were able to significantly increase their own testing capacity.

Despite formidable efforts and progress, supply issues have complicated response capabilities and remain unresolved to this day. While the shortages were seen in every aspect of testing, swabs, reagents, tips on processing, every imaginable aspect of the testing process, ultimately the system was crushed by the numbers, due in no small part to less than universal adoption of public health measures by large parts of the country. As a result, the burden on the diagnostic testing system was overwhelming given the need to screen large numbers of asymptomatic people, causing significant delays in returning results in a timely manner.

With the need to test significant numbers of individuals for surveillance/screening purposes, other deficits came to light. One was the lack of effective point of care testing that could produce a quality and timely result, followed by the overall lack of infrastructure which supports decentralised testing, as well as public health initiatives that seek to fill the same void. In this context, the different available technologies offer additional challenges. While PCR testing offers higher sensitivity, they are associated with central laboratories, higher cost and longer turn-around time for results. When used for diagnostic purposes alone, meaning when the suspicion of infectivity is great due to close exposure or symptoms, they remain the gold standard. In some cases, if the purpose is to test for 'infectiousness' in asymptomatic patients, they may be too sensitive, meaning finding the virus at levels that are probably not consistent with passing on the disease (Alemany et al, 2021). Most point of care assays test for viral fragments or antigens. By and large, these are available in many modalities and configurations; they are also less costly, easy to operate, and can be adapted to lower resourced areas. The trade-off is that they are often less sensitive and therefore not really applicable for use in a 'diagnostic setting'.

COVID-19 testing started at point zero, meaning that entirely new assays had to be developed. The approach that all testing is the same created undue expectations. We have learned that the key to any programme is to match the specific application with the most appropriate technology (Mina and Andersen, 2020). The usual standards of efficacy, like sensitivity and specificity, have to be considered under specific circumstances, which is why WHO recently recommended that 80% sensitivity and 97% specificity is adequate for antigen testing, a conclusion that is reflective of the application, practicality and cost. Even other measures of positive and negative predictive value, measures that have long been used to evaluate the adequacy of testing, will markedly change if testing is conducted in communities with 1–2% of active infections rather than those with 5–10% or greater (Peeling et al, 2021).

Sequencing of the COVID-19 virus is relatively straightforward, however it is more expensive, takes greater technical skill and sophistication, and requires dedicated specialised informatics, as do most sequencing-based technologies. Sequencing is not a routine test, but it is critical that a percentage of positives are routinely sequenced to discover new variants and assess their potential resistance to antibody treatments and existing or newly developed vaccine candidates. Without attention to these questions and a full understanding of the available technology, their limitations, the scope of their application, and the diagnostic aspect of pandemic responsiveness will remain problematic.

2.5.5   Special Considerations for Children

When compared to other populations, children are not as likely to face severe health risks from COVID-19 – clinical presentations of COVID-19 in children have most often been mild or asymptomatic (Yasuhara et al, 2020). Paediatric patients may develop Multisystem Inflammatory Syndrome in Children (MIS-C) as a result of severe COVID-19 infection; MIS-C presents with generalised symptoms that are seen in other paediatric systemic illnesses, such as Kawasaki Disease or Toxic Shock Syndrome (American Academy of Pediatrics, 2021). Though paediatric patients with MIS-C are commonly treated with Intravenous Immunoglobin (IVIG) and usually started on aspirin for anti-coagulation (if clinically appropriate), the care of MIS-C patients is not dramatically different from the treatment of severe adult COVID-19 infections (Larson et al, 2020).

Children do, however, face unique challenges, such as decreased access to childhood vaccination and medications to manage chronic conditions, particularly in the developing world; gaps in education due to school closures; threats to adequate nutrition in the face of economic downturn; and an increased risk of child abuse due to financial hardships, overcrowding, and stress (Chandan et al, 2020). These issues will require special attention from governments and humanitarian aid organisations.

Organisations such as UNICEF, UNESCO, Gavi, CEPI, and the WHO are mounting efforts such as the Access to COVID-19 Tools (ACT), an accelerator set up to ensure the needs of vulnerable groups such as children are met. A recent study by Abbas et al, found that the potential loss of life resulting from suspending routine childhood immunisation during the pandemic far outweighs the mortality risk posed to children by SARS-CoV-2 (Abbas et al, 2020). For this reason alone, efforts must be made to ensure that a steady supply of standard childhood vaccinations remains intact for the duration of the pandemic. Humanitarian efforts must also focus on supplying adequate nutrition to pregnant women and children in developing countries.

Decisions to close schools have been made internationally, and with good cause – it is difficult to implement effective social distancing protocols and mitigate pathogen spread in traditional school settings. As a result, many children face significant gaps in education due to the challenges posed by remote learning; they also face adverse social and economic effects due to the strain put on parents and teachers during the transition to distance education (UNESCO, 2020a). In order to meet these challenges, innovative solutions are necessary. Efforts should be made to maximise accessibility to the technology necessary to access online materials (UNESCO, 2020b).

Children and women also face an increased risk of domestic violence, as many families are now being confined together at home for extended periods. Child abuse is most commonly detected at school and during medical appointments. Due to school closures and an increased use of telemedicine, it is likely that many instances of abuse are going undetected (Roca et al, 2020).

While children are less likely to become seriously ill or die from COVID-19, they nevertheless spread the virus when infected. More attention needs to be paid to the potential direct and indirect benefits of childhood immunisation with a COVID-19 vaccine. Immunising children would contribute to herd immunity and likely accelerate a return to normal, including a return to school (Barber, 2020).

2.6 CONCLUSION AND RECOMMENDATIONS

As the COVID-19 crisis begins to resolve, the threat of novel emerging infectious diseases is ever-present. The consensus among epidemiologists and infectious disease experts is that a novel influenza virus with high transmissibility and mortality could result in human and economic destruction on the scale of a thermonuclear war (Barrett and Stanberry, 2009) (Morse, 1996). Improving the infrastructure of global health security is paramount to preparedness for future pandemics. Globalisation has led to an increase in international trade and travel, allowing a novel respiratory pathogen to spread quickly across borders and among continents if the initial outbreak is not promptly reported and contained. If the international response to such a disease outbreak is delayed, uncoordinated, and inadequate, as it has been with COVID-19, the human and economic consequences of the disease could be devastating. The deliberate weaponisation of pathogens and biological agents also remains a threat, therefore future planning must include the strengthening of existing biosecurity and biosafety practices and legislation.

In order to strategically invest in preparedness and to strengthen the existing legislation and institutions that support global health security, we make the following recommendations:

- The UN Security Council and the G7 and G20 country processes should declare pandemic prevention and response high-priority issues in geopolitics.
- A permanent unit should be established in the Office of the UN Secretary-General to monitor and coordinate multilateral responses to all high consequence infectious diseases and biological events, whether they are natural, accidental or deliberate.
- The Global Preparedness Monitoring Board should be strengthened in order to substantially improve accountability for epidemic and pandemic preparedness.
- Greater investments should be made in UNICEF to care for the welfare of children, especially during disasters.
- A robust and diverse financing mechanism for a reformed World Health Organisation that shields it from opportunistic shocks should be developed.
- A catalytic global health security challenge fund should be established to specifically drive sustainable, measurable investments in pandemic preparedness.

Even with the aforementioned recommendations, the key factor towards the success of the global health security ecosystem is coordination among all its members. Whether from governmental, philanthropic, or other entities, various organisations are making substantial contributions. The political will of all nations of varying wealth will always be problematic in a global endeavour whose beneficiaries may be far away. COVID-19 has illustrated to a frightening extent the global risk posed by a new pandemic, as well as the need for a united response to such threats from a global community. How we react to this moment, to institutionalise these advances to combat future outbreaks, will define our response as much as that to the COVID-19 pandemic itself.

2.7   SELF-ASSESSMENT QUESTIONS

1. Discuss the role of the Global Alliance for Vaccines and Immunisation with reference to its resource allocation and pricing of vaccines.
2. Discuss some of the country level deficiencies that contributed to the spread of COVID-19 globally.

2.8   REFERENCES

Abbas, K., Procter, S.R., Van Zandvoort, K., Clark, A., Funk, S., Mengistu, T., Hogan, D., Dansereau, E., Jit, M., Flasche, S., Rein M G J Houben, Edmunds, W.J., Villabona-Arenas, C.J., Atkins, K.E., Knight, G.M., Sun, F.Y, Auzenbergs, M., Rosello, A., Klepac, P., Hellewell, J., Russell, T.W., Tully, D.C., Emery, J.C., Gibbs, H.P., Munday, J.D., Quilty, B.J., Diamond, C., Pearson, C.A.B., Leclerc, Q.J., Nightingale, E.S., Liu, Y., Akira Endo, Deol, A.K., Kucharski, A.J., Abbott, S., Jarvis, C.I., O'Reilly, K., Jombart, T., Gimma, A., Bosse, N.I., Prem, K., Hué, S., Davies, N.G., Eggo, R.M., Clifford, S. and Medley, G. 2020. Routine Childhood Immunisation During the COVID-19 Pandemic in Africa: A Benefit–Risk Analysis of Health Benefits Versus Excess Risk of SARS-CoV-2 Infection. *The Lancet Global Health*. Available at: http://www.sciencedirect.com/science/article/pii/S2214109X20303089.

Alemany, A., Baró, B., Ouchi, D., Rodó, P., Ubals, M., Corbacho-Monné, M., Vergara-Alert, J., Rodon, J., Segalés, J., Esteban, C., Fernández, G., Ruiz, L., Bassat, Q., Clotet, B., Ara, J., Vall-Mayans, M., G-Beiras, C., Blanco, I. and Mitjà, O. 2021. Analytical and Clinical Performance of the Panbio COVID-19 Antigen-Detecting Rapid Diagnostic Test. *Journal of Infection* 82(5). Available at: https://www.journalofinfection.com/article/S0163-4453(21)00004-9/fulltext.

American Academy of Paediatrics (2021). Multisystem Inflammatory Syndrome in Children (MIS-C) Interim Guidance. services.aap.org. Available at: https://services.aap.org/en/pages/2019-novel-coronavirus-covid-19-infections/clinical-guidance/multisystem-inflammatory-syndrome-in-children-mis-c-interim-guidance/.

Barber, G. 2020. Making a Covid-19 Vaccine Is Hard. Making One for Kids Is Harder. *Wired*. Available at: https://www.wired.com/story/making-a-covid-19-vaccine-is-hard-making-one-for-kids-is-harder/.

Barrett, A. and Stanberry, L.R. 2009. *Vaccines for Biodefense*. 1st ed. Amsterdam: Elsevier.

Beasley, D. and O'Donnell, C. 2021. Merck Pill Seen as "huge advance," Raises Hope of Preventing COVID-19 Deaths. *Reuters*. Available at: https://www.reuters.com/business/healthcare-pharmaceuticals/mercks-covid-19-pill-cuts-risk-death-hospitalization-by-50-study-2021-10-01/.

Benn, C.S., Fisker, A.B., Rieckmann, A., Sørup, S. and Aaby, P. 2020. Vaccinology: time to change the paradigm? *The Lancet Infectious Diseases* 20(7). Available at: https://www.sciencedirect.com/science/article/pii/S147330991930742X.

Bernasconi, V., Kristiansen, P.A., Whelan, M., Román, R.G., Bettis, A., Yimer, S.A., Gurry, C., Andersen, S.R., Yeskey, D., Mandi, H., Kumar, A., Holst, J., Clark, C., Cramer, J.P., Røttingen, J.-A., Hatchett, R., Saville, M. and Norheim, G. 2020. Developing vaccines against epidemic-prone emerging infectious diseases. *Bundesgesundheitsblatt, Gesundheitsforschung, Gesundheitsschutz* 63(1), pp. 65–73. Available at: https://www.ncbi.nlm.nih.gov/pmc/articles/PMC6925075/.

Bollyky, T.J. and Bown, C.P. 2020. The Tragedy of Vaccine Nationalism. *Foreign Affairs.* Available at: https://www.foreignaffairs.com/articles/united-states/2020-07-27/vaccine-nationalism-pandemic/.

Cahan, E. 2020. Drug recently shown to reduce coronavirus death risk could run out, experts warn. *Science | AAAS.* Available at: https://www.sciencemag.org/news/2020/06/corticosteroid-drug-recently-shown-reduce-coronavirus-death-risk-could-run-out-experts.

Cameron E.E., Nuzzo J.B. and Bell J.A. Global health security index: building collective action and accountability. October 2019. *GHS Index.* Available: https://www.ghsindex.org/wp-content/uploads/2019/10/2019-Global-Health-Security-Index.pdf.

Cameron, E., Katz, R., Konyndyk, J. and Nalabandian, M. 2019. A Spreading Plague: Lessons and Recommendations for Responding to a Deliberate Biological Event. *NTI Paper.* Available at: https://media.nti.org/documents/NTI_Paper_A_Spreading_Plague_FINAL_061119.pdf.

CDC. 2019. Advancing the Global Health Security Agenda: CDC Achievements & Impact. Centers for Disease Control and Prevention. Available at: https://www.cdc.gov/globalhealth/security/ghsareport/2018/jee.html.

CDC. 2019c. CDC Global Health – Global Health Security Agenda: Action Packages. Centers for Disease Control and Prevention. Available at: https://www.cdc.gov/globalhealth/security/actionpackages/default.htm.

CDC. 2020a. Coronavirus Disease 2019 (COVID-19) Testing In US. Centers for Disease Control and Prevention. Available at: https://www.cdc.gov/coronavirus/2019-ncov/cases-updates/previous-testing-in-us.html.

CDC. 2020b. COVIDView, Key Updates for Week 33. Centers for Disease Control and Prevention. Available at: https://www.cdc.gov./coronavirus/2019-ncov/covid-data/covidview/index.html.

Chandan, J.S., Taylor, J., Bradbury-Jones, C., Nirantharakumar, K., Kane, E. and Bandyopadhyay, S. 2020. COVID-19: A Public Health Approach to Manage Domestic Violence is Needed. *The Lancet Public Health*, 309(5), p.6.

Chiotos, K., Hayes, M., Kimberlin, D.W., Jones, S.B., James, S.H., Pinninti, S.G., Yarbrough, A., Abzug, M.J., MacBrayne, C.E., Soma, V.L., Dulek, D.E., Vora, S.B., Waghmare, A., Wolf, J., Olivero, R., Grapentine, S., Wattier, R.L., Bio, L., Cross, S.J. and Dillman, N.O. 2020. Multicenter Interim Guidance on Use of Antivirals for Children with COVID-19/SARS-CoV-2. *Journal of the Paediatric Infectious Diseases Society* 13(10).

Clinton, C. and Devi Lalita Sridhar. 2017. *Governing Global Health : Who Runs the World and Why?* 1st ed. New York, NY: Oxford University Press, pp. 86–87.

European Leadership Network (2020). COVID-19 shows that the Biological Weapons Convention must be strengthened. Available at: https://www.european leadershipnetwork.org/commentary/covid-19-shows-that-the-biological-weapons-convention-must-be-strengthened/.

FDA. 2020. Emergency Use Authorization for Remdesivir. US Food and Drug Administration. Available at: https://www.fda.gov/media/137564/download.

Frat, J-P., Thille, A.W., Mercat, A., Girault, C., Ragot, S., Perbet, S., Prat, G., Boulain, T., Morawiec, E., Cottereau, A., Devaquet, J., Nseir, S., Razazi, K., Mira, J-P., Argaud, L., Chakarian, J.-C., Ricard, J.-D., Wittebole, X., Chevalier, S. and Herbland, A. 2015. High-Flow Oxygen through Nasal Cannula in Acute Hypoxemic Respiratory Failure. *New England Journal of Medicine* 372(23), pp. 2185–2196. Available at: https://www.nejm.org/doi/full/10.1056/NEJMoa1503326.

GAVI (2021). *COVAX: the Forecast for Vaccine Supply.* [online] www.gavi.org. Available at: https://www.gavi.org/vaccineswork/covax-forecast-vaccine-supply.

Gavi. 2020. COVAX Facility. Gavi – Vaccine Alliance. Available at: https://www.gavi.org/covid19/covax-facility.

Gavi. 2020. World Leaders Make Historic Commitments to Provide Equal Access to Vaccines for All. Gavi – Vaccine Alliance. Available at: https://www.gavi.org/covid19/covax-facility.

GHSA. 2018. Global Health Security Agenda (GHSA) 2024 Framework Overview. Global Health Security Agenda. Available at: https://ghsagenda.org/wp-content/uploads/2020/06/ghsa2024-framework.pdf.

GHSA. 2020. Sustainable Financing. Global Health Security Agenda. Available at: https://ghsagenda.org/sustainable-financing/.

Global Preparedness Monitoring Board. 2019. Annual Report on Global Preparedness for Health Emergencies. Global Preparedness Monitoring Board: A World at Risk. Available at: https://www.gpmb.org/annual-reports/overview/item/2019-a-world-at-risk.

Gostin, L.O. 2020. COVID-19 Reveals Urgent Need to Strengthen the World Health Organization. *JAMA Health Forum* 1(4), p.e200559.

Gouglas, D., Thanh Le, T., Henderson, K., Kaloudis, A., Danielsen, T., Hammersland, N.C., Robinson, J.M., Heaton, P.M. and Røttingen, J.A. 2018. Estimating the Cost of Vaccine Development Against Epidemic Infectious Diseases: A Cost Minimisation Study. *The Lancet Global Health* 6(12), pp. e1386–e1396.

Gupta, V., Kraemer, J.D., Katz, R., Jha, A.K., Kerry, V.B., Sane, J., Ollgren, J. and Salminen, M.O. 2018. Analysis of Results from the Joint External Evaluation: Examining its Strength and Assessing for Trends Among Participating Countries. *Journal of Global Health* 8(2). Available at: https://www.ncbi.nlm.nih.gov/pmc/articles/PMC6204750/.

Harvard Health Publishing. 2020. Treatments for COVID-19. *Harvard Health.* Available at: https://www.health.harvard.edu/diseases-and-conditions/treatments-for-covid-19.

Islam, M.S., Sarkar, T., Khan, S.H., Mostofa Kamal, A.H., Hasan, S.M.M., Kabir, A., Yeasmin, D., Islam, M.A., Amin Chowdhury, K.I., Anwar, K.S., Chughtai, A.A. and Seale, H. 2020. COVID-19–Related Infodemic and Its Impact on Public Health: A Global Social Media Analysis. *The American Journal of Tropical Medicine and Hygiene*, 103(4).

Jenkins, B. 2020. Now Is the Time to Revisit the Global Health Security Agenda. *Brookings.* Available at: https://www.brookings.edu/blog/order-from-chaos/2020/03/27/now-is-the-time-to-revisit-the-global-health-security-agenda/.

Larson, D.T., Sherner, J.H., Gallagher, K.M., Judy, C.L., Paul, M.B., Mahoney, A.M. and Weina, P.J. 2020. Clinical Outcomes of Coronavirus Disease 2019 With Evidence-based Supportive Care. *Clinical Infectious Diseases: An Official Publication of the Infectious Diseases Society of America.* Available at: https://www.ncbi.nlm.nih.gov/pmc/articles/PMC7314121/.

Lazer, D., Baum, M.A., Ognyanova, K. and Della Volpe, J. 2020. The State of the Nation: A 50-State COVID-19 Survey. Available at: http://www.kateto.net/COVID19%20CONSORTIUM%20REPORT%20April%202020.pdf.

Market Dynamics. 2021. COVID-19 Oxygen Needs Tracker. PATH. Available at: https://www.path.org/programs/market-dynamics/covid-19-oxygen-needs-tracker/.

Mcneil, D.G. 2016. *Zika the Emerging Epidemic.* 1st ed. New York W.W. Norton & Company, pp. 149–150.

Médecins Sans Frontières. 2011. *GAVI Money Welcome but Could it Be More Wisely Spent?.* Available at: https://www.msf.org/gavi-money-welcome-could-it-be-more-wisely-spent.

Médecins Sans Frontières. 2019. *Gavi Must Stop Giving Millions in Subsidies to Pfizer and GSK for Pneumonia Vaccine*. Doctors Without Borders – USA. Available at: https://www.doctorswithoutborders.org/what-we-do/news-stories/news/gavi-must-stop-giving-millions-subsidies-pfizer-and-gsk-pneumonia.

Metcalf, C.J.E., Viboud, C., Spiro, D.J. and Grenfell, B.T. 2020. Using Serology with Models to Clarify the Trajectory of the SARS-CoV-2 Emerging Outbreak. *Trends in Immunology* 41(10), pp. 849–851.

Mimche, H., Squires, E., Miangotar, Y., Mokdad, A. and El Bcheraoui, C. 2018. Resource Allocation Strategies to Increase the Efficiency and Sustainability of Gavi's Health System Strengthening Grants. *The Paediatric Infectious Disease Journal* 37(5), pp. 407–412. Available at: https://www.ncbi.nlm.nih.gov/pmc/articles/PMC5916462/.

Mina, M.J. and Andersen, K.G. 2020. COVID-19 Testing: One Size Does Not Fit All. *Science* 371(6525), pp. 126–127.

Ministry of Foreign Affairs. 2020. *Norway to increase support for vaccine development by NOK 2.2 billion*. Government.no. Available at: https://www.regjeringen.no/en/aktuelt/norge-oker-bistanden-til-vaksineutvikling-med-22-milliarder-kroner/id2695577/.

Morse, S.S. 1996. *Emerging Viruses*. New York: Oxford University Press.

Nature Biotechnology. 2020. The COVID-19 Testing Debacle. *Nature Biotechnology*, 38(653). Available at: https://www.nature.com/articles/s41587-020-0575-3#citeas.

NIH. 2021. COVID-19 Treatment Guidelines. COVID-19 Treatment Guidelines. Available at: https://www.covid19treatmentguidelines.nih.gov/table-of-contents/.

Nkengasong, J.N., Maiyegun, O. and Moeti, M. 2017. Establishing the Africa Centres for Disease Control and Prevention: Responding to Africa's Health Threats. *The Lancet Global Health* 5(3), pp. e246–e247. Available at: https://www.thelancet.com/journals/langlo/article/PIIS2214-109X(17)30025-6/fulltext.

NTI. 2011. Convention on the Prohibition of the Development, Production and Stockpiling of Bacteriological (Biological) and Toxin Weapons (BTWC) | Treaties & Regimes. Available at: https://www.nti.org/learn/treaties-and-regimes/convention-prohibition-development-production-and-stockpiling-bacteriological-biological-and-toxin-weapons-btwc/.

Nuclear Threat Initiative. 2001. *Biological Weapons Convention (BWC) Compliance Protocol*. Available at: https://www.nti.org/analysis/articles/biological-weapons-convention-bwc/.

Peeling, R.W., Olliaro, P.L., Boeras, D.I. and Fongwen, N. 2021. Scaling up COVID-19 Rapid Antigen Tests: Promises and Challenges. *The Lancet Infectious Diseases, Published Online.*

RAPS. 2021. COVID-19 Vaccine Tracker. Available at: https://www.raps.org/news-and-articles/news-articles/2020/3/covid-19-vaccine-tracker.

REMAP-CAP Investigators (2021). Interleukin-6 Receptor Antagonists in Critically Ill Patients with Covid-19. New England Journal of Medicine, April 2021(384).

Risch, J.E. 2020. Text - S.3829 - 116th Congress (2019–2020): Global Health Security and Diplomacy Act of 2020. congress.gov. Available at: https://www.congress.gov/bill/116th-congress/senate-bill/3829/text?q=%7B%22search%22%3A%5B%22s+3829%22%5D%7D&r=1&s=1.

Roca, E., Melgar, P., Gairal-Casado, R. and Pulido-Rodriguez, M.A., 2020. Schools That 'Open Doors' to Prevent Child Abuse in Confinement by COVID19. *Sustainability* 12(11), pp. 4685.

Shear, M.D. and Jr, D.G.M. 2020. Criticized for Pandemic Response, Trump Tries Shifting Blame to the W.H.O. *The New York Times*. 14 Apr. Available at: https://www.nytimes.com/2020/04/14/us/politics/coronavirus-trump-who-funding.html.

Siji, D. 2020. The Truth About 'Dramatic Action'. *China Media Project*. Available at: http://chinamediaproject.org/2020/01/27/dramatic-actions/.

The Global Fund (2020). COVID-19 Situation Report #24. Available at: https://www.theglobalfund.org/media/10026/covid19_2020-08-04-situation_report_en.pdf?u=637321610110000000.

The Global Fund. 2019. Global Fund Overview. Available at: https://www.theglobalfund.org/en/overview/.

The Lancet Infectious Diseases. 2017. A New Day for African Public Health. *The Lancet Infectious Diseases* 17(3), p.237.

The RECOVERY Collaborative Group (2020). Dexamethasone in Hospitalized Patients with Covid-19 – Preliminary Report. *New England Journal of Medicine*, 384(11).

Tonti, L. 2020. The International Health Regulations: The Past and the Present, But What Future? *Harvard International Law Journal*. Available at: https://harvardilj.org/2020/04/the-international-health-regulations-the-past-and-the-present-but-what-future/.

UNESCO. 2020a. Adverse Consequences of School Closures. Available at: https://en.unesco.org/covid19/educationresponse/consequences.

UNESCO. 2020b. Distance learning solutions. Available at: https://en.unesco.org/covid19/educationresponse/solutions.

UNICEF. 2020. *UNICEF – Humanitarian Action for Children – Coronavirus (COVID-19) Global Response*. Available at: https://www.unicef.org/appeals/covid-2019.html#:~:text=Improve%20IPC%20and%20provide%20critical.

Von Tigerstrom, B. and Wilson, K. 2020. COVID-19 Travel Restrictions and the International Health Regulations (2005). *BMJ Global Health* 5(5), p.e002629.

Wee, S.L. and Simões, M. 2020. In Coronavirus Vaccine Race, China Strays From the Official Paths. *The New York Times*. 16 Jul. Available at: https://www.nytimes.com/2020/07/16/business/china-vaccine-coronavirus.html.

World Bank. 2019. World Bank and Global Fund Deepen Partnership with Co-Financing Agreement. Available at: https://www.worldbank.org/en/news/press-release/2019/10/22/world-bank-and-global-fund-deepen-partnership-with-co-financing-agreement.

World Health Assembly. 2019. Seventy-Second World Health Assembly A72/48 Provisional Agenda Item 18.1 WHO Reform Processes, Including the Transformation Agenda, and Implementation of United Nations Development System Reform. Available at: https://apps.who.int/iris/bitstream/handle/10665/328884/A72_48-en.pdf?sequence=1&isAllowed=y.

World Health Organization. 2019. *How WHO Is Funded*. Available at: https://www.who.int/about/planning-finance-and-accountability/how-who-is-funded.

World Health Organization. 2020. *Timeline of WHO's response to COVID-19*. Available at: https://www.who.int/news-room/detail/29-06-2020-covidtimeline.

World Health Organization. 2020a. *Access to COVID-19 Tools (ACT) Accelerator*. Available at: https://www.who.int/publications/m/item/access-to-covid-19-tools-(act)-accelerator.

World Health Organization. 2020c. WHO | Joint External Evaluations. Available at: https://www.who.int/ihr/procedures/joint-external-evaluations/en/.

World Health Organization. 2020c. COVAX: Working for Global Equitable Access to COVID-19 Vaccines. Available at: https://www.who.int/initiatives/act-accelerator/covax.

World Health Organization. 2020e. WHO Recommends Against the Use of Remdesivir in COVID-19 Patients. Available at: https://www.who.int/news-room/feature-stories/detail/who-recommends-against-the-use-of-remdesivir-in-covid-19-patients.

World Health Organization. 2021. Draft landscape of COVID-19 candidate vaccines. Available at: https://www.who.int/publications/m/item/draft-landscape-of-covid-19-candidate-vaccines.

World Health Organization. 2021a. COVID-19 Oxygen Emergency Impacting More Than Half a Million People in Low-and Middle-Income Countries Every Day, As Demand Surges. Available at: https://www.who.int/news/item/25-02-2021-covid-19-oxygen-emergency-impacting-more-than-half-a-million-people-in-low--and-middle-income-countries-every-day-as-demand-surges#_ftn2.

World Health Organization. 2021b. First COVID-19 COVAX Vaccine Doses Administered in Africa. Available at: https://www.who.int/news/item/01-03-2021-first-covid-19-covax-vaccine-doses-administered-in-africa.

Yamey, G. 2002. WHO in 2002: Interview With Gro Brundtland. *BMJ* 325(7376), pp. 1355–1355.

Yasuhara, J., Kuno, T., Takagi, H. and Sumitomo, N. 2020. Clinical Characteristics of COVID19 in Children: A Systematic Review. *Paediatric Pulmonology* 15(10). Available at: https://doi.org/10.1002/ppul.24991.

CHAPTER 3

AN OVERVIEW OF ETHICAL ISSUES IN THE CONTEXT OF PANDEMICS AND HEALTH CARE

Ames Dhai

Melodie Labuschaigne

David McQuoid-Mason

3.1 INTRODUCTION

Difficult choices need to be made during pandemics. COVID-19 has affected a substantial proportion of the global population. Significant social, economic and personal disruption and hardships have arisen. It may last for some time, resulting in sustained pressure on essential services such as health, food supplies and pharmaceutical production and distribution (BMA, 2020; Dhai, 2020). Historically, resource distribution principles in the inter-pandemic years usually focused on prioritising individuals at most risk of serious negative health consequences. However, when managing a pandemic, principles guiding preservation of the functioning of society must, of necessity, be drawn upon as well (Kinlaw and Levine, 2007). Therefore incorporating diverse voices, including those of citizens in general, in pandemic planning is essential. Special attention should be paid to vulnerable communities. Cultural, ethnic, religious, community and other values need to be considered. Importantly, transparent procedures for decision-making are essential (Kinlaw and Levine, 2007; UNESCO, 2020). Mutual trust and social solidarity are vital during these challenging times and pandemic planning must be mindful of these values (Thompson et al, 2006). Both substantive values, which inform decision-making, and procedural values that guide implementation are necessary (Tuohey, 2007). Ethical processes are essential as they enable ethical outcomes. This chapter provides an overview of the ethical considerations (substantive values) that merit being taken into account when reflecting on pandemics.

3.2 OBJECTIVES

The objectives of this chapter are:

- To describe and discuss the ethical issues that arise during pandemic situations in the context of healthcare.
- To identify the pertinent principles and their application relevant to healthcare during pandemics.
- To discuss prioritisation in the context of treatment, diagnostics and prevention during pandemics.
- To explore ethical issues that have arisen specifically related to COVID-19 vaccines.

3.3 ETHICAL VALUES AND PRINCIPLES

The values and principles described below are valuable tools for ethical decision-making in the context of pandemics.

3.3.1 Social Solidarity

Bonds unifying a community, and structures like schools, hospitals and other organisations that support and maintain these bonds, epitomise the value of social solidarity. A person's interdependence with others and among others, a person's attachment to or interest in others and their concerns, a person's commitment to or support for the social structures that make social life possible, and a person's personal involvement or engagement in the community's social life are some characteristics of social solidarity. Shared beliefs and convictions allow the community to contribute to achieving consensus on significant issues of great concern. While these characteristics are challenged in a pandemic, decision-making must take them into account if decisions are to promote the common good, i.e., the moral requirement of subsidiarity, such that all people are able to lead full and productive lives, albeit during a pandemic (Tuohey, 2007). The COVID-19 pandemic brought about an acute awareness of the interdependence of South Africa's two-tier health systems, with social solidarity being necessary across systemic and institutional boundaries for curtailment of the contagion. A framework for social solidarity, as we move forward with preparations for future pandemics, requires *inter alia*, respectful, open and honest communication, candid collaboration in a spirit of common purpose, timely and truthful sharing of reliable public health information, coordinating healthcare delivery, food and water supplies and other social amenities to prevent the spread of infection, and overcoming territoriality between healthcare, other facilities, and government departments. In this manner, a sense of common purpose will be achieved and equitable care across the social determinants of health provided (Thompson et al, 2006).

The importance of community engagement in the solidarity response to an infectious disease outbreak cannot be adequately emphasised. For example, during the Ebola epidemic in West Africa, the World Health Organization (WHO) guidance initially prohibited traditional burial practices for containment purposes, but these guidelines had to be changed and modified in collaboration with the affected communities (Gillespie et al, 2016). South Africa has already learnt from the HIV experience that prevention, testing and treatment campaigns must involve the community in order to achieve results (Hanson et al, 2015; Newman et al, 2015). For any measures during a pandemic to succeed, it is necessary to know *what* different communities need to meet these measures, and key to this is engaging these communities. A community-centred response for managing a pandemic is thus of critical importance (UNAIDS, 2020). Although President Ramaphosa stated in his March 2020 address to the nation that he had consulted with business and industry, no consultation took place with those living in cramped informal settlements where it was impossible to comply with restrictive measures as a result of their location and physical environment. A public health crisis approach should be people-centred and ensure public empowerment with information and resources, as well as public participation in policy responses (Merten, 2020).

3.3.2   Fair Allocation Principles

Pandemics lead to severe resource constraints even in the world's richest countries with rapidly growing imbalances between supply and demand, leading to normative questions of how medical resources should be allocated fairly. It is necessary to prioritise and fairly allocate these resources, which range from preventative measures like N-95 masks and vaccines to clinical supplies and management like diagnostics, therapeutics interventions, ICU admission and ventilator allocation. In addition, effective vaccines, take time to manufacture, distribute and administer (Emanuel et al, 2020). Many countries do not have the purchasing power to acquire vaccines for the entire population, and tough choices have to be made. Existing health system capacity plays a pivotal role in how resources are allocated. While a scramble can be made for equipment and medications, an important capacity is healthcare workers and particularly nurses and trained critical care staff, who are already in short supply in many low- and middle-income countries (LMICs). The healthcare workforce is also vulnerable to illness caused by the pandemic and doctors and nurses do end up having to go into quarantine, isolate, and many even succumb to the disease (Emanuel et al, 2020).

Setting limits on access to treatment and preventative interventions is a necessary response to the overwhelming effects of a pandemic and must be done ethically. The processes must be transparent, inclusive, consistent and those making these limit-setting decisions must be accountable and held responsible for them (WHO, 2020a). The fundamental values to guide fair allocation of resources are: treating people equally; maximising the benefits of these resources; giving priority to the worst off; and promoting and rewarding social usefulness. Competing ethical principles exist within these values, allowing for a tailoring of the fair allocation process to accommodate differing resources like therapeutics or vaccines (Persad et al, 2009; Emanuel et al, 2020; Sheehan and Hope, 2002).

Treating people equally allows people to have equal opportunities to receive a medical intervention. The principles emanating from this value are that of (a) Lottery or Random Selection where people have an equal probability of obtaining a given medical resource, regardless of other circumstances; and (b) First-Come, First-Served where people who arrive first receive the limited resource first, irrespective of the differences between people and their circumstances.

Maximising the benefits of the resources is a utilitarian-based ethical value where the objective is to maximise the potential good that can be achieved. The ethical principles from this value are: (a) Saving the most lives where saving the most individual lives are prioritised and each life is of equal worth regardless of factors like age and comorbidity; and (b) Saving the most life-years is prioritised irrespective of how this distribution is concentrated or spread (Persad et al, 2009; Emanuel et al, 2020).

Giving priority to the worst off is an ethical value which characterises 'prioritarianism' where individuals who are worse off are given priority access to needed medical resources. Examples of ethical principles emerging from this ethical value are: (a) Sickest first where those with the worst chance of survival are considered to be the worst off and are therefore prioritised to receive the scarce medical intervention; (b) Youngest first where those who have lived fewer life years and who have yet to benefit from living longer are prioritised (Persad et al, 2009; Emanuel et al, 2020); and (c) Those most at risk first as has been seen with prioritisation for the COVID-19 vaccines where healthcare workers, people over 60 and people with comorbidities have been prioritised to receive the vaccine first in several countries.

The ethical value of promoting and rewarding social usefulness prioritises people who have previously provided or will provide, in the future, benefit to society. Societal and cultural norms will need to be considered when defining the benefits to society and hence who to prioritise. The ethical principles encompassed in this value are: (a) Instrumental value where people with current and future usefulness are prioritised, for example, prioritising healthcare workers because of their added value for treating patients during the pandemic and in the future; and (b) Reciprocity where people who previously were useful or had to sacrifice are prioritised. Examples here include healthcare workers and research participants (Persad et al, 2009; Emanuel et al, 2020; WHO, 2020a; WHO, 2020b).

The WHO (WHO, 2020a) concludes the following on fair allocation of scarce resources within countries during the COVID-19 outbreak:

1. It is justifiable to prioritise healthcare workers caring for patients and first responders when allocating some resources because of their contribution to the health and well-being of the community. This is because their health is necessary to help preserve the health of others.

2. Some priority should be given to participants of research aimed at developing vaccines, therapies or other critical interventions because they have also helped save others by their participation. This should not be considered an absolute priority and should not take precedence over giving priority to those most at risk in the case of certain resources such as vaccines.

3. The principle of first come, first served is helpful when allocating resources in healthcare settings but is rarely appropriate in an emergency because it is very likely to favour certain groups, such as those closest to a distribution centre, those with access to better information, or those who are most well-off.

4. Because younger populations appear to be at lower risk in the COVID-19 context, the principle of youngest first should have low priority for vaccine, but perhaps may have more weight if they do become sick and need critical care resources.

5. Different principles or values may be used to justify the allocation of different resources, for example, should a novel vaccine be found to be safe and effective, a lottery-based allocation may be justified among those at highest risk, the old and those with comorbidities, if they outnumber available vaccines.

6. Maximising utility should be balanced with the principle of priority to the worst-off. If resources are concentrated in larger centres, their benefits may extend to more people, but isolated populations may be excluded hence challenging our concerns for those at highest risk.

Most countries have drawn from this WHO guidance as they developed their country-level, contextually relevant policies on resource allocation for both the management and prevention of COVID-19. Although South Africa has derived its guidance from African traditional values and Ubuntu principles to guide its allocation of COVID-19 vaccines (see 3.7.1 below) there is resonance in its policies with the WHO norms as outlined above.

An additional resource allocation quandary is that of denying ongoing non-pandemic care to patients in need with resultant morbidity and mortality. During pandemics authorities at local and national levels make decisions to suspend medical care unrelated to the outbreak emergency. At times, facilities are closed prematurely when there is no pandemic-related shortage of beds and resources.

It has been noted in several countries, that admissions for non-COVID-19-related illnesses decreased dramatically and mortality rates increased for these conditions (Appleby, 2020). Adequate effort into planning and consultation on how to downscale services when the pandemic escalates and how to prioritise resources appropriately, to ensure that patients who require necessary care are not prejudiced because their care is compromised unfairly, is necessary to prevent this 'out-of-site-out-of-mind' phenomenon (Brannigan and Botha, 2020; Kola, 2020; Garcia, 2020; Liebensteiner, 2020).

3.3.3   Respect for Persons

People have intrinsic worth, dignity and sense of value (HPCSA, 2016). All persons are to be respected, and this includes patients and healthcare professionals. In the context of COVID-19, while privacy remains important, some aspects of confidentiality must be limited in order to halt the spread of the virus (Constitution, 1996; NHA, 2003; SA Government, 2020). It is prudent to bear in mind that limiting confidentiality can result in social harms like stigmatisation and discrimination. Hence, any limitation must be instituted with care to avoid these adverse consequences. Evidence of the stigmatisation of people, including healthcare professionals who have been infected with the disease did emerge during the COVID-19 pandemic. The World Medical Association (WMA) reported that in some countries physicians and other healthcare workers were stigmatised, ostracised, discriminated against and even attacked because of the perception that they were carriers of the virus (World Medical Association, 2020). In South Africa, in early April 2020, two doctors who were infected by SARS-CoV-2, but were asymptomatic and were in isolation at their home, were forcibly removed and quarantined in a provincial hospital by the health authority of that province, despite this being contrary to both international and local guidelines. Of note, the health official issuing the order was herself a healthcare professional and, in addition, the order was contrary to the terms of the COVID-19 pandemic disaster regulations (SA Government, 2020), which stipulated that any information obtained through the regulations was to be treated as confidential and was not be disclosed unless one was authorised to do so, or if the information was necessary to address, prevent or combat the spread of the virus. The reported reason for the action was that this official blamed these doctors for 'bringing the virus into [her] province to infect [her] rural people' (Medical Brief, 2020). Not only did her action result in extensive media coverage impacting on the doctors' privacy, but it also portrayed disregard for their dignity and sense of value, and exposed them to the risk of social harm. Stigmatisation of COVID-19 positive staff and students was also reported in healthcare facilities, with demands to identify those who were infected (Dhai and Veller et al, 2020). This raises concerns about the protection of privacy and respect for individuals' rights. Moreover, such behaviour reflects poorly on the professionalism of the healthcare workers involved.

3.3.4   Duty of Care

Promoting the common good entails a move from patient-centred care to patient care guided by public health duties. Patient-centred care is contained within the scaffold of duty of care, where the focus is that of maintaining fidelity to the individual patient such that suffering is relieved, the rights and preferences of the patient are respected and the patient is not abandoned. On the other hand, a focus on community recognises the moral equality of persons, thereby promoting equity in the distribution of risks and benefits. Hence, public safety is promoted, community health is protected and limited resources are fairly allocated relative to need. This inevitably creates conflicts for healthcare workers. It is therefore not surprising that in the context of resource limitations moral distress could result. Moral distress is amplified during pandemics. Moral distress is the emotion experienced when one is not able to do the right thing. It is the sense of being helpless to avoid wrongdoing or harm. Moral distress was first identified in the 1980s. In this situation, the healthcare worker is aware of the moral problem, concedes to moral responsibility, recognises what the morally correct action should be, but participates in the perceived moral wrongdoing because of institutional, procedural or social constraints, which make doing the right thing nearly impossible (Rushton and Schoonover-Shoffner, 2017; American Nurses Association, 2015). Core values and moral integrity are threatened and people and systems are negatively affected. During pandemics, burnout and lack of empathy at the individual level and reduced quality of care with poor patient outcomes at the organisational level could ensue because of moral distress. Moral resilience, i.e. the ability to sustain or restore moral integrity and exercise moral agency in response to moral distress is exceedingly difficult to attain during these stressful times. It is therefore not surprising that moral distress impacts negatively on professionalism during pandemics.

3.4   PROFESSIONALISM

Duty of care is closely aligned to professionalism. Through the centuries, healthcare professionals have shared a common heritage – that of caring for the sick and suffering, with professionals applying their skills and knowledge competently, altruistically and, often heroically (Dhai and Veller et al, 2020). The practice of healthcare is viewed as a social contract with humanity (AMA, 2001). However, questions that repeatedly arise during pandemics are: whether healthcare professionals have obligations to work during the pandemic irrespective of the level of personal risk and risk to their families; whether healthcare professionals have a right to refuse to provide care; whether there are reciprocal obligations on governments and society; and whether healthcare professionals should be absolved of their obligations in the event of these reciprocal obligations not being honoured (Blackmer, 2009). The reality is that under these circumstances healthcare professionals do experience some challenges to the dynamic of the traditional patient–professional relationship because the patient is not only the victim, but also the vector of the disease and therefore, also a danger to others (Kotalik, 2006). Inherent in this dilemma is that their availability is essential in order to provide an effective response to the pandemic and to continue to provide healthcare for conditions not related to the pandemic. A strong case can be made for a moral obligation to provide care because of the skills obtained during their training that cannot be provided by others (WHO, 2007). Moreover, there is a definite line between self-protection, the dereliction of duty (Kotalik, 2006) and fidelity, i.e. non-abandonment of the patient (Berlinger et al, 2020). Challenges to professionalism are not new and not confined to pandemics. Several substantial challenges to professionalism in healthcare have existed in the inter-pandemic periods. These include the fact that political, social and economic factors together with advances in science and technology, medical negligence and adverse media coverage have reshaped the attitudes and expectations of the public and healthcare professionals (Dhai and McQuoid-Mason, 2020). The COVID-19 period has witnessed fear, misinformation and a detachment from one's calling, putting professionalism even more strongly to the test. Further compounding the challenge is that even a caring response may not always translate into pragmatic ends (Afolabi, 2018).

3.5   TRANSPARENT PROCESSES AND CORRUPTION

Both institutions and individuals entrusted with governance over scarce resources will need to make difficult decisions over their allocation and the collateral damage that may result. They should be guided by the notion of stewardship which encompasses trust and ethical decision-making. Trust is indispensable in relationships at the different levels of healthcare decision-making and delivery. When access to care is denied or collateral damage suffered because of social distancing measures, this could be perceived as a betrayal of trust and abandonment at a time of greatest need. Faced with the challenge of maintaining public trust while simultaneously stemming the pandemic through various control measures, decision-makers need to be trustworthy by ensuring early engagement with stakeholders and decision-making processes must be ethical and transparent (Thompson et al, 2006). For this, integrity, which reflects the need to act with honesty, reliability, and fairness, and a willingness to be held accountable to explain one's actions, is critical (Tuohey, 2007). Evidence from pandemics, however, reveals otherwise.

Lived experiences during the COVID-19 pandemic are that the pandemic itself has given rise to unethical processes with little to no openness and very significant risks of corruption. Massive resources mobilised to respond to health and economic crises, coupled with the suspension of many prevention and enforcement mechanisms, including procurement oversight, due to social distancing have created fertile ground for opportunities for corruption or for the rapid perpetuation of these immoral activities in already existing corrupt regimes. The pandemic response is compromised by corruption, trust in public institutions is undermined, supplies and resources squandered and access to care impeded for those in need. Corruption remains a global problem and persists in almost every part of the world despite a robust global attempt over the past twenty years to address the situation (World Justice Project, 2020), including the United Nations Convention against Corruption (UN, 2003) and the OECD Anti-bribery Convention (OECD, 1997). Fraudulent charities, government and private sector benefit fraud, identity theft, government contract and procurement fraud plagued the United States during Hurricane Katrina, Rita, and Wilma (World Justice Project, 2020). In West Africa, during the Ebola crisis, funds and supplies were diverted and containment measures were compromised as citizens bribed their way around restrictions on their movements as a result of corrupt practices (Dupuy and Divjak, 2015). During COVID-19, price gouging and lucrative contracts being awarded without proper procurement processes have been seen in countries like Colombia, Italy and South Africa. In addition, funds aimed at addressing the economic crisis have also fallen prey to corruption, with evidence of fraud in the distribution of unemployment benefits (US Department of Labour, 2020). Trading off accountability for speedily procuring supplies needed during pandemics is morally offensive and transparency during the processes is necessary so that perpetrators are held accountable without foregoing timelines.

3.6   RESTRICTIONS ON PERSONAL FREEDOM FOR MANAGING PANDEMICS

When managing a pandemic, procedures and interventions that limit the freedom of movement of individuals or create conditions of social distancing are usually employed. These include isolation, quarantine, closing of schools, cancellation of public events, closing public venues and limiting travel. An unforeseen adverse effect of restrictions emerged early during the COVID-19 pandemic when families were not allowed to visit their loved ones who had been admitted into hospital. Healthcare workers managing these patients grappled with the ethical complexities that appeared as a result of this separation. Many patients who were admitted into intensive care when they developed severe complications spent several weeks there. The psychological trauma and negative effects on the mental health of patients, survivors and families cannot be underestimated and should be factored into the care of patients effected during infectious disease outbreaks.

Ideally, any interventions that restrict freedoms should be in the form of recommendations for voluntary action. Mandatory liberty-limiting and social distancing interventions should be imposed where voluntary actions are unlikely to be effective (Kinlaw and Levine, 2007). It is essential that these interventions are based on the best available scientific evidence. Legitimate restrictions on individual freedom may be imposed if, in exercising one's freedom, one places others at risk and poses grave harm to the functioning of society or to the wellbeing of the public. The least restrictive effective measure should be taken when limiting personal freedom. The liberty-limiting measure should achieve its intended goal with the limitation being proportional and no other restrictive measure would be likely to be as effective. Notwithstanding the principle of respect for individual freedom remaining a priority throughout the process of restriction (Kinlaw and Levine, 2007), legal impositions limiting choice become necessary to curb the spread of pandemic outbreaks. The negative implications of such legal restrictions must also be recognised.

3.7   ETHICAL ISSUES SPECIFIC TO COVID-19 VACCINES

As the development of COVID-19 vaccines evolved, so did ethical issues specific to the vaccines emerge. With demand outstripping supply, ethical considerations of equitable access to vaccines arose both within and between countries. In addition, reluctance to accept a vaccine based on a number of different reasons added to the challenges.

3.7.1   Prioritisation for vaccine access – an approach based on indigenous African values and Ubuntu principles

The imbalance between the supply and the demand for COVID-19 vaccine resulting in the high likelihood of vaccine scarcity, with the scaling up of supply taking time, was recognised early on in the pandemic. Equitable distribution of COVID-19 vaccines within countries, across countries within the African continent and globally is especially important to ensure containment of the virus and control the pandemic thereby allowing for the rebuilding of societies and economies. The Ubuntu philosophy of inter-relatedness and interdependence was utilised during an African consultation on the continent, spearheaded by the Africa Centre for Disease Control and Prevention (Africa CDC) and the South African Medical Research Council (SAMRC) to inform prioritisation decisions for the vaccine. The following framework was developed to inform allocation decisions guided by indigenous African values (Africa CDC, 2021 p. 8):

a. **'Affirming the humanity of others**: Allocation decisions must be for societal benefit and promote common good while respecting human dignity. Every person has equal dignity, worth, and value, hence allocation decisions must be non-discriminatory. Characteristics such as ethnicity, nationality, gender, sexual orientation, race and religion are not to play a role in allocation decisions. People are to be treated fairly and equally. Allocation decisions are to be impartial and in accordance with fair criteria.

b. **Survival of the community**: Allocation decisions are to be based on the best available evidence. In addition, essential service workers and those that contribute towards the prevention and treatment of diseases could be considered as essential for the survival of the community. Furthermore, those at greatest risk of severe illness and death could be included in the priority groups. In this way, benefits will be maximised, the risks of severe morbidity and mortality caused by transmission due to SARS-CoV-2 reduced, and the community will survive.

c. **Social Solidarity**: Allocation decisions are to take into consideration the bonds unifying communities, their interdependence, attachment to or interest in others and the significant social, economic and personal disruptions and hardships experienced. The possibility that the pandemic may widen existing inequities and create new inequalities should be taken into account.

d. **Meaningful community engagement:** Allocation decisions must be trusted. Active community engagement allows for authenticity, and promotes accountability and ownership of the decisions made about allocation thereby engendering trust. Active community engagement is needed to address vaccine hesitancy, maintain public trust and simultaneously, control the pandemic. For these reasons, integrity, which reflects the need to act with honesty, reliability, and fairness, and a willingness to be held accountable to explain one's actions, is crucial.'

3.7.2 Vaccine Nationalism impeding access to COVID-19 Vaccines as a Public Good

Inequalities in vaccine access mean that many poor regions in the world could be last in the queue for effective vaccines. Advance purchase agreements between vaccine manufacturers and several rich countries for vaccines far in excess of their populations' requirements had already been signed early in the second half of 2020 (Launch and Scale Speedometer, 2020). This is reminiscent of the H1N1 influenza pandemic in 2009 when rich countries bought nearly all the vaccines that were available. It was only after these countries received adequate supplies that low- and middle-income countries managed to get access, with the vaccines arriving in most of these countries when the pandemic was over (Usdin, 2020).

Within four months of the WHO approving a COVID-19 vaccine for emergency use, one billion vaccinations had been administered globally. This global milestone was an unprecedented scientific achievement; never before had so many in the world been vaccinated only 6 months after a vaccine had been discovered. As of 27 April 2021, 7.3% of the world's population of 7.79 billion had received at least one dose. However, 75% of the population globally will need to be vaccinated if the pandemic is to be contained. Moreover, while some celebrated this unparalleled success, what is stark is that as many as 75% of these doses had been administered in only 10 countries during that time, highlighting the huge global disparities between high-income countries (HICs) and LMICs. Furthermore, Africa had at this stage received only 2% of the total doses (Kreier, 2021). The global nature of the problem has been shockingly overlooked and the most vulnerable continue to be affected the most (Dhai, 2021).

According to the United Nations, vaccine equity affirms human rights, vaccine nationalism denies it and vaccines must be a global public good, accessible and affordable to all (UN, 2021). A global public health good is a good where the impacts are equitably spread across the globe without causing division. A price cannot be placed on the benefits of these goods and hence the principle of exclusion cannot be applied to them. The use of these goods by one individual cannot be allowed to reduce their availability to others. Moreover, these goods are not marketable and the goods and their benefits must be available at negligible or zero cost to all in the global village (Van den Berg, 2015). Therefore, the two criteria that determine a public good are: non-rival in consumption and being non-excludable. Non-rivalry denotes that the consumption by one person must not interfere with the goods being available to others equally and non-excludable denotes that suppliers cannot deny it to those who are unable to pay its market price. There are transboundary implications with most public goods, and hence international cooperation and action are necessary (Van den Berg, 2015). The vaccine nationalism displayed by rich countries undermines equitable access to the vaccine, hence the notion of COVID-19 vaccines being a public good.

Internationally, as countries introduce vaccine programs, and despite vaccines being in short supply, many HICs have proposed, and several have implemented, digital and/or physical health passes, which are also called 'vaccine passports' or 'vaccine certificates' (also referred to as 'passes'). These passes are potential tools for recording and sharing the immune status of individuals. With these passes, people are able to demonstrate that they are unlikely to transmit the virus, hence the documents could play an essential role in re-opening societies, civil freedoms and hence positively impact livelihoods. Furthermore, such passes could function as 'passports' internationally opening travel between countries. While COVID-19 certificates/passports could play a critical role in establishing relative normality, they raise several ethical concerns (Gostin and Cohen, 2021; Hall and Studdert, 2021; Brown and Kelly et al, 2021).

Possible Benefits of Vaccine Passports/Certificates: (SAMRC, 2021)

- During lockdowns, it would be possible for immune individuals to follow less stringent requirements with regard to physical distancing and travel, including international travel (both business and leisure).

- Broader society could benefit if immune individuals are allowed to return to their work and care obligations, which include attending international meetings and conferences.
- There could be a safe return to normal life and a gradual re-opening of the economy in key sectors like food, retail, entertainment and travel, especially with regard to import and export.
- With time, the use of the passes for travel could assist with academia and research returning to normal, in particular in the context of international collaborative research.
- Countries may require such vaccine passports/certificates at the entry point to assist with international travel.

Possible Challenges Associated with Vaccine Passports/Certificates: (SAMRC, 2021)

- There could be possible infringements of civil rights of those individuals who are not vaccinated based on medical, religious, personal and other reasons.
- Unjust forms of discrimination and exclusions with not having a passport/certificate resulting in stigmatisation and societal divides could arise. This may include technological or algorithmic discrimination based on private information.
- Uncertainties remain with regard to the degree and duration of vaccine protection. The WHO recommends an efficacy value higher than 50% with a lower limit of 30%. Based on clinical trial data, the range of protection with vaccines thus far is between 65.5% to 94.6% in preventing symptomatic COVID-19. Because of this variability, the usefulness of the passes could be affected and some regions could limit their passports/documents to only certain vaccines resulting in deepening inequities in particular between HICs and LMICs.
- The reality of the scarcity of supply means that the passes would automatically unfairly exclude anyone who does not have access to the vaccines while societies are being re-opened, resulting in the privileged continuing to enjoy privileges while others are excluded.
- If a vaccination is premised on a system of prioritisation, some will be able to receive their vaccine passports sooner than others, thereby limiting the passports for younger age groups who are arguably more active in the labour market with a greater need for international and national mobility.
- There could be possible infringements of privacy, especially where the passes are digital.

- Technical challenges could emerge with the use of digital passes, including authentication of vaccine status. In South Africa, the Electronic Vaccine Delivery System (EVDS) is being used to register vaccinees. Implementation of this system started with the commencement of the Sisonke Trial. Research participants who have been involved in successful vaccine studies prior to the EVDS being used are not registered on the system and may not be recognised as having received the vaccine. They would hence suffer social harms that are associated with exclusionary policies.

With the potential for corruption as discussed above, an effective vaccine passport system should be implemented in a manner that will prevent fraud.

3.7.3   Vaccine Hesitancy and Vaccine Confidence

Once vaccines are available for use, containment of the virus is largely dependent on its willing uptake. Initiatives to allocate the vaccines fairly will not be successful if people are not willing to receive them. A survey conducted on behalf of the World Economic Forum in August 2020 revealed that only 64% of South Africans surveyed would accept a COVID-19 vaccine if it became available. This was lower than the 74% global average of adults surveyed in 27 countries that said they would accept a vaccine. Only 29% of the 64% agreed strongly to a vaccine, while 71% 'somewhat' agreed. Fear of adverse events, concerns about safety and a lack of confidence in the effectiveness of the vaccine were the two most cited reasons. Distrust in the vaccines mirrored lack of trust in public health institutions, with 32% of South Africans saying they had no trust in hospitals and clinics. The overall figure for Africa was 27% (Ballet, 2020). This one-third deficit in accepting the vaccine could severely compromise the effectiveness of any COVID-19 vaccine rollout programme. The surveys were repeated in October and December 2020. Similar results were obtained in October (Ipsos, 2020a) but in December, only 53% said they would get a vaccine when it became available (Ipsos, 2020b). The University of Johannesburg together with the Human Sciences Research Council conducted the largest survey in the country on vaccine hesitancy (Cooper, 2021). The main findings were that 67% said they would definitely or probably take a vaccine; 18% said they would definitely not or probably not take the vaccine and 15% were unsure if they would take the vaccine. Factors influencing vaccine acceptance included race (white South Africans were less accepting); education (those with less than matric education were more accepting); age (people over 55 years were more likely to take the vaccine); and political (supporters of the ruling party were more accepting of the vaccine and those that were politically disillusioned were less supportive of the vaccine).

Generally, reasons for vaccine hesitancy include: the novelty of the disease; the unusually rapid speed of vaccine development; mistrust of science and health experts by some; emotional detachment due to fatigue as a result of the 'infodemic', and the uncontrollable nature and prolonged uncertainty of the pandemic; politicisation of the vaccine and its safety and efficacy standards by some groups; and conspiracy theories by anti-vaxxers. In addressing vaccine hesitancy and fostering vaccine confidence, it is critical that evidence-based communication strategies are used (Chou and Budenz, 2020). Increasing vaccine disinformation is of concern. It is essential that trust is built up to offset high levels of public health misinformation and anti-vaccination sentiment. Critical to this is that communities are able to access accurate information that is backed by evidence in order to make informed decisions on the vaccines.

3.8   CONCLUSION

Infectious disease outbreaks give rise to a number of ethical issues and dilemmas ranging from specific considerations at the point of patient management to broader public health matters. Many challenges during pandemics are of a global nature and hence global solutions are necessary. This means that international cooperation and global solidarity are critical for the infective agent to be defeated. As has been seen during the COVID-19 pandemic, for containment of the virus to be realised, everyone in the world must have access to vaccines, and interventions developed to combat the virus and disease must be recognised as global public health goods.

3.9   SELF-ASSESSMENT QUESTIONS

1. What are the benchmarks in the framework based on indigenous African values that guide prioritisation of COVID-19 vaccines?
2. Discuss some of the challenges to professionalism in healthcare during pandemics.

3.10 REFERENCES

Afolabi M.O. 2018. Pandemic Influenza: A Comparative Ethical Approach. In: Public Health Disasters: A Global Ethical Framework. Advancing Global Bioethics. Volume 12. Springer Cham, pp. 59–96.

Africa Centre for Disease Control and Prevention. 2021. Framework for the Fair, Equitable and Timely Allocation of COVID-19 Vaccines in Africa. Available at: https://africacdc.org/download/framework-for-fair-equitable-and-timely-alloca tion-of-covid-19-vaccines-in-africa/.

American Medical Association. AMA Declaration of Professional Responsibility. 2001. Available at: https://www.ama-assn.org/delivering-care/public-health/ama-declaration-professional-responsibility.

American Nursing Association. Codes of Ethics for Nurses With Interpretive Statements. Development, Interpretation and Application. 2015. Available at: https://slideplayer.com/slide/10173441/.

Appleby, J. 2020. What is Happening to Non-Covid Deaths? BMJ, 369:m1607. Available at: http://dx.doi.org/doi:10.1136/bmj.m1607.

Balet, A. 2020. What We Know About Vaccine Hesitancy in South Africa. Spotlight. Available at: https://www.spotlightnsp.co.za/2020/10/07/what-we-know-about-vaccine-hesitancy-in-south-africa/.

Berlinger, N., Wynia, M., Powell, T., Hester, M., Milliken, A., Fabi, R., Cohn, F., Guidry-Grimes, L.K., Watson, J.K., Bruce, L., Chuang, E.J., Oei, G., Abbott, J. and Jenks, N.P. Guidelines for Institutional Ethics Services Responding to COVID-19 Managing Uncertainty, Safeguarding Communities, Guiding Practice. The Hastings Centre. 2020. Available at: https://www.thehastings center.org/ethicalframeworkcovid19/.

Blackmer, J. 2009. Current Global Trends in Medical Professionalism. *World Med Health Pol* 1(1) Article 2. Available at: https://doi.org/10.2202/1948-4682.1006.

BMA. 2020. British Medical Association. COVID-19 Ethical Issues. A Guidance Note. Available at: https://www.bma.org.uk/media/2360/bma-covid-19-ethics-guidance-april-2020.pdf.

Brannigan, L. and Botha, J. 2020. In Service of the Patient and not the Virus: A Pragmatic Assessment of the Approach to Transplantation in South Africa during the COVID-19 Pandemic. *Wits Journal of Clinical Medicine* 2(2), pp. 153–156. Available at: http://dx.doi.org/10.18772/26180197.2020.v2n2a8.

Brown, R.C.H., Kelly, D., Wilkinson, D. and Savulescu, J. 2021. The Scientific and Ethical Feasibility of Immunity Passports. *Lancet Infect Dis* 21, pp. e58–63.

Chou, W.S. and Budenz, A. 2020 Considering Emotion in COVID-19 vaccine communication: addressing vaccine hesitancy and fostering vaccine confidence. *Health Communication* 35(14). Available at: https://www.tandfonline.com/doi/full/10.1080/10410236.2020.1838096.

Constitution of the Republic of South Africa, 1996. Available at: http://justice.gov.za/legislation/constitution/SAConstitution-web-eng.pdf.

Cooper, S. 2021. Vaccine Hesitancy in South Africa: Summary of Existing Studies. Available at: https://sacoronavirus.co.za/wp-content/uploads/2021/04/Report_Covid-19-vaccine-hesitancy_SA-studies_1April2021.pdf.

Dhai, A. 2020. The Need to Invest In Pandemic Preparedness: COVID-19 is not the First Pandemic, Neither Will it be the Last. *S Afr J Bioethics Law* 13(1), pp. 3–4. Available at: https://doi.org/10.7196/SAJBL.2020.

Dhai, A. 2021. Access to COVID-19 Vaccines as a Global Public Good: A Coordinated Global Response Based on Equality, Justice and Solidarity is Key. *S Afr J Bioethics Law* 14(1), pp. 2–3. Available at: https://doi.org/10.7196/SAJBL.2021.v14i1.768.

Dhai, A., Veller, M., Ballot, D. and Mokhachane, M. 2020. Pandemics, Professionalism and The Duty of Care: Concerns From the Coalface. *S Afr Med J* 110(6), pp. 450–452. Available at: https://doi.org/10.7196/SAMJ.2020.v110i6.14901.

Dhai, A. and McQuoid-Mason, D.J. 2020. *Bioethics, Human Rights and Health Law.* 2 ed. Kenilworth: Juta & Co Ltd, pp. 73–93.

Dupuy, K. and Divjak, B. 2015. Ebola and Corruption: Overcoming Critical Governance Challenges in a Crisis Situation. Bergen: Chr. Michelsen Institute (U4 Brief 2015:04), p. 4.

Emanuel, E.J., Persad, G., Upshur, R., Thome, B., Parker, M., Glickman, A., Zhang, C., Boyle, C., Smith, M. and Phillips, J. 2020. Fair Allocation of Scarce Medical Resources in the Time of COVID-19. *N Eng J Med* 382(21), pp. 2049–2055. Available at: https://doi.org/10.1056/NEJMsb2005114.

Gillespie, A.M. et al. 2016. Social Mobilization and Community Engagement Central to the Ebola Response in West Africa: Lessons for Future Public Health Emergencies. *Global Health: Science and Practice* 4(4), pp. 626–646.

Garcia, S., Albaghdadi, M.S., Meraj, P.M., Schmidt, C. et al. 2020. Reduction in ST-Segment Elevation Cardiac Catheterization Laboratory Activations in the United States During COVID-19 Pandemic. *Journal of the American College of Cardiology* 9; 75(22), pp. 2871–2872. Available at: https://doi.org/10.1016/j.jacc.2020.04.011.

Lawrence, O., Gostin, I. Cohen, G. and Shaw, J. 2021. Digital Health Passes in the Age of COVID-19 Are "Vaccine Passports" Lawful and Ethical? *JAMA*, published online 7 April 2021. Available at: https://jamanetwork.com/.

Hall, M.A, and Studdert, D.M. 2021. "Vaccine Passport" Certification — Policy and Ethical Considerations. *The New England Journal of Medicine.* Available at: nejm.org.

Hanson, S., Zembe, Y. and Ekström, A.M. 2015. Vital Need to Engage the Community in HIV Control in South Africa. Global Health Action 8, p. 27450. Available at: https://doi.org/10.3402/gha.v8.27450.

HPCSA. Booklet 1. 2016. General Ethical Guidelines For Healthcare Professionals. Available at: https://www.hpcsa.co.za/Uploads/Professional_Practice/Conduct%20%26%20Ethics/Booklet%201%20Guidelines%20for%20Good%20Practice%20%20September%202016.pdf.

Ipsos. 2020a. COVID-19 Vaccination Intent is Decreasing Globally, 5 November; Available from: https://www.ipsos.com/en/global-attitudes-covid-19-vaccine-october-2020.

Ipsos. 2020b. U.S. and U.K. are Optimistic Indicators for COVID-19 Vaccination Uptake, 29 December. Available at: https://www.ipsos.com/en/global-attitudes-covid-19-vaccine-december-2020.

Kinlaw, K. and Levine, R. 2007. Ethical Guidelines in Pandemic Influenza. Recommendations of the Ethics Subcommittee of the Advisory Committee to the Director, Centre for Disease Control and Prevention. Available at: https://www.cdc.gov/os/integrity/phethics/docs/panFlu_Ethic_Guidelines.pdf.

Kola, L. 2020. Global mental health and COVID-19. *The Lancet Psychiatry* 7(8), pp. 655-657. Available at: https://doi.org/10.1016/S2215-0366(20)30235-2.

Kotalik, J. 2006. Ethics of Planning for and Responding to Pandemic Influenza. Literature review. Swiss National Advisory Commission on Biomedical Ethics. Available at: https://www.nekcne.admin.ch/inhalte/Externe_Gutachten/gutachten_kotalik_en.pdf.

Kreier, F. 2021. "Unprecedented achievement": Who Received the First Billion COVID Vaccinations? *Nature News*, 29 April. Available at: https://www.nature.com/articles/d41586-021-01136-2.

Launch and Scale Speedometer. 2020. Africa: New Study Shows Rich Country Shopping Spree for COVID-19 Vaccines Could Mean Fewer Vaccinations for Billions in Low-Income Countries. Available at: https://allafrica.com/stories/202011020103.html.

Liebensteiner, M.C., Khosravi, I., Hirschmann, M.T. et al. 2020. Massive Cutback In Orthopaedic Healthcare Services Due to the COVID-19 Pandemic. *Knee Surg Sports Traumatol Arthrosc* 28, pp. 1705–1711. Available at: https://doi.org/10.1007/s00167-020-06032-2.

Medical Brief. 8 April 2020. Forced quarantine of two Limpopo Doctors. Available at: https://www.medicalbrief.co.za/archives/forced-quarantine-of-2-limpopo-doctors-causes-dismay/.

Merten, M. 17 July 2020. Lockdown Level 3, Version 3: Policymaking On The Hoof Amid War Talk. *Daily Maverick*. Available at: https://www.dailymaverick.co.za/article/2020-07-17-lockdown-level-3-version-3-policymaking-on-the-hoof-amid-war-talk/.

National Health Act 61 of 2003. Available at: www.gov.za/documents/national-health-act.

OECD. 1997. Convention on Combatting Bribery of Foreign Public Officials in International Business Transactions and Related Documents. Available at: http://www.oecd.org/daf/anti-bribery/ConvCombatBribery_ENG.pdf.

Newman, P.A. et al. 2015. Towards a Science of Community Stakeholder Engagement in Biomedical HIV Prevention Trials: An Embedded Four-Country Case Study. PLOS ONE, 10(8), p. e0135937. Available at: https://doi.org/10.1371/journal.pone.0135937.

Persad, G., Wertheimer, A. and Emanuel, E.J. 2009. Principles for Allocation of Scarce Medical Interventions. *The Lancet* 373.9661, pp. 423–431. Available at: https://doi.org/10.1016/s0140-6736(09)60137-9.

Rushton, C.H., Schoonover-Shoffner, K. and Kennedy, M.S. 2017. A Collaborative State of the Science Initiative: Transforming Moral Distress into Moral Resilience in Nursing. *American J of Nursing* 117(2), pp. S2–S6. Available at: https://doi.org/10.1097/01.NAJ.0000512203.08844.1d.

Sheehan, M. and Hope, T. 2002. Allocating healthcare resources in the UK: putting principles into practice. *Medicine and Social Justice: Essays on the Distribution of Healthcare,* pp. 219–230.

South African Government. Disaster Management Act: Regulations to Address, Prevent And Combat The Spread of Coronavirus COVID-19: Amendment (as amended by Gazette 43168 of 26 March 2020 and Gazette 43199 of 2 April 2020, Gazette 43232 of 16 April and Gazette 43240 of 20 April 2020). www.gov.za/documents/disaster-management-act-regulations-address-prevent-and-combat-spread-coronavirus-covid-19.

South African Medical Research Council. 2021. Advisory: COVID-19 Vaccine Health Certificates and Passports (Passes). Available at: https://www.samrc.ac.za/sites/default/files/attachments/2021-08-04/Advisory%20vaccine%20passports.pdf.

Thompson, A., Faith, K., Gibson, J. and Upshur, R. 2006. Pandemic Influenza Preparedness: An Ethical Framework to Guide Decision-Making. *BMC Medical Ethics* 7, p. 12. Available at: https://bmcmedethics.biomedcentral.com/articles/10.1186/1472-6939-7-12.

Tuohey, F. 2007. A Matrix for Ethical Decision Making in a Pandemic. The Oregon Tool for Emergency Preparedness. Available at: https://www.chausa.org/publications/health-progress/article/november-december-2007/a-matrix-for-ethical-decision-making-in-a-pandemic.

United Nations. 2021. UN Security Council demands COVID-19 Vaccine Ceasefires; WHO Pushes for More Actions to Speed Up Inoculations. 26 February. Available at: https://news.un.org/en/story/2021/02/1085942.

United Nations Convention Against Corruption. 2003. Available at: https://www.unodc.org/pdf/corruption/publications_unodc_convention-e.pdf.

United Nations Educational, Scientific and Cultural Organisation. 2020. Statement on COVID-19: Ethical Considerations From a Global Perspective. 26 March. Available at: https://unesdoc.unesco.org/ark:/48223/pf0000373115.

U.S. Department of Labor, Office of Inspector General. CARES Act: Initial Areas of Concern Regarding Implementation of Unemployment Insurance Provisions. REPORT NUMBER: 19-20-001-03-315, 21 April 2020. Available at: https://www.oversight.gov/sites/default/files/oig-reports/19-20-001-03-315.pdf.

Usdin, S. 2020. COVAX Created to Try to Avoid Global Bidding Frenzy for COVID-19 Vaccines. *Biocentury*, 1–3.

Van den Berg, R.D. 2015. Evaluation of the Funding of Global Public Goods Note For the OECD/DAC Evaluation Network. 27 May. Available at: https://www.oecd.org/dac/evaluation/Evaluation-of-Global-Public-Goods-Evalnet-note.pdf.

World Health Organization. 2007. Ethical Considerations in Developing a Public Health Response to Influenza. Available at: https://www.who.int/csr/resources/publications/WHO_CDS_EPR_GIP_2007_2c.pdf.

World Health Organization. 2020a. Ethics and COVID-19: Resource Allocation and Priority Setting. WHO reference number: WHO/RFH/20.2. Available at: https://www.who.int/ethics/publications/ethics-covid-19-resource-allocation.pdf?ua=1.

World Health Organization. 2020b. Rational Use of Personal Protective Equipment For Coronavirus Disease (COVID-19) and Considerations During Severe Shortages. Interim Guidance: 6 April. Geneva: WHO, 2020. Available at: www.http://WHO-2019-nCov-IPC_PPE_use-2010.3-eng.pdf.

World Justice Project. 2020. Corruption and the COVID-19 Pandemic. Available at: https://worldjusticeproject.org/sites/default/files/documents/Corruption%20Design%20File%20V4.pdf.

World Medical Association Condemns Attacks on Healthcare Professionals. 21 April 2020. Available at: https://www.wma.net/news-post/world-medical-association-condemns-attacks-on-health-care-professionals/.

CHAPTER 4

SELECTED MEDICO-LEGAL ISSUES RELATING TO SOUTH AFRICA'S RESPONSE TO THE COVID-19 PANDEMIC

Melodie Labuschaigne
David McQuoid-Mason
Ames Dhai

4.1 INTRODUCTION

Following the WHO's declaration of COVID-19 as a pandemic on 11 March 2020 and the first reported case of community transmission in South Africa, President Cyril Ramaphosa declared a National State of Disaster on 15 March 2020. Since the first reported case in March 2020, the total number of confirmed cases on 28 September 2021 stood at 2 898 888, and 87 417 reported deaths (National Department of Health, 2021). South Africa was fortunate as it took almost three months for COVID-19 to arrive in 2020. It was clear from the beginning that the COVID-19 pandemic in South Africa was always going to play out against the backdrop of other pandemics necessitating quick and decisive action.

An effective pandemic response requires a very robust legal framework that is not only able to curb and limit the number of infections, but also one that is able to balance many competing societal and individual interests. Extreme measures must be taken which may result in the limitation of certain human rights and freedoms, such as bodily integrity, privacy, freedom of association and freedom of movement. In constitutional democracies such as South Africa, however, such limitations have to be consistent with the limitation provision in the Constitution (Constitution of the Republic of South Africa, 1996, section 36). A consideration of rationality is important, not only as a requirement of the principle of legality, but to ensure that a decision, whether legislative or executive, must be rationally related to a legitimate governmental purpose, otherwise it will be arbitrary and inconsistent with the Constitution (*Pharmaceutical Manufacturers: In re Ex parte Application of the President of the Republic of South Africa*, 2000).

In terms of international law, states have legal obligations to affirmatively protect the right to health of their populations during a pandemic. This is particularly clear for States Parties to the International Covenant on Economic, Social and Cultural Rights (ICESCR, 1996), which include South Africa who ratified the Covenant in 2015. In a statement on 11 April 2020, the ESCR Committee reiterated its guidance from General Comment No. 14 that States Parties establish urgent medical care systems in pandemics. The Committee called on States Parties to 'make all efforts to mobilize the necessary resources to combat COVID-19 in the most equitable manner' (ICESCR, 2020). In so doing, it outlined several recommendations for States Parties in addressing the current pandemic. States are urged to mobilise healthcare resources and ensure 'a comprehensive, coordinated health-care response to the crisis', and to pay close attention to marginalised and vulnerable groups most likely to suffer disproportionate negative effects of the pandemic (ICESCR, 2020). It further stated that workers should be protected from risks of contagion at work, measures should be adopted to address profiteering, and accessible information about the pandemic be disseminated.

Against this backdrop and turning the focus to South African, this chapter will focus on some common medico-legal situations that arise in the legal framework of constitutional democracies during pandemics. The chapter concludes with some observations and lessons learnt from the South African government's response to the pandemic.

4.2   OBJECTIVES

The objectives of the chapter are to:
- Consider the relationship between law and ethics during pandemics.
- Discuss the limitations on informed consent and confidentiality during pandemics.
- Explore healthcare personnel's access to personal protective equipment and COVID-19 vaccines when there are shortages of resources.
- Discuss the legal implications of frontline healthcare personnel refusing to treat infected patients despite being issued with proper PPE.
- Apply legal principles to delayed test results during pandemics.
- Examine the need to dispense with the consent requirements for the extraction of human tissue samples or the holding of autopsies to determine if deceased patients have died from the infection causing the pandemic.
- Explore the lack of clarity on whether extended ICU COVID-19 care could be seen as emergency medical treatment.
- Consider the intellectual property rights in COVID-19 vaccines in the context of so-called vaccine 'apartheid' vs the public good.

4.3 RELATIONSHIP BETWEEN LAW AND ETHICS DURING PANDEMICS

The bioethical principles of patient autonomy, beneficence, non-maleficence and justice or fairness provide a convenient framework for illustrating the relationship between law and ethics during pandemics (Dhai and McQuoid-Mason, 2020). Healthcare practitioners who follow the bioethical principles will generally be acting in accordance with the Constitution, the statute law and the common law of constitutional democracies. During pandemics the constitutional rights of patients may be limited provided it is reasonable and justifiable to do so, as is required by the South African Constitution (Constitution, 1996). Problems arise when, during pandemics, it is necessary to limit certain rights in the Constitution, which limitations for clarity should be set out clearly in the pandemic regulations. For example, if informed consent (McQuoid-Mason, 2020a) or confidentiality (McQuoid-Mason, 2020b) are limited by pandemic regulations, such limitations may be a violation of the constitutional rights to bodily integrity and privacy; the national health legislation provisions regarding informed consent and confidentiality; and the common-law rights to bodily integrity and privacy (Dhai and McQuoid-Mason, 2020). In South Africa, it would also violate the rules of professional conduct of the Health Professions Council of South Africa's (HPCSA, 2006) and the South African Nursing Council (SA Nursing Council, 1985).

Furthermore, with the increased demand on access to healthcare services during a pandemic, triage of critically ill patients becomes a high priority and clear and practical guidelines should exist which take into account the country's limited human and medical resources such as ICU beds and ventilators (Singh and Moodley, 2020). However, if it can be shown that such limitations in the regulations are reasonable and justifiable in order to halt the pandemic and save lives, the breaches of the bioethical principles and various legal provisions would not be actionable in law (McQuoid-Mason, 2020a).

4.4 LIMITATIONS ON INFORMED CONSENT

As mentioned, during pandemics, governments may need to impose strict measures to combat their spread. Some of these measures impact on the patient's right to give informed consent for screening, testing and treatment of the disease concerned (McQuoid-Mason, 2020a), as occurred during the COVID-19 pandemic in South Africa (Disaster Management Regulations, 2020).

Patients need to be reassured that wherever possible, healthcare practitioners are ethically bound to obtain informed consent from patients before they subject them to diagnostic testing and treatment, but have to comply with the demands of the law. Healthcare practitioners, therefore, need to explain the ethical and legal situation to their patients, and the consequences of refusing to comply with any relevant pandemic regulations for both themselves and their patients (McQuoid-Mason, 2020a).

In the case of COVID-19 related research, consent requirements may need to be adapted for safety reasons. Although the right to informed consent for research participation as a core principle is entrenched in the Constitution, the consent process may need to be adapted for practical or safety concerns (De Vries et al, 2021). This could mean turning to telephonic or electronic means to collect informed consent, and in exceptional instances, e.g. where a patient's competence is compromised, researchers would be justified to consider proxy consent from next of kin for the collection of samples. Delayed consent from participants who survive should be obtained. A waiver of informed consent should be accepted only in highly exceptional cases and where this has been fully justified to the research ethics committee (De Vries et al, 2021).

4.5   LIMITATIONS ON CONFIDENTIALITY

When the right to confidentiality of patients has been limited during a pandemic to halt the spread of the virus or disease, patients must be reassured that healthcare practitioners are ethically bound to continue to respect such confidentiality, while also complying with the demands of the law (McQuoid-Mason, 2020b).

For instance, it was suggested that during the COVID-19 pandemic in South Africa, healthcare practitioners who sent patients for testing and/or who tested patients for COVID-19 should have informed them that although, according to the Disaster Management Act regulations, they had to send personal information about their patients and copies of their patients' documents to the Director-General of Health for inclusion in the COVID-19 Tracing Database, such information would be kept confidential (Disaster Management Regulations, 2020; McQuoid-Mason, 2020b). The information was captured on the database and sent to a designated judge, to ensure that it was used for the purposes of the COVID-19 regulations only. Furthermore, the information could not be disclosed by persons not authorised to do so unless it was necessary to prevent the spread of the pandemic (Disaster Management Regulations, 2020).

In such circumstances, healthcare practitioners should also tell their patients that any other information from their consultations that are not relevant to the pandemic preventive measures, or necessary to be disclosed in terms of any other law, will be kept confidential (McQuoid-Mason, 2020b). The importance of confidentiality is underscored by the risk of stigmatisation of patients testing positive for COVID-19, as has emerged in South Africa (Spotlight, 2020). The stigmatisation of and unfair discrimination of HIV-positive persons in South Africa in many contexts are well-documented, and also acknowledged by the Constitutional Court of South Africa in the case of *Hoffmann v South African Airways* (2001). Following the findings of a recent study focusing on a hospital in KwaZulu-Natal that indicated that HIV positivity increased the chances of refusal of ICU access more than two-fold (Joynt et al, 2019), contrary to

South African guidelines on ICU triage and rationing, it is reasonable to assume that HIV positive patients' access to ICU beds may be compromised in the context of a pandemic (Labuschaigne, 2020).

4.6 PROVIDING HEALTHCARE PERSONNEL WITH PERSONAL PROTECTIVE EQUIPMENT AND ACCESS TO VACCINES WHEN THERE ARE SHORTAGES OF RESOURCES

The question of ensuring that frontline healthcare personnel have sufficient personal protective equipment (PPE), as well as priority access to the relevant vaccines, is a major concern during pandemics – particularly where there is a shortage of resources (McQuoid-Mason, 2020c). The World Medical Association (WMA, 2014), World Health Organization (WHO, 2020), and in South Africa, the HPCSA guidelines (HPCSA, 2020) regarding the use of PPE, for instance, during the COVID-19 pandemic, all state that the safety of healthcare workers is a priority if they are to care for their patients properly. Mitigation measures are suggested but do not extend to failing to provide PPE to those healthcare workers who deal directly with patients. Healthcare personnel continue to be on the frontline of the nation's fight against COVID-19. As they will be responsible for providing critical care to those who are or might be infected with the virus that causes COVID-19, they are at an increased risk of infection from the virus. By the end of May 2021, the Sisonke trial (often mistaken for phase one of South Africa's national vaccination plan), whose target was to vaccinate 500 000 healthcare workers out of a total of 1.2 million, ended up vaccinating 479 768 healthcare workers (Discovery, 2021). The Sisonke trial, as a phase 3b implementation study, was primarily instituted because of the urgency to get healthcare workers vaccinated before the arrival of the third wave or surge of COVID-19 in South Africa. The rest of the healthcare workers not yet vaccinated would be included under the national vaccine roll-out system. Initially, the limited availability of vaccines also exacerbated the sluggish roll-out of vaccinations to healthcare workers. To compound the problem, one million doses of AstraZeneca received in February 2021 to kick start phase 1 of the national roll-out programme were found to be ineffective against the South African COVID-19 variant. Vaccine hesitancy (Dhai, 2021a; Cooper, 2021) also plays a role in the low number of healthcare personnel being vaccinated.

The law in most countries usually protects workers' constitutional and statutory rights to a working environment that is not harmful and which threatens their health and safety (Occupational Health and Safety Act, 1983). It has been suggested that if advocacy attempts by frontline healthcare personnel to persuade health establishments to provide PPE protection against infection from the pandemic fail, they can, as a last resort, ethically and legally refuse to work, if such healthcare workers are exposed to a disease such as COVID-19

(McQuoid-Mason, 2020d). It is submitted that mandatory vaccination for South African healthcare workers, as happened in Italy (Paterlini, 2021), would pass constitutional muster as a reasonable and justifiable limitation on the right to freedom and security of the person. The reason for this is that such limitation would be regarded as rational and proportional considering the significance of the reason for the limitation, which is public health. Since health care workers are most likely more exposed to potential COVID-19 infection, it would be in both their interests, as well as those of other patients, to require that they are vaccinated.

Regulations were also promulgated to enable healthcare players to cooperate to ensure that adequate PPE capacity and stock at healthcare facilities are maintained throughout the country in response to COVID-19 (COVID-1 Block Exemption for the Health Care Sector, 2020). The purpose of these block exemption regulations for the healthcare sector is to exempt a category of agreements or practices from the application of section 4 of the Competition Act (Competition Act, 1998), which prohibits restrictive horizontal practices, including cartel conduct between competitors, as well as from section 5 of the same Act, which prohibits restrictive vertical practices, including minimum resale price maintenance. These will assist in ensuring that private and public healthcare service providers cooperate and provide the necessary care to citizens without fear of falling foul of the Competition Act. However, the cooperation envisaged between competitors in the healthcare sector does not extend to communication and agreements in respect of prices charged to the public (i.e. price-fixing). The cooperation will take place at the request of and in coordination with the Department of Health. Healthcare players covered by this exemption include those between hospitals or healthcare facilities, medical suppliers, medical specialists or radiologists, pathologists or laboratories, pharmacies and healthcare funders.

4.7   FRONTLINE HEALTHCARE PERSONNEL REFUSING TO TREAT PANDEMIC PATIENTS DESPITE BEING ISSUED WITH PROPER PPE OR AFTER BEING VACCINATED

A problem that may occur, and has occurred in South Africa during the health COVID-19 pandemic, is that some healthcare practitioners may refuse to treat patients despite being provided with the required PPE (McQuoid-Mason, 2020c) or after being vaccinated against COVID-19. For instance, in South Africa, during the COVID-19 pandemic at some health establishments, doctors and nurses employed there refused to treat COVID-19 patients – even when they had been provided with the necessary personal protective equipment. Such conduct, including refusing to treat patients after being vaccinated against COVID-19, is in breach of the World Medical Association International Code of Medical Ethics (WMA, 1949), the International Council of Nurses Code of Ethics for Nurses (International Code of Conduct for Nurses, 2020), the Rules of Conduct of the Health Professions Council of South Africa (HPCSA, 2006), the SA Nursing Council (Nursing Council, 1985), and some of the provisions of the SA Constitution (Constitution of the Republic of South Africa, 1996) and some relevant labour legislation provisions (Labour Relations Act, 1995). Such healthcare practitioners need to be informed that not only are they breaching the ethical rules of their professions, but they may also be in breach of the law.

4.8 DELAYED TEST RESULTS

During the early and subsequent stages of pandemics there may be delays in obtaining test results and this may cause ethical and legal dilemmas for healthcare practitioners who need to know the results for treatment purposes. For instance, a patient may need to be referred to a specialist who requires the patient's pandemic status in order to treat the person properly (McQuoid-Mason, 2020e).

If it is not a medical emergency, and the specialist treatment can be delayed, there is the problem that if at the time of the test the patient's results were negative, (s)he could subsequently contract the virus. Hence, the test will need to be repeated prior to the specialist commencing the elective treatment. Where the emergency treatment can be delayed for a short period of time (e.g. 24 hours), it may be possible to have a new test done at a laboratory with a very quick turnaround time. However, if it is a medical emergency that cannot be delayed even for a short period of time, the specialist will have to make a judgement call on how to treat the patient, using a clinical diagnosis to determine whether or not the patient may have the particular disease or virus concerned. In such circumstances, provided the specialist acts as a reasonably competent colleague would have done in a similar situation, (s)he will not be legally liable for any harm caused to the patient or their family as a result of a wrong call (McQuoid-Mason, 2020e).

4.9 DISPENSING WITH CONSENT REQUIREMENTS FOR THE EXTRACTION OF HUMAN TISSUE SAMPLES OR THE HOLDING OF AUTOPSIES TO DETERMINE IF DECEASED PATIENTS HAVE DIED FROM A PANDEMIC

It may be that during pandemics it is necessary to conduct autopsies or remove samples of tissue from deceased persons to determine whether or not they have died from a pandemic-related illness. Usually, this requires some form of consent either by the deceased beforehand, by a proxy mandated by the patient in writing, authorised by law or a court order, or in terms section 7(1)(*a*) of the National Health Act (National Health Act, 2003). The South African experience is instructive in this respect. It has been suggested that ethically and legally obtaining biological samples for research after death during the COVID-19 pandemic in South Africa justified a waiver of consent followed by a deferred proxy consent (Moodley K et al, 2020).

In South Africa, deceased persons are not protected by the Constitution (Constitution, 1996) and only partially protected by the common law crime of interfering with a corpse (*S v Coetzee,* 1993) and statute law governing the removal of tissue (National Health Act, 2003). Therefore it has been submitted that consent and the need for consent to autopsies may be dispensed with altogether under the common law doctrine of 'necessity' (Neethling et al, 2001) during pandemics.

Such information is in the public interest because it will inform critical care facilities on how to save the lives of future patients and assist government in responding to a pandemic by adequate planning. It is also reasonably justifiable in the public interest to ascertain the health status of deceased persons who have been exposed to the risk of the pandemic, in order to protect their family, their friends, healthcare practitioners, undertakers and their staff members, and members of the public with whom they have been in contact. Finally, it is suggested that the law can be clarified by including in the pandemic regulations that consent may be done away with for autopsies or tissue sample collections from deceased persons who were exposed to the risk of contracting the pandemic disease or virus, subject to certain conditions (McQuoid-Mason, 2020f).

4.10 EXTENDED ICU CARE: EMERGENCY MEDICAL TREATMENT?

Healthcare services are put under severe pressure during pandemics, and South Africa, with 13,8 million people living on less than R19 a day (PMBEJD, 2020) and the majority reliant on an already under-resourced public healthcare sector, is no exception. Inequalities relating to ill-health and disability, with the burden of communicable diseases such as TB, HIV and diarrhoeal diseases particularly high for poorer groups (Gopalan and Vasconcellos, 2019), are exacerbated by social and economic factors, such as inequitable access to housing, sanitation, potable water, educational attainment, employment and regular income (Gopalan and Vasconcellos, 2019). Although the right of 'access to healthcare services' is guaranteed in section 27 of the South African Constitution (Constitution, 1996), this right is not absolute and may be limited (Constitution, 1996, section 36). Section 27 furthermore provides that the state must take 'reasonable legislative and other measures, within its available resources, to achieve the progressive realisation' of this right. No limitation appears to apply to emergency medical care, as section 27(3) states that no one 'may be refused emergency medical treatment'. If one has regard for the Constitutional Court judgment in *Soobramoney v Minister of Health (Kwazulu-Natal)* (Soobramoney, 1998), which held that continuous dialysis treatment for chronic disease does not constitute emergency medical treatment, the continued and extended ICU care for COVID-19 patients may arguably by analogy also not be seen as emergency medical treatment. The Constitutional Court referred to the standard of 'reasonableness' in evaluating the relevant measures, in a judgment that dealt with a vulnerable group's right of access to housing and whether the government's measures to address the progressive realisation of the right of access to housing were adequate (Grootboom, 2001 paras [40]–[44]). Any measure that would significantly exclude a (vulnerable) segment of society 'whose needs are most urgent' and 'whose ability to enjoy all rights is therefore most in peril' would hence be viewed as unreasonable (Grootboom, 2001 paras [43]–[44]).

Whether COVID-19 patients in need of extended care in an intensive care unit qualify for 'emergency medical treatment' is answered by considering the Constitution, the meaning of emergency medical treatment, and whether such patients are in an incurable chronic condition (McQuoid-Mason, 2021). Ethical guidelines for the withholding and withdrawal of treatment may guide courts in deciding whether a healthcare practitioner has acted with the degree of skill and care required of a reasonably competent practitioner (McQuoid-Mason, 2021).

4.11 INTELLECTUAL PROPERTY RIGHTS IN COVID-19 VACCINES: VACCINE 'APARTHEID' VS THE PUBLIC GOOD

In February 2021, UNESCO's International Bioethics Committee (IBC) and the World Commission on the Ethics of Scientific Knowledge and Technology (COMEST) made a call for a change of current COVID-19 vaccination strategies, urging that vaccines be treated as a global public good to ensure they are made equitably available in all countries, and not only to those who bid the highest for these vaccines (UNESCO, 2021). While many HICs have secured enough vaccines to protect their entire population up to five times over, the global south faces a bleak future. At the current rate, many developing countries will not have access to sufficient vaccines until well into 2022. The application by South Africa and India to the World Trade Organisation (WTO) for a temporary waiver of IPR for COVID-19 vaccines during the pandemic, was met with resistance (Dhai, 2021a). UNESCO's statement on global vaccine equity and solidarity, referring to COVID-19 vaccines as a 'global common good' (article 3), strongly condemns vaccine nationalism as a 'predatory rush' and calls for responses to the pandemic to be built on equality, justice and solidarity. The statement rightly points out that true equity in global access to vaccines requires a shared understanding of health as a global common good without territorial limits, including new global legal instruments for economic and political treaties. As the Agreement on Trade-Related Aspects of Intellectual Property Rights (TRIPS) and the agreements of the WTO were not drafted with pandemics in mind, vaccine 'apartheid' (ENCN, 2021) or vaccine nationalism, will lead to further inequitable erosion of global public health principles. In the absence of firm and binding international law instruments addressing such inequity during pandemics, the call for international solidarity, fairness and multilateral support is critical if South Africa is to win the COVID-19 war (Dhai, 2021a).

4.12 CONCLUSION

An effective response to a pandemic requires a robust, yet flexible legal framework in order to balance a range of competing individual and societal interests in a rational, justified and transparent manner. By focusing on a selection of relevant medico-legal issues arising from this context, this chapter has clarified some critical pandemic-specific medico-legal issues by proposing practical recommendations aligned with South Africa's constitutional framework, medico-legal jurisprudence in general, as well as relevant ethical guidelines.

4.13 SELF-ASSESSMENT QUESTIONS

1. Discuss the legal protection of workers during pandemics.
2. Why is consent not a legal requirement for autopsies during pandemics?

4.14 REFERENCES

Bosch, R. 2021. Ramaphosa warns of 'vaccine apartheid'. *ENCA*, 28 May. Available at: https://www.enca.com/news/ramaphosa-warns-vaccine-apartheid.

Cooper, S. 2021. COVID-19 Vaccine hesitancy in South Africa: Summary of existing studies. Available at: http://www.health.gov.za/wp-content/uploads/2021/04/Report_Covid-19-vaccine-hesitancy_SA-studies_1April2021.pdf.

De Vries, et al. 2020. Research on COVID-19 in South Africa: Guiding principles for informed consent. *South African Medical Journal* 110(7), pp. 635–639. Available at: https://doi.org/10.7196/SAMJ.2020.v110i7.14863.

Dhai. 2021a. Access to COVID-19 vaccines as a global public good: A co-ordinated global response based on equality, justice and solidarity is key. *South African Journal of Bioethics and Law* 14(1), pp. 2–3. Available at: https://doi.org/10.7196/SAJBL.2021.v14i1.768.

Dhai. 2021b. COVID-19 vaccines: Equitable access, vaccine hesitancy and the dilemma of emergency use approvals. *South African Journal of Bioethics and Law* 13(2), pp. 77–78. Available at: https://doi.org/10.7196/ SAJBL.2020. v13i2.754.

Dhai, A. and McQuoid-Mason, D.J. 2020. *Bioethics, Human Rights and Health Law*. 2 ed. Kenilworth: Juta & Co Ltd, pp. 45–64.

Discovery. 2021. Understanding the progress of SA's vaccine rollout plan. Available at: https://www.discovery.co.za/corporate/covid-19-understanding-sa-vaccine-rollout-plan.

Health Professions Council of South Africa. 2006. Ethical Rules of Conduct for Practitioners Registered under the Health Professions Act, 1974: GN R717 of 4 August 2006.

Health Professions Council of South Africa. 2020. COVID-19 Outbreak in South Africa: Guidance to health practitioners. Pretoria: HPCSA.

Hoffmann v South African Airways 2001 (1) SA 1 (CC).

ICESCR. 2020. Statement on the coronavirus disease (COVID-19) pandemic and economic, social and cultural rights. 11 April. Available at: http://unsr. vtaulicorpuz.org/?p=2808.

International Council of Nurses. 2012. Code of Conduct for Nurses. Geneva: ICN. Available at: https://www.icn.ch/sites/default/files/inline-files/2012_ICN_ Codeof ethicsfornurses_%20eng.pdf.

International Covenant on Economic, Social and Cultural Rights. Adopted by the United Nations General Assembly on 16 December 1966 through GA. Resolution 2200A (XXI), entering in force on 3 January 1976.

Joynt, G.M., Gopalan, D.P., Argent, A.A., et al. 2019. The Critical Care Society of Southern Africa Consensus Statement on ICU Triage and Rationing (ConICTri). *South African Medical Journal* 109(8b), pp. 613–629. Available at: https://doi. org/10.7196/SAMJ.2019.v109i8b.13947613.

Labuschaigne, M. 2020. Ethicolegal issues relating to the South African government response to COVID-19. *South African Journal of Bioethics and Law* (13)1, pp. 23–28.

McQuoid-Mason, D.J. 2020a. COVID-19 and its impact on informed consent: What should health professionals tell their patients or their proxies? *South African Journal of Bioethics Law* 13(1), pp. 7–10.

McQuoid-Mason, D.J. 2020b. COVID-19 and patient-doctor confidentiality. *South African Medical Journal* 110(6), pp. 37–38.

McQuoid-Mason, D.J. 2020c. COVID-19: What should employers do if health practitioner employees registered with the HPCSA refuse to treat COVID-19 patients despite being provided with the required PPE? *South African Journal of Bioethics and Law* 13(1), pp. 11–14. Available at: https://doi.org/10.7196/ SAJBL.2020.v13i1.720.

McQuoid-Mason, D.J. 2020d. COVID-19: May healthcare practitioners ethically and legally refuse to work at hospitals and health establishments where frontline employees are not provided with personal protective equipment? *South African Journal of Bioethics and Law* 13(1), pp. 11–14. Available at: https://doi.org/10.7196/ SAJBL.2020.v13i1.720.

McQuoid-Mason, D.J. 2020f. May a sample be legally removed or an autopsy undertaken without an advance directive or proxy consent to determine if a critical care patient at risk of COVID-19 infection has died as a result of the virus? *South African Medical Journal* 110 (online first: COVID-19 in South Africa). Available at: https://doi.org/10.7196/SAMJ.2020.v110i10.15190.

McQuoid-Mason, D.J. 2020e. What should referring doctors do if there is a delay in receiving COVID-19 test results and specialists require them for proper treatment of patients referred to them? *South African Journal of Bioethics and Law* 13(1), pp. 5–6. Available at: https://doi.org/10.7196/SAJBL.2020.

McQuoid-Mason, D.J. 2021. Do COVID-19 patients needing extended care in an intensive care unit fall under the 'emergency medical treatment' provisions of the South African Constitution? *South African Medical Journal* 111(1), pp. 23–25. Available at: https://doi.org/10.7196/SAMJ.2021.v111i1.15424.

National Department of Health. 2021. COVID-19 statistics. Available at: http://health.gov.za/covid19/index.html.

Neethling, J., Potgieter, J.M. and Visser, P.J. 2001. *Law of Delict*. Durban: Butterworths, pp. 86–92.

Paterlini, M. 2021. COVID-19: Italy makes vaccination mandatory for healthcare workers. *British Medical Journal* 373, p. n905. DOI:10.1136/bmj.n905 pmid:33824155.

Pharmaceutical Manufacturers: In re Ex parte Application of the President of the Republic of South Africa 2000 (2) SA 674 (CC) at para [85].

Pietermaritzburg Economic Justice and Dignity Group (PMBEJD). Household Affordability Index. March 2020. Available at: https://za.boell.org/sites/default/files/2020-04/ March-2020-Household-Affordability-Index-PMBEJD.pdf.

S v Coetzee 1993 2 SACR 191 (T).

Singh, J.A. and Moodley, K. 2020. Critical care triaging in the shadow of COVID-19: Ethics considerations. *South African Medical Journal* 110(5), pp. 355–359.

Soobramoney v Minister of Health (KwaZulu-Natal) 1998 (1) SA 765 (CC) at para 44.

South Africa. Competition Act No 89 of 1998. COVID-19 Block Exemption for the Health Care Sector, 2020. Regulations published in GN R. 349 of Government Gazette No 43114 of 19 March 2020, expanded on 8 April 2020 (*GG* 43215, GN R. 456. Available at: https://openbylaws.org.za/za/act/gn/2020/r349/eng/resources/eng.pdf.

South Africa. Constitution of the Republic of South Africa, 1996.

South Africa. Disaster Management Act No 57 of 2002. Available at: https://www.gov.za/sites/default/files/gcis_document/201409/a57-020.pdf.

South Africa. Disaster Management Act No 57 of 2002. Regulations issued in terms of section 27(2) of the Disaster Management Act, 2002.

South Africa. Labour Relations Act No 66 of 1995. Available at: www.gov.za/ documents/ labour-relations-act.

South Africa. National Health Act No 61 of 2003. Available at: www.gov.za/ documents/national-health-act.

South Africa. Occupational Health and Safety Act No 85 of 1993. Available at: www. gov.za/sites/default/files/gcis_document/201409/act85of1993.pdf.

South African Nursing Council. Rules of the South African Nursing Council (SANC) setting out the Acts or Omissions in Respect of which the Council may take Disciplinary Action. GN R 387 of 15 February 1985, as amended by GN R 866 of 24 April 1987 and GN R 2490 of 26 October 1990. Available at: https://www.sanc. co.za/regulat/ Reg-act.htm.

Spotlight. 2020. COVID-19: Concerns mount over COVID-19 stigma in KZN. 21 May. Available at: https://www.spotlightnsp.co.za/2020/05/21/covid-19-concerns-mount-over-covid-19-stigma-in-kzn/.

UNAIDS. 2020. Rights in the time of COVID-19 — Lessons from HIV for an effective, community-led response. Available at: https://www.unaids.org/sites/default/files/ media_asset/human-rights-and-covid-19_en.pdf.

UNESCO. 2021. Ethical commission's call for global vaccine equity and solidarity. Available at: https://ngomigration.files.wordpress.com/2021/02/unesco-call-ethics-solidarity-vaccine3.pdf

UNESCO. 2020. United Nations Educational, Scientific and Cultural Organisation. Statement on COVID-19: Ethical considerations from a global perspective. 26 March. Available at: https://unesdoc.unesco.org/ark:/48223/pf0000373115.

World Health Organization. 2007. Ethical considerations in developing a public health response to influenza. Available at: https://www.who.int/csr/resources/ publications/WHO_CDS_EPR_GIP_2007_2c.pdf.

World Health Organization. Ethics and COVID-19: Resource allocation and priority setting WHO reference number: WHO/RFH/20.2. Available at: https://www.who. int/ethics/publications/ethics-covid-19-resource-allocation.pdf?ua=1.

World Health Organization. 2020. Rational use of personal protective equipment for coronavirus disease (COVID-19) and considerations during severe shortages. Interim guidance. 6 April. Geneva: WHO. Available at: www.http://WHO-2019 -nCov-IPC_PPE_use-2010.3-eng.pdf.

World Medical Association. 2014. Declaration on the protection of health care workers in situations of violence. Ferney-Voltaire: WMA. Available at: https:// www.wma.net/policies-post/wma-declaration-on-the-protection-of-health-care-workers-in-situation-of-violence/.

World Medical Association. International Code of Medical Ethics (adopted by the 3rd General Assembly of the World Medical Association, London, England, October 1949; amended by the 22nd World Medical Assembly, Sydney, Australia, August 1968; the 35th World Medical Assembly, Venice, Italy, October 1983; and the 57th WMA General Assembly, Pilanesberg, South Africa, October 2006). Available at: https://www.wma.net/policies-post/wma-international-code-of-medical-ethics/.

CHAPTER 5

HEALTH RESEARCH, ETHICS AND PANDEMICS: CHALLENGES AND RECOMMENDATIONS

Ames Dhai

Glenda Gray

Mantoa Mokhachane

Mongezi Mdhluli

5.1　INTRODUCTION

Infectious disease outbreaks and emergencies associated with high mortality and a lack of safe and efficacious interventions are fundamental characteristics of pandemics. Pandemics result not only in significant numbers of lives being lost, but increased morbidity has a concomitant strain on the public health system. In addition, the accompanying economic and social adversities place a huge strain on livelihoods and the well-being of households. During this period of mounting uncertainty, resources are inevitably constrained. This is exacerbated in regions where resources and capacities are already severely limited even prior to the onset of the pandemic. While the primary obligation will be to respond to the medical need of those affected, there is a parallel obligation to conduct health research. Moral urgency for research that responds to this public health need is critical. Moreover, research must be expedited to allow for the timely production of evidence on the safety and efficacy of preventative and therapeutic interventions. Research also enables the building of an evidence base for pandemics that may follow. The research that is required during a global health emergency is wide-ranging and includes clinical trials of novel treatments and vaccines, epidemiological research, socio-behavioural studies, implementation research and health systems research. Although the valuable role of research in this context cannot be denied, several accompanying challenges emerge that require a careful balancing of the obligation for evidence-based interventions with the obligation for protecting the interests and rights of research participants and communities. These two obligations may often conflict. Vulnerability increases or may appear for the first time during a pandemic and unanticipated ethical issues may emerge. Without both scientific and ethical rigour, it would be difficult to justify using the research results and, furthermore, respect for human dignity and social justice would be denied. The authors of this chapter have been actively involved in COVID-19 research, either as researchers or ethics reviewers. Their collective experience has informed many of the sections that follow.

5.2 OBJECTIVES

The objectives of this chapter are to:

- Discuss the challenges that arise in health research during infectious disease outbreaks.
- Explore ethical principles specific to health research in the context of pandemics.
- Discuss why community consultation and engagement are essential components of health research during pandemics.
- Consider the complexities associated with sample and data sharing during pandemics.
- Describe ethical issues that have arisen in the context of publications during the COVID-19 pandemic.
- Examine ethical issues specific to vaccine research during pandemics.

5.3 GLOBAL PUBLIC HEALTH EMERGENCIES AND HEALTH RESEARCH: GENERAL ETHICAL CHALLENGES

Experience from pandemics in the past and the current severe acute respiratory syndrome coronavirus 2 (SARS-CoV-2) outbreak allow for the recognition of the many challenges to conducting research in this context. A pandemic itself puts pressure on the need to conduct research, especially where the mortality rate is high and treatment options are limited, as has been the case with the COVID-19 disease. Ethically conducted research needs to be supported and promoted and the risk of unethically conducted health research during these emergencies must be vigorously curtailed. All people during this time deserve their health to be promoted. Hence there is an ethical imperative for the meticulous collection of robust and good data. This must be coupled with respecting dignity and upholding rights. Expedience will not justify unethical practice. Careful ethical reflection is essential, albeit the urgency. What is required is balance, and this balance must be informed by voices from the community and other relevant stakeholders. Local contexts need to be understood (O'Mathúna and Siriwardhana, 2017).

Ethical challenges to health research during global health emergencies include:

- Disruption from stable situations or disruption from the norm resulting in increased vulnerability. Infrastructure supporting health services provision and research is unavoidably undermined while there is a simultaneous increase in demand for research. In addition, affected populations may raise questions about the value of research at this time (Nuffield Council, 2020).

- Significant risks to physical and/or mental well-being at both individual and population levels result in increased vulnerability and may make it difficult for people to protect their own rights and interests (Nuffield Council, 2020).

- Pressures of time because the effectiveness of the research is directly linked to the timeliness in which the research is undertaken and the window of research cannot be lost. Planning, conducting and producing research results are often in conflict with the short timeframes for response efforts (Nuffield Council, 2020).

- Evolving uncertainty creates challenges for decision-making at several levels, including that of research governance and research participants. Scientific uncertainty in the face of experimental interventions where no effective vaccines or treatments exist may result in premature use of products where knowledge is deficient. This will need to be balanced with the risks associated with delaying or not acting within the time-limited window for action (Nuffield Council, 2020).

- Fear, distress, and panic created by the emergency may affect individuals' and populations' inclination to participate in research, potentially erode trust in researchers and create further demands on fair recruitment procedures (Nuffield Council, 2020).

- Limited health infrastructure in many resource-limited regions of the world can challenge the implementation of preferred study designs and data collection. In addition, efforts to make interventions developed from the research as quickly as possible to communities in remote and rural areas could be particularly challenging (CIOMS, 2016).

- The multi-country, multi-agency, and multi-sectoral nature of responses will probably give rise to tensions and competing interests with regard to cooperation between participants, researchers and relevant stakeholders, governments, intergovernmental agencies, research funding bodies, and research institutions. Furthermore, values and priorities between the different role players may also be in conflict (Nuffield Council, 2020).

A major and complex challenge that unfolded during the COVID-19 pandemic was the neglect of other non-COVID-19 health research initiatives and already established research programmes (Singh, Bandewarb and Bukusi, 2020). This was because of highly restrictive lockdowns and other containment initiatives coupled with a rapid and massive COVID-19 research response. Recruitment and retention of participants into non-COVID-19 studies were almost impossible due to the restrictions on freedom of movement. With funding for research being prioritised to COVID-19 enquiry, and with the global economy being substantially affected, funding for other types of research was negatively affected as well.

5.4   SPECIFIC ETHICAL PRINCIPLES REQUIRING SPECIAL ATTENTION DURING PANDEMICS

Generally, ethics in research is concerned with protecting vulnerable research participants and communities against exploitation and other forms of harm. It also serves to guide researchers and other role players on the most appropriate way to conduct research and implement the research findings so that ethical norms and standards are included throughout the process. There are two components to ethics in research: the ethical principles and regulatory requirements. The latter include obtaining the necessary permissions, and approvals and complying with legal requirements and will not be discussed further in this chapter save to say that the Research Ethics Committee (REC) review involves both components (Dhai, 2019a). While all ethical principles must be upheld, some require special attention during a pandemic (CIOMS, 2016).

5.4.1   Scientific Validity and Social Value

Lessons learnt from the SARS-CoV-2 outbreak is that it has rapidly evolved, necessitating the use of alternative study designs to yield meaningful data. Study designs, while feasible, must also be appropriate in order to ensure scientific validity. Where the science is deficient, the research will lack social value and should not be conducted. For research to have social value, it must be responsive to the health needs and priorities of those communities in which the research is being conducted (CIOMS, 2016). In a pandemic situation, social value would apply to the global community and the responsiveness requirement will be violated globally. Nevertheless, given that some interventions may have features that would make them difficult to implement in some low- and middle-income countries (LMICs), local contexts must be considered as well, and designs will need to be modified to ensure interventions from research during pandemics are truly global public goods. While the randomised-controlled trial design is often considered the gold standard for obtaining robust data in clinical trials, alternate trial designs that may increase efficiency while still maintaining scientific validity must be explored. It is essential that the methodological and ethical merits of these designs be carefully assessed prior to the research being conducted.

5.4.2   Distributive Justice: Equitable Distribution of Risks and Benefits

Burdens and benefits of participation must be equitably distributed. Interventions developed during emergency infectious disease outbreaks, when being implemented, are usually limited initially. Fair selection of participants is requisite and there is an ethical obligation to ensure that privileged, well-off or well-connected individuals are not further privileged, and selection is not politicised.

Where vulnerable populations are excluded, there must be sound justification for this (CIOMS, 2016). It is important to remember that there are degrees of vulnerability, and once safety concerns have been addressed in less vulnerable adults, it is ethically imperative that research designs include children, pregnant and lactating women and other vulnerable individuals and groups. As has been seen with COVID-19, it may be acceptable to prioritise certain populations when enrolling into the study. An example is frontline healthcare workers who put themselves at risk during infectious disease outbreaks while attending to infected patients. If experimental interventions have been proven to be effective, they could be prioritised for enrolment in, for instance, an implementation study so they are readily available to help more patients (CIOMS, 2016). The principles of utility and reciprocity would both justify them being prioritised. In South Africa, emerging evidence of the lack of efficacy of the ChadoX/AstraZeneca vaccine against the dominant beta (B1.351) variant strain circulating curtailed the roll-out of this vaccine to healthcare workers that had been prioritised in the national programme. The lack of available vaccines authorised for use in South Africa and the emerging evidence of the efficacy of the Ad26 SARS-CoV-2 vaccine created an opportunity to rapidly translate this evidence into practice utilising a phase 3B open-label study design, the Sisonke Study, which thus enabled healthcare workers early access to an efficacious vaccine before emergency use authorisation. This rapid translation of evidence in practice is instructive of the speed required in emergency or pandemic situations.

5.4.3 Beneficence and Nonmaleficence: Safety, Risks, Emergency Use of Investigational Interventions

In the context of infectious disease outbreaks research, reducing risks of harms includes providing participants non-pharmaceutical prevention methods that have already been proven to be effective. The question here is what the standard of prevention should be in the research setting. The standard of prevention refers to the package of comprehensive tools provided or made available to participants in the trial. This would mean the aggregate services and interventions available to help reduce the risk of acquiring the virus. The principle of beneficence places an obligation on researchers and sponsors to minimise risk to participants in the trial. This translates to participants having access to effective means to minimise their risk of acquiring the infection during the research. The approach by researchers should be both pragmatic and aspirational (HPTN, 2020). The necessary conditions for the interventions in the prevention package are: the intervention is a known effective means of prevention; it is practically achievable as a standard in the local setting, and it is reasonably accessible to those at risk of infection. The standard of prevention should not replicate substandard prevention services in the community. It is necessary for researchers to consult with community stakeholders on the standard of prevention. The locally available standard of prevention in an emergency setting may be lower than the best-proven global standard. However, determining what level of prevention a trial will offer requires deliberation with relevant stakeholders about how best to achieve the highest level possible and what ethical justifications are required to support a trial providing a higher standard or a lower one that is aligned with that available to others in the population. Helping trial participants reduce their risk of acquiring the infection is a key ethical obligation of research teams. Providing a standard of prevention package in trials conducted in underserved contexts is a challenge that must be addressed. The components of the prevention package will vary with the degree of risk of exposure. Researchers must work with relevant stakeholders, including community representatives in establishing the type, scope, and process by which participants are provided with the full prevention package as relevant (UNAIDS, 2012)

Infectious disease outbreaks can be highly contagious, life-threatening and can cause excessive mortality as has been seen with Ebola and COVID-19. It is therefore not surprising that many people react by being willing to take high risks and use unproven interventions within and outside the trial context. Furthermore, emergency use may compromise recruitment of research participants and undermine the conclusion of the trial. Researchers, sponsors and RECs have an ethical obligation to meticulously assess the potential individual benefits and risks of the experimental interventions and communicate these clearly and in language that is understandable to potential participants and individuals. In addition, extensive emergency use with inadequate data collection on patient outcomes must be avoided (CIOMS, 2016). The ongoing accumulation of safety reports pertaining to the occurrence of rare thrombotic events related to vaccine use after emergency use authorisation highlights the need for ongoing pharmacovigilance and safety evaluation. The reports of vaccine-induced thrombotic thrombocytopaenia led to the pause of the roll-out of the Ad26 COVID-19 vaccine in the USA, and a concomitant pause in all Ad26 COVID-19 vaccine research. The Sisonke study was paused for 14 days with the regulators initially barring pregnant and lactating healthcare workers from being enrolled into the study. Following an outcry by interest groups, the regulatory authorities allowed the study to be amended to include this group.

5.4.4   Autonomy: Informed Consent

Infective disease outbreaks cause enormous amounts of anxiety, distress and even mental ill-health in populations at large. This could result in a challenge to the informed component of informed consent as many would not be in the proper frame of mind to make well-informed choices. Nevertheless, the principle of autonomy requires that both the liberty and agency elements are satisfied for consent to be truly informed. Hence, being under duress cannot be used as an excuse for people not making voluntary decisions. Therefore potential participants must be assisted in understanding the study and the true implications of their enrolment in it. The notion that informed consent is a process does not change just because the research is being conducted in a pandemic. Where individuals are incapable of giving informed consent, for example, patients in intensive care units on ventilation, special protections apply in that RECs could be approached to allow for proxy or deferred/delayed consent to be obtained.

There were challenges in the execution of protocol amendments, trial processes and unblinding processes in COVID-19 vaccine research. In the ChadoX/AstraZeneca study conducted in South Africa, there were delays in unblinding participants because of differences of opinion at RECs in the country. This resulted in differential offers of access to the active vaccine. Some sites were delayed in being unblinded as RECs tousled with investigators as to who should receive the vaccine post-unblinding. Disgruntled participants petitioned one of the RECs regarding their lack of access to information and autonomy infringements, with respect to knowing their treatment allocation, and access to the active vaccine should they have received the placebo arm. Despite the low vaccine efficacy of the ChadoX/AstraZeneca vaccine, participants felt they should be offered the vaccine post unblinding.

When the Food and Drug Administration (FDA)/Centre for Disease Control (CDC) paused the roll-out of the Johnson & Johnson vaccine in the USA, this resulted in a near-global pause to the Ad26 SARS CoV-2 vaccine trials. Countries had to wait weeks for amendments to protocols that met the FDA requirements. The delay in unblinding of participants and access to the active vaccine caused distress to participants. The slowness in drafting protocol amendments, and regulatory authority and REC approvals frustrated participants. Although regulatory authorities and RECs have worked under severe pressure to fast-track approvals, participants have felt frustrated at their lack of power to be unblinded and/or receive the active vaccine.

5.4.5   Building Trust: Community Consultation and Engagement

It is critical that local communities are consulted and engaged at an early stage during the planning of the research. This is essential to build and maintain trust so that the research can be legitimised by the communities. In this way, recruitment and retention can be optimised as well. Respecting community leadership and input is important. Of essence, however, the potential for conflict of interest at this level must be recognised (CIOMS, 2016). By asserting their authority, community leaders could attempt to use the research to provide services for the communities and in this way make researchers responsible for what would actually be government's responsibilities. (See section 5.5 below for more detail on community engagement). Often, communities are not engaged early enough in processes of trial conduct. Advocacy should be employed to accelerate the delays in decisive action of RECs that have frustrated trial participants. Advocacy regarding unblinding and access to the treatment group requires organisation. Clearly, implementing structures like the Community Advisory Groups that were fundamental to HIV studies, may have supported researchers and participants, who often felt helpless by the to-ing and fro-ing in COVID-19 vaccine trials.

5.4.6   Protectionism: Ethics Review and Oversight

Soon after COVID-19 was declared a pandemic by the World Health Organisation (WHO), there was an explosion of research activities, including clinical trials with the objective of finding cures and vaccinations. Most of these were initially occurring at a local level and it soon became clear that there was a need for coordination of international efforts and the formulation of a common understanding of the ethical review process. In a pandemic, untested interventions need to be tested in several countries as multiple small trials with different methodologies may not provide the evidence needed (UNESCO, 2020). Standard mechanisms for ethical review are too time-consuming to enable full research ethics applications to be prepared and reviewed at the outset and procedures need to be developed to facilitate and accelerate ethics review and continued oversight where significant ethical concerns are raised by the research (CIOMS, 2016). Rapid review and approval of novel approaches are necessary to avoid delays in research during this time. When the nature of the global threat is considered, it becomes understandable that new practices will be embarked upon in the emergency context. Nevertheless, any such decisions will require ethical justification, and it is important to bear in mind that ethical principles cannot be transgressed but can be adjusted to exceptional circumstances. The urgency to find a cure cannot be used as a justification to preclude responsible research practice (UNESCO, 2020). REC over-reach is also a concern that may lead to delays in the implementation of studies or amendments to protocols. Paternalism has restricted participation, especially in the area of pregnant women and lactating women. Other examples include a REC's ruling that post-unblinding of the ChadoX/AstraZeneca study at one of the sites in South Africa, people under 30 years of age were to be excluded from receiving the investigational product. This deviation was contrary to the regulatory and other RECs approval.

5.5   COMMUNITY CONSULTATION AND ENGAGEMENT

Engaging with relevant communities is pivotal to the success of ethical research. While this is an accepted norm generally in research, its significance in the context of infectious disease outbreaks is substantially emphasised. Difficulties with defining a community are well recognised. Definitions and types vary based on locations, settings, age and other variables, including urban, rural or suburban.

To complicate issues further, there exist communities within communities. These are people that are brought together by types of disease, characteristics, actions, preferences or goals (Douglas, 2010).

Douglas provides a useful definition of community as follows (Douglas, 2010 p. 539):

> A community may be defined as a set of meaningful social connections in a group of any size where members have something in common. A community is social. It is a web of some kind of relationships. A community operates within certain boundaries that are agreed among members either tacitly or explicitly. Each community establishes traditions and patterns of behavior which may be implied or written as rules. Members of a community share some kind of a bond such as location, interests, background or identity, situations or experiences.

5.5.1   Ethical Goals of Community Consultation

The primary ethical goal is respect. Respecting communities and individuals within communities and being sensitive to their cultures is of ethical consequence. In an African setting, the notion of Ubuntu/Botho emphasises that a community is the collective, not an individual. It is a belief that 'I am because you are' and decisions are made as a collective, followed by an individual's decision-making (Seehawer, 2018; Metz, 2010; Dhai, 2019b).

According to Dieckert, the ethical goals of community consultation are four-fold (Dieckert, 2005):

1. Enhanced benefits, where the community could recommend that the trial include referral programmes for participants including empowering the community with research skills;
2. Legitimacy, where the community express their views and concerns;
3. Shared responsibility, where consultations may lead to active involvement by community who assume active roles in the research; and
4. Enhanced protection by identifying what risks may be encountered by the participants.

5.5.2   Stages and Process of Consultation

Consultation may be approached in stages and should be tailored to the communities with whom research will be conducted. Consultation and engagement should be non-judgmental nor paternalistic. Each stage of consultation may be met with challenges and difficulties. Researchers first need to decide which community they are interested in working with. It is recommended that initial consultation should be with the broader community, even where the research will need to be conducted in a community within communities.

This is because identifying some of these communities within communities can be challenging (Dieckert, 2005).

Challenges with community emerge during pandemics, especially in the face of an unknown disease with no known treatment. The rush for evidence needed for prevention and cure could result in communities being excluded from the processes giving rise to conflict and tension. Researchers and sponsors need to remember that during a pandemic there is heightened fear, confusion, lack of trust for those in power, including researchers, hope for survival, therapeutic misconceptions and confusion about goals of the research (Busta, 2017).

It is crucial to engage and consult with communities on all facets of the pandemic from the outset, whether or not the researchers know or understand what is going on. They need to walk the journey with the communities and participants. Complete trust amongst all involved is highly valuable (Busta, 2017). In African countries where there has been abuse of power by researchers in the past, communities are very suspicious of foreigners who embark on doing research especially where there is no cure nor known treatment (Okonta, 2014), hence the importance of communication every step of the way. Furthermore, foreign nationals who have arrived specifically to conduct research during this period must endeavour to co-create with communities, including native researchers.

The San Community of South Africa developed their own Code of Research Ethics with four principles: respect, honesty, fairness and care. The San are one of the first indigenous groups to develop their own Research Ethics Code (Schroeder, 2019).

The San Code of Research Ethics is a valuable tool for use during pandemics due to lack of trust in foreign nationals, as mentioned above (Schroeder, 2019). The Code underscores respect for communities; being honest throughout the process, the proposal, the challenges you are facing and admitting to not knowing everything; practice justice and fairness; care for all those involved; and follow process as set out in the protocol.

Communities need to be involved from the conception of the research question. It is important to plan and co-create the research protocol where possible or allow the community into the protocol development process through community advisory boards, respected leaders or other role players that the community recognise and respect. Their participation in and contribution to the development of the informed consent process is essential as they will be able to advise *inter alia* on the accepted language and the level at which this language is utilised across the community. Community members also contribute meaningfully to the ethics approval process, the research itself, analysis of data, write-up and dissemination of the findings. Researchers should not use the public health emergency as an excuse to exclude the community from this process.

5.6   SHARING OF BIOLOGICAL SAMPLES AND DATA

For research in global health emergencies to be effective, the collection, storage, and sharing of biological samples and data are essential (Nuffield Council, 2020). Most of these samples and data are used for genomic research through which large data sets are generated. There has been a shift in practice towards open science, and a drive for sharing of biological samples, data and research results (Mahomed and Staunton, 2021). Given that the use of data can drive rapid response and informed decision-making during public health emergencies, timely and accurate collection, reporting and sharing within and between research communities, public health practitioners, clinicians and policymakers are necessary (K Littler et al, 2017). Open research data is currently strongly supported as a key component of pandemic preparedness and response. Accurate and rapid availability of data will inform assessment of the severity, spread and impact of a pandemic and assist in implementing efficient and effective response strategies (Research Data Alliance, 2020). Early on during the COVID-19 pandemic, both local and international consortia were established to assist with the understanding of the genetic determinants of susceptibility to SARS-CoV-2 and COVID-19 disease. Results and data have been shared from the outset. A global infectious disease outbreak deserves a global response and it is therefore necessary that as many countries as possible participate in the sharing and research (Mahomed and Staunton, 2021). Sharing data and samples for current or for future research use, can significantly help in reducing suffering, both during emergencies and in the routine surveillance that forms part of emergency preparedness (Nuffield Council, 2020).

These activities have also resulted in several challenges. Samples are resources that may get depleted; hence it is imperative that serious consideration is given to which research should be prioritised. The social, cultural and religious status of samples could also lead to disquiet and researchers need to be sensitive to these issues. Risks of harm and exploitation, particularly in already disadvantaged and vulnerable communities are a reality and often result in undermining trust. Access and governance arrangements may not be adequate to protect sample and data donors from social and other forms of harm (Nuffield Council, 2021). Privacy considerations around participant and patient data are significant. Individual, community and societal interests and benefits must be balanced with the need to address public health concerns and objectives. It is important that access to data is as open as possible and as closed as necessary, to protect privacy and reduce the risk of data misuse (Research Data Alliance, 2020).

Efficient information and communication technology is relatively easily available. While this has improved the global capacity to implement systems to share data during pandemics, lack of harmonisation across these systems is a major limitation (Research Data Alliance, 2020). Nevertheless, the unprecedented spread of the SARS-CoV-2 virus triggered a rapid and massive research response with diverse outputs challenging interoperability. Implementing legal frameworks that promote sharing data across jurisdictions and sectors is key. Data custodianship/ownership, publication rights and arrangements, consent models, and permissions around sharing data and exemptions must be unambiguously delineated in emergency data-related legislation that is enacted during a pandemic (Research Data Alliance, 2020).

5.7   UPHOLDING PUBLICATION ETHICS WHILE RESPONDING TO THE DEMANDS OF PANDEMICS

There has been a phenomenal increase in publications during the COVID-19 pandemic, with manuscripts focused predominantly on issues around the novel virus. Observational research became a common phenomenon in intensive care medical journals (Citero, 2020). This period has also created some positives, which include open access to COVID-19 studies, enhanced collaboration, expedited REC approvals of new clinical studies, expedited governance and use of preprints on a larger scale (Glasziou, 2020). The flip side to these gains has been major ethical challenges at various levels; the research process and design, ethics review and journal publications. As stated by Glasziou, out of more than a thousand publications, only a few are scientifically sound to add to the body of knowledge. Using the hydroxychloroquine trial as an example, Glasziou illustrated that out of the 145 registered trials, 32 had a sample size of less than 100; 10 studies had no control group and 12 were non-randomised (Glasziou, 2020). Scientific validity, a critical element for ethical research (as discussed above) was highlighted by Emanuel in 2000 (Emanuel, 2000). However, it has become rapidly clear that during the COVID-19 pandemic, especially during the earlier days, scientific validity of the research, albeit published in peer-reviewed journals, was questionable. This may have occurred because the unprecedented nature of the outbreak led to researchers trying to do as much as they could to understand the disease. Hence, a flurry of observational studies as a consequence (Citero, 2020).

In order to mitigate against poor research being produced and subsequently published during pandemics, leading to the harm of communities at large, stakeholders need to interrogate what the fundamental issues are. Problems may arise in three areas: the research process, the research ethics approval process and the publication process. The first two have already been discussed earlier on in this chapter. The publication process needs to follow the Committee on Publication Ethics (COPE) Guidelines even though challenges have surfaced with the pandemic. Journals are committed to adhering to strict COPE guidelines and should not relax them because of the pandemic (Citero, 2020). A public health emergency does not justify lowering standards during any of the approval processes.

5.8   ETHICAL CONCERNS SPECIFIC TO RESEARCH ON VACCINES DURING PANDEMICS

The primary ethical requirement is to ensure that safe, effective and affordable vaccines are made available to all people in all countries during a pandemic. To this end, studies must comply with sound, scientific methodology. Despite the enormous pressure to develop an effective vaccine as soon as possible, the primacy of the safety and well-being of each trial participant and the quality of the research results should not be undermined by these time demands. In addition, regulators should not compromise the quality of their evaluations and follow-up in particular during the transition from research to industrial-scale production and distribution (UNESCO, 2021).

As vaccines get approved, issues with regard to the use of placebos emerge. Towards the end of the first year of the COVID-19 pandemic, phase 3 trials found some vaccines to be efficacious resulting in emergency use authorisation being granted by regulators (CBS News, 2020). A WHO ad hoc consultation determined that ongoing studies and those that were yet to start should use directly randomised comparisons against placebos in order to collect high-quality information and also address as many of the data requirements as possible. It was further stated that because vaccine supplies were limited, available vaccines were still investigational and public health recommendations to use those vaccines had not been made, it was ethically appropriate to continue blinded follow-up of participants that had received placebos in existing trials and to randomly assign new participants to vaccine or placebo (WHO, 2021). However, UNESCO, in its call for Global Vaccine Equity and Solidarity, rejected this stance by the WHO, asserting that it characterised a double-standard situation and that researchers would take advantage of the unequal distribution of vaccines to conduct trials in countries where there was no access to vaccines thereby exploiting disadvantaged populations (UNESCO, 2021).

In advance of a clinical trial, provisions must be made for post-trial access for all participants who still need an intervention identified as beneficial in the research (WMA, 2015; CIOMS, 2016). In the context of SARS-CoV-2 vaccine trials, this would entail unblinding participants at the end of the trial and offering all those in the placebo arm the vaccine if proven to be efficacious, in keeping with the principles of justice and reciprocity. As many of the participants could be young and healthy volunteers, it is recommended that they are given a choice to offer the vaccine to individuals at greater risk and in more immediate need of the intervention.

The COVID-19 pandemic has been witness to unconscionable vaccine nationalism (Yamey, 2021). Within four months of the WHO approving a COVID-19 vaccine for emergency use, one billion doses had been administered globally. This global milestone was an unprecedented scientific achievement as never before had so many in the world been vaccinated only sixteen months after a virus had been discovered. As of 27 April 2021, 7.3% of the world's population of 7.79 billion had received at least one dose. However, according to a number of scientists, 75% of the population globally would require to be vaccinated if the pandemic is to be contained. Moreover, while some may have celebrated this unparalleled success, what is stark is that as many as 75% of these doses had been administered in only ten countries, highlighting the huge global disparities between high-income countries (HICs) and low- and middle-income countries (LMICs). Furthermore, just 2% of the total doses had come to Africa (Kreier, 2021). The vaccine nationalism was possible because, through advanced purchase agreements, rich countries were able to secure many times more vaccines than required by their populations which, consequently, undermined global equitable access and solidarity. Most clinical trials for these vaccines were conducted globally in several countries, including LMICs. Given that research participants were enrolled from all these countries, and that they all contributed to the development of the vaccines, justice as in fairness would demand that all countries contributing to the research ought to be given a fair chance to access these interventions if proven efficacious at the end of the study. The principle of proportionality could facilitate the application of fairness with countries being given the opportunity to purchase the vaccines in line with the proportion of research participants enrolled.

With the emergence of rapidly spreading variants, the need to speed up the vaccine development process and to have as many alternatives as possible became clear. Discussion and debate ensued on the feasibility and ethics of human challenge trials. The WHO defines controlled human infection studies as research that involves the deliberate infection of healthy volunteers (WHO, 2020). These studies can be conducted substantially faster than vaccine field studies as far fewer participants will be required to provide estimates of safety and efficacy. In addition, the studies can be used to compare the efficacy of multiple vaccine candidates thereby selecting the most promising vaccines for larger studies. This type of research can also be used to study processes of infection and immunity from their inception and validate tests for immunity, identify correlates of immune protection and investigate the risks for transmission posed by infected individuals. Hence, the overall public health response to a pandemic could be significantly improved.

According to WHO, while research involving the deliberate infection of individuals may seem intuitively unethical, these studies could be ethically acceptable under certain conditions. They need to be carefully designed to minimise harms to participants and also to ensure that public trust in research is not undermined. In addition, particularly high standards will be required where healthy participants are exposed to relatively high risks; studies involve first-in-human interventions or high levels of uncertainty; and the context is such that public trust in research is particularly crucial, e.g. in public health emergencies caused by pandemics.

In the context of COVID-19, WHO present eight criteria that need to be satisfied for SARS-CoV-2 challenge studies:

- There must be strong scientific justification.
- The potential benefits must outweigh the risks.
- The studies should be informed by consultation and engagement with the public, relevant experts and policymakers.
- There should be close coordination between researchers, funders, regulators and policymakers.
- The sites selected should be where the research can be conducted to the highest scientific, clinical and ethical standards.
- Researchers need to ensure that participant selection criteria limit and minimise risk.
- A specialised independent committee of experts should review this research.
- Informed consent must be rigorous.

Concerns with regard to the ethics of human challenge trials in the context of the COVID-19 pandemic have been raised (Kahn, 2020).

- Typically there is a requirement that the disease for which a challenge is introduced either has rescue therapy available for those who become infected or the disease is self-limiting. Currently, with the SARS-CoV-2 infection, there is no rescue therapy.
- The acceleration argument is flawed in that comparative speed is an accepted scientific justification for human challenge studies, but its conventional application is to circumstances where conducting field studies would be prohibitively difficult as the target pathogen is rarely transmitted in the natural environment. Given that SARS-CoV-2 transmission has been so widespread, several vaccine trials were already underway early in the outbreak and with all the field studies that rapidly followed, the necessity and relative speed argument were less convincing.
- Ethically sound research mandates that the relationship between risks and potential benefits must be reasonable. However, with human challenge studies, uncertainties remain with regard to knowledge about infection and potential resulting COVID-19 illness because of the continuously evolving disease. Because of this uncertainty, adequate disclosure during the informed consent process may be almost impossible.

- Human challenge studies in the context of the SARS-CoV-2 outbreak also risk fuelling and potentially worsening public mistrust in scientific research especially as they do not meet the basic principles of research ethics and vaccine development.

5.9   CONCLUSION

The importance of research in the context of infectious disease outbreaks is underscored. This research must take into consideration the several ethical challenges that will inevitably emerge. The evolutionary nature of pandemics means that alternate research designs and methodologies will need to be utilised and the ethical issues specific to these designs will need to be recognised. Furthermore, appropriate study designs that ensure scientific validity and social responsiveness are critical. The voices of those most affected by the outbreak must be heard and incorporated into the planning and execution of the research. Regulatory and ethics review systems must be flexible. Community consultation and engagement are essential to building trust and legitimising research initiatives. Community and individual interests must be respected. There is an ethical obligation for research to build in strategies to address future pandemics.

5.10   SELF-ASSESSMENT QUESTIONS

1. What are the specific ethical principles requiring special attention during pandemics?
2. Name the four principles of the SAN Code of Research Ethics.

5.11   REFERENCES

Busta, E.R., Mancher, M. and Cuff, P.A., et al (Eds). 2017. Integrating clinical research into epidemic response: The Ebola Experience. National Academies of Sciences, Engineering, and Medicine; Health and Medicine Division; Board on Health Sciences Policy; Board on Global Health; Committee on Clinical Trials During the 2014–2015 Ebola Outbreak; Washington (DC): National Academies Press (US). Available at: https://www.ncbi.nlm.nih.gov/books/NBK441673/.

CBS News. 2020. UK approves emergency use of AstraZeneca COVID-19 Vaccine. Available at: https://www.cbsnews.com/news/covid-vaccine-oxford-astrazeneca-approved-uk-emergency-use/.

Citero, G., Bakker, J. and Brochard, L. 2020. Critical journals during the Covid-19 pandemic: challenges and responsibilities. *Intensive Care Med* 46, pp. 1521–1523. https://doi.org/10.1007/s00134-020-06155-7.

Council for International Organisations of Medical Sciences. 2016. International Ethical Guidelines for Health-Related Research Involving Humans. Available at: https://cioms.ch/wp-content/uploads/2017/01/WEB-CIOMS-Ethical Guidelines.pdf.

Dhai, A. 2019a. Guiding principles of ethical research. In *Health research ethics. Safeguarding the interests of research participants*. 1 ed. JUTA, Cape Town, pp. 60–83.

Dhai, A. 2019b. Understanding ethics with specific reference to health research. In *Health research ethics. Safeguarding the interests of research participants*. 1 ed. JUTA, Cape Town, pp. 3–30.

Dieckert, N. and Sugarman, J. 2005. Ethical goals of community consultation in research. *American Journal of Public Health* 95(7).

Douglas, H. 2010. Types of Community. In H. Anheier and S. Toepler (Eds). *International Encyclopedia of Civil Society*. New York: Springer, pp. 539–544.

Emanuel, J.E., Wendler, D. and Grady, C. 2000. What makes clinical research ethical? *JAMA* 283, pp. 2701–2711. doi:10.1001/jama.283.20.270.

Glasziou, P.P., Sanders, S. and Hofmann, T. 2020. Waste in covid-19 research. *BMJ* 369. 12 May. m1847. https://doi.org/10.1136/bmj.m1847. PMID: 32398241.

HPTN. 2020. Ethics Guidance for Research. Available at: https://www.hptn.org/sites/default/files/inline-files/HPTNEthicsGuidanceDocument_2.26.20.pdf.

Kahn, J.P., Henry, L.M., Mastroianni, A.C., Chen, W.H. and Macklin, R. 2020. Opinion: For now, it's unethical to use human challenge studies for SARS-CoV-2 vaccine development. *Proceedings of the National Academy of Sciences, USA* 117(46), pp. 28538–28542.

Kreier, F. 2021 'Unprecedented achievement': who received the first billion COVID vaccinations? *Nature News*, 29 April. Available at: https://www.nature.com/articles/d41586-021-01136-2.

Littler, K., Boon, W.M., Carson, G., Depoortere, E., Mathewson, S., Mietchen, D., Moorthy, V.S., O'Connor, D., Roth, C. and Segovia, C. 2017. Progress in promoting data sharing in public health emergencies Bull World Health Organ 95, p. 243. doi: http://dx.doi.org/10.2471/BLT.17.192096.

Mahomed, S. and Staunton, C. 2021. Ethico-legal analysis of international sample and data sharing for genomic research during COVID-19: A South African perspective. *BioLaw Journal* – Rivista di BioDiritto, Special Issue 1/2021. Available at: http://rivista.biodiritto.org/ojs/index.php?journal=biolaw& page= article&op=view&path%5B%5D=785&path%5B%5D=654.

Metz, T. and Gaie, J.B. 2010. The African ethic of Ubuntu/Botho: implications for research on morality. *Journal of Moral Education* 39(3), pp. 273–90.

Nuffield Council of Bioethics, 2020. Research in global health emergencies: ethical issues. Available at: https://www.nuffieldbioethics.org/publications/research-in-global-health-.emergencies.

O'Mathúna, D. and Siriwardhana, C. 2017. Research ethics and evidence for humanitarian health. *Lancet* 390, pp. 228–2229. Published Online, 8 June 2017. doi: http://dx.doi.org/10.1016/ S0140-6736(17)31276-X.

Okonta, P.I. 2014. Ethics of clinical trials in Nigeria. *Nigerian Medical Journal* 55(3), pp. 188–194.

Research Data Alliance COVID-19 Recommendations and Guidelines on Data Sharing, 30 June 2020. Available at: https://www.rd-alliance.org/system/files/ RDA%20COVID-19%20Recommendations%20and%20Guidelines%2C%20 30%20June%202020_Endorsed-Final_0.pdf.

Schroeder, D., Chatfield, K., Singh, M., Chennells, R., Herissone-Kelly, P. 2019. The San Code of Research Ethics. In *Equitable Research Partnerships. SpringerBriefs in Research and Innovation Governance*. Springer, Cham. Doi: dhttps://doi. org/10.1007/978-3-030-15745-6_7.

Seehawer, M.K. 2018. Decolonising research in a Sub-Saharan African context: Exploring Ubuntu as a foundation for research methodology, ethics and agenda. *International Journal of Social Research Methodology* 21(4), pp. 453–66.

Singh, J.A., Bandewarb, S.V.S. and Bukusi, E.A. 2020. The impact of the COVID-19 pandemic response on other health research. *Bull World Health Organ* 98, pp. 625–631. doi: http://dx.doi.org/10.2471/BLT.20.257485.

UNAIDS, AVAC. 2011. Good Participatory Practice. Guidelines for Biomedical HIV Prevention Trials. 2011. Available at: https://www.unaids.org/en/resources/ documents/2011/20110629_JC1853_GPP_Guidelines_2011%20OK.

UNESCO's Ethics Commissions' Call for Global Vaccine Equity and Solidarity. Available at: https://unesdoc.unesco.org/ark:/48223/pf0000375608.

United Nations Educational, Scientific and Cultural Organisation. 2020 UNESCO IBC & COMEST statement on COVID-19: Ethical considerations from a global perspective. Available at: https://en.unesco.org/inclusivepolicylab/e-teams/ ethical-considerations-covid-19-responses-and-recovery/documents/unesco-ibc-comest-statement.

Wellcome Trust. 2020. Sharing of data and findings relevant to the novel coronavirus (Covid-19) outbreak. Available at: https://wellcome.ac.uk/coronavirus-covid-19/ open-data.

WHO. 2020. Key criteria for the acceptability of COVID-19 human challenge studies. Available at: WHO-2019-nCoV-Ethics_criteria-2020.1-eng.pdf.

WHO. 2021. Ad hoc expert group on the next steps for COVID-19 vaccine evaluation. Placebo-controlled trials of COVID-19 vaccines–why we still need them. *New England Journal of Medicine* 384(2), p. e2.

World Medical Association. 2015. Declaration of Helsinki, art 34. Available at: https://www.wma.net/policies-post/wma-declaration-of-helsinki-ethical-principles-for-medical-research-involving-human-subjects/.

Yamey, G. 2021. No to vaccine nationalism. Available at: https://sanford.duke.edu/media/no-vaccine-nationalism.

CHAPTER 6

THE ROLE OF THE NEWS MEDIA DURING PANDEMICS

Mia Malan

6.1 INTRODUCTION

The news media has the power to make or break communication during public health crises; it can empower people with crucial, lifesaving information that holds governments accountable for the implementation of sound strategies, or it can disseminate incorrect facts which can potentially lower the uptake of health services and lead to loss of life.

But epidemics, particularly those with a sudden onset, such as Ebola and COVID-19, come with huge challenges: journalists with little understanding of medical science are forced to become health reporters overnight and report on complex, fast-moving research. This frequently results in the unintentional publication of misinformation in the form of confusing, contradictory stories, as the Ebola, COVID-19 and HIV epidemics have demonstrated.

The value of well-trained health journalists during such outbreaks is therefore enormous. But can the media industry afford to train – and maintain – specialist journalists?

Where personal communication was used in this chapter, permission was obtained from the respective individuals to use their comments.

6.2 OBJECTIVES

The objectives of this chapter are:
- To evaluate the role of the news media during pandemics by unpacking the public service role of journalists in disseminating accurate scientific information and holding governments accountable for the implementation of evidence-based responses.
- To discuss the ethical issues that reporters and editors should consider when covering pandemics, as well as the mental health impact on, and the support required for, media professionals who report on outbreaks for extended periods.

- To consider the ramifications of pandemics on the financial sustainability of news media – and their consequent ability to adequately cover sustained outbreaks, as well as the journalistic training needs that pandemics highlight.

These issues are addressed by appraising examples of news media coverage of the world's most recent pandemic, COVID-19, but also, to a lesser extent, reporting on the HIV and Ebola epidemics.

6.3   WHAT IS THE NEWS MEDIA AND WHAT DO PEOPLE WANT FROM IT?

For the purposes of this chapter, the news media is defined as the elements of mass media, such as newspapers, radio, television and online publications, that deliver news to the public.

'The word news, for most people, primarily means content produced by professional journalists from media organisations,' stated Rasmus Nielsen, the director of the Reuters Institute for the Study of Journalism at Oxford University, in an interview on 3 December 2020. Nielsen noted that there is something clear-cut about professional journalism. 'I would maintain a distinction between things that are simply novel and interesting and perhaps relevant [for instance, social media posts of influencers] and then things that are news reported by journalists to seek truth in reporting.'

Most people want simple, basic things from the news media (Newman et al, 2019): '[They want the news] to keep them up to date, help them understand what is going on and keep an eye on those in a position of power' (Kalogeropoulos and Fletcher, 2019). Many journalists and news media organisations would argue that they're already fulfilling these functions, but studies show there is still a significant gap to close in terms of public perception (Newman et al, 2019).

It was against the background of a decline in trust in the news media that the COVID-19 pandemic emerged.

Although research (Nielsen, Cherubini and Angi, 2020) shows that many independent news media organisations' audiences increased markedly between May and September 2020, the pandemic simultaneously had a devastating financial impact on an already financially constrained industry.

A survey among 165 media organisations found that respondents, particularly commercial media, on average expected a decline of between 20–30% drop in revenues for 2020. 'Such a drop would have dramatic consequences for the number of journalists employed, especially at the local level and in poorer communities and countries' (Nielsen, Cherubini and Angi, 2020).

6.4 THE NEWS MEDIA'S PUBLIC SERVICE ROLE IN DISSEMINATING ACCURATE SCIENTIFIC INFORMATION AND TO COUNTER FEAR

6.4.1 The 'Infodemics' Pandemics Create

Pandemics, particularly fast-moving outbreaks such as COVID-19 and the Ebola epidemic, are almost always accompanied by what the World Health Organisation calls massive 'infodemics': an overabundance of information – some accurate and some not – that makes it difficult for people to find trustworthy sources and reliable advice when they need it (World Health Organisation, 2020a).

What has made the COVID-19 infodemic worse than its predecessors is the fact that the coronavirus disease was the first pandemic in history in which technology and social media were being used on a massive scale to keep people informed. But the technology was simultaneously also enabling the amplification of incorrect, and potentially harmful, information (World Health Organisation, 2020b).

One of the most dangerous potential repercussions of the large-scale spread of misinformation is 'the prospect of audiences downgrading their trust in all information because they're finding it harder to discern facts from falsehoods, legitimate publications from fraudulent ones and hyper-partisan content from critical independent journalism' (Posetti and Matthews, 2020).

The result? The undermining of public health, the destabilisation of democratic processes (Posetti and Matthews, 2020) and endangering countries' ability to stop pandemics (World Health Organization, 2020).

6.4.2 The Science Communication Role of Journalists During Pandemics

The news media's enormously influential role in shaping public health responses and people's uptake of public health interventions is well recognised (Leask, Hooker and King, 2010). News media organisations – print, television, radio and internet – have an extraordinary reach as a communication mechanism (Gunther, 1998) and media houses have considerable power in setting agendas with regard to the issues we should be worried about and take action on and how we should think about them (McCombs and Shaw, 1972).

During pandemics, the media therefore has the potential ability to influence whether members of the public adhere to government regulations or public health measures and whether they embrace or reject science. A six-country survey of the Reuters Institute conducted during the first wave of COVID-19, for instance, found that people who used news organisations as a source of information about coronavirus had a statistically significant higher level of coronavirus knowledge (Nielsen et al, 2020).

But the news media's role as a partner in fighting a pandemic goes beyond 'putting facts on the table', stated Salim Abdool Karim, the co-chair of South Africa's scientific advisory committee on COVID-19, during an interview on 7 December 2020. 'It's about creating a consistent narrative that enables people to understand why things are happening the way they are.'

Reuters Institute research (Nielsen et al, 2020) found that the public wanted information [on protection measures, government measures and what the future holds] that is independently verified and assessed by someone who doesn't have a direct stake in the outcome of the pandemic. 'When somebody who has no expertise in the subject is given a platform, it has to be within the context that they have no expertise – and that has to be clarified,' stated Abdool Karim (Abdool Karim, 2020, personal communication, 7 December 2020).

Journalists' responsibility to provide context in their stories, Nielsen said, goes even beyond quoting credible sources – it's as important not to over-represent unscientific and potentially harmful minority views (Nielsen, 2020, personal communication, 3 December 2020).

For instance, Reuters Institute research (Nielsen et al, 2020) showed that only 2% of the United Kingdom public gave any credence to a COVID-related conspiracy theory that 5G mobile phone signals transmit the coronavirus or reduce our defences to it. 'But the issue received quite a lot of news coverage, creating the risk that people who are undecided about the theory would be drawn to it because of the news coverage' (Nielsen, 2020, personal communication, 3 December 2020).

Nielsen noted that the same argument could be applied to anti-vaxxers or politicians who were opposed to wearing masks for protection during COVID-19: 'When the views of small, dissident groups are overrepresented in the news, it can be harmful for public understanding of pandemic-related issues and also to public health in general – because it creates the impression that large numbers of people are opposed to evidence-based interventions when it's in fact a small minority' (Nielsen, 2020, personal communication, 3 December 2020).

6.4.3 The Challenges Pandemics Create for Reporters to Accurately Report on Data and Science

Slow-moving pandemics such as HIV make it possible for journalists to become specialists in a relevant field over time, but in the case of fast-moving viruses such as SARS-CoV-2, the virus that causes COVID-19, as well as the Ebola virus, the situation is entirely different. With COVID-19, political, sports and business reporters without any background in health journalism had to start reporting on complex, evolving pandemic science almost overnight. One survey, for instance, showed that only 4% of COVID-reporters were specialist health journalists (Selva, 2020a).

This situation created numerous caveats for uninformed reporting and consequent misinformation, especially because editors too, had no health reporting background. One of South Africa's foremost political and investigative journalists, the engagement editor of the *Daily Maverick*, Ferial Haffajee, explained: 'When I heard on the radio that Russia had come up with the world's first working vaccine, it wasn't really true at all, but my colleagues and I had initially thought it was news, because we didn't understand how clinical trials worked and that the vaccine had not been tested on nearly enough subjects to produce reliable results' (Haffajee, 2020).

Additionally, governments often get defensive during pandemics, limiting access to information to journalists, which makes it close to impossible to accurately report on the true extent of the outbreak and the impact of a country's pandemic response. In an International Centre for Journalists (ICFJ) survey conducted among 1 406 media professionals across 125 countries in May and June 2020, 28% of respondents reported that they were denied access to government representatives or other official sources and one out of five said they were excluded from government press conferences (Posetti, Bell and Brown, 2020).

In Kenya, these scenarios played out frequently during the first wave of COVID-19. Daily briefings by the health ministry were restricted to a very small number of media houses and 'big name' journalists who had a limited understanding of science. This resulted in the mainstream media 'appearing to "hide" the story, regurgitation of case numbers given by government without interpretation, and no explanation of where government's COVID-19 dedicated funds were going' (Sulcas, 2020).

COVID-19 also happened against the background of fast-tracked research, which was often published as preprint studies that bypassed the traditional peer-reviewed process during which results are vetted. This complicated journalists' reporting processes even further, because many did not have the skills to analyse whether study methodologies and results were credible, and, because of their lack of background in health reporting, the majority of media professionals did not have a contact list of scientists to ask for help. The research results of preprint studies were therefore often reported as the 'truth' when there was in fact great uncertainty about them.

Finally, pandemics present a dilemma to reporters, who operate within an industry that mostly simplifies complex issues to make them more understandable to audiences, in their attempts to communicate risk. 'Figuring out the right degree of alarm to sound [during a pandemic] is a basic problem for journalists,' *MSNBC* host Chris Hayes told the US online news publication, *Vox* in April 2020.

'In a fundamental, definitional way, news is bad at communicating risk... Telling you about a plane crash is new, but it doesn't convey the risk of flying – it overstates it, by giving it prominence. The same with local crime stories. Meanwhile, telling you about a pandemic that's about to overtake the country, kills tens of thousands of people and craters the economy is very hard to do when it hasn't happened yet, but there's a chance it could' (Kafka, 2020).

6.4.4   How Misinformation and Disinformation Spread During Pandemics

Misinformation, false information that is spread, regardless of whether there is intent to mislead (University of Washington, 2020), and disinformation, deliberately misleading or biased information such as manipulated narratives or propaganda (University of Washington, 2020), are rampant during 'infodemics'.

Four out of five of the media respondents in the ICFJ's survey reported that they encountered disinformation connected to COVID-19 at least once a week (Posetti, Bell and Brown, 2020).

'Disinformation purveyors seek out the most vulnerable aspects of the information ecosystem – from small [news] publications with poorly trained staff and limited resources, to those with weak defenses, suffering from complacency and niche, impressionable audiences,' ICFJ researchers Julie Posetti and Alice Matthews stated (Posetti and Matthews, 2020). 'That's why it's vital that editors, publishers and reporters are aware of the growing sophistication of disinformation tactics, including fraudulent sources, faux think tanks, inauthentic social media accounts, polluted datasets and fake publications.'

The consequences of pandemic disinformation can be deadly, particularly because many people find it hard to judge whether a message is true or false (Morosoli et al, 2020).

For instance, almost two decades into South Africa's HIV pandemic, during the late 1990s and early 2000s, the country's then-president, Thabo Mbeki, spread false information that antiretroviral drugs – which prevent HIV from replicating in infected people's bodies and as a result can lead to a life expectancy equal to that of non-infected people – were poisonous and did not work (Malan, 2003). Consequently, some private-sector patients who could afford the treatment (the government did not provide it in the public sector at the time), stopped taking their drugs and died, including Mbeki's own spokesperson (Mail & Guardian, 2000).

Another crucial example is that of an elderly man in the United States who died in March 2020 after the country's former president, Donald Trump, falsely promoted the drugs chloroquine and hydroxychloroquine as both a treatment and prevention of COVID-19. There was no solid scientific evidence that the medicines, which are ordinarily used for the treatment of lupus, malaria and rheumatoid arthritis, had any preventive or curative benefits pertaining to COVID-19. On the contrary, studies have shown that the drugs could be harmful to COVID-19 patients (Food and Drug Administration, 2020). However, when a man and his wife from Arizona heard the president endorsing the medication and announcing that he was using it himself, they decided to ingest a form of chloroquine that is used to treat parasites in fish, to protect themselves from contracting SARS-CoV-2, which then led to the man's death (Haelle, 2020).

Politicians such as Mbeki and Trump are not uncommon begetters of false news.

In the ICFJ's survey, media professionals identified politicians and elected officials (46%), as well as government agencies and their spokespeople (23%), as top sources of disinformation (Posetti, Bell and Brown, 2000).

At times journalists amplify such messages as well.

'There are some situations where parts of the news media end up being complicit with these problems, either by giving uncritical news coverage to unfounded and potentially harmful views or in the form of opinion columns and commentary from guests on broadcast shows who are not held to the same standards of fact-checking and verification as news reporters,' Rasmus Nielsen stated (Nielsen, 2020, personal communication, 3 December 2020).

For example, although large parts of the South African news media opposed Mbeki's HIV views during his presidency (Malan, 2006), several news publications and television programmes gave a platform to HIV denialists, who shared the president's views, by allowing them to publish guest columns or by quoting them without providing any accompanying information that their views were not supported by science (Malan, 2003).

Also, as COVID-19 ran its initial course in the United States, conservative, Republican-orientated media houses such as the television channel, *Fox News*, regularly reported uncritically on many of the unscientific falsehoods that Trump announced during press conferences or on social media. 'That apparatus simply provided an echo chamber and feedback loop for Trump's messaging, so that when Trump said he expected the virus to "miraculously" disappear, they said the same, and when he said it was time to take it seriously, they did the same. This did a deadly disservice to an enormous swath of the country, which takes its cues from those outlets' (Kafka, 2020).

However, many news organisations also responded proactively to counter false information about COVID-19 in their countries, including in the United States. The ICFJ's survey shows that 70% of US respondents said that their media outlets had created a specific COVID-19 disinformation beat and almost a third indicated that they were producing fact-checks and debunks and were using digital verification tools to expose false video, images and memes connected to COVID-19. Moreover, one out of five media professionals who participated in the survey reported that they had collaborated with other news organisations and non-governmental organisations to investigate COVID-19 disinformation and 12% said they had engaged their audiences in fact-checking or media literacy projects to combat the spread of false content (Posetti, Bell and Brown, 2020).

6.5 THE NEWS MEDIA'S ROLE IN HOLDING GOVERNMENTS ACCOUNTABLE FOR THE IMPLEMENTATION OF EVIDENCE-BASED POLICIES

Accountability journalism – investigative journalism that holds people and institutions responsible for their words and actions (Elizabeth, 2016) – is crucial during pandemics, because it helps to ensure that governments implement effective pandemic responses based on sound science. But this journalistic role becomes complicated when the science of a disease is still evolving. '[In the case of COVID-19], science is not [always] giving us the kind of unambiguous guidance that we can then use to take policymakers to task if they don't follow it,' said Edward Wasserman, professor and dean Emeritus of the Graduate School of Journalism at the University of California, Berkeley in a webinar about the role of the media in pandemics (Wasserman, 2020). Wasserman pointed out that in the United States, for instance, arguments about whether states should reopen the economy and schools, and the speed at which it should be done, were complicated by the fact that the science around it was not clear-cut, resulting in the media, and even scientists, being ambiguous about it.

Moreover, many governments withhold information from the news media during pandemics and misuse state of disaster laws which target disinformation to curb media freedom and limit reporters' ability to investigate state policies and budgets. In Eswatini, for example, the Swaziland Editors Forum reported that the country's state of emergency laws during COVID-19 'confined journalists to reproducing official statements in a copy and paste manner' and in Botswana and Zambia, restrictions were placed on the use of sources outside of government (Mawarire, 2020).

The ICFJ's survey revealed that one in ten media respondents said they had been publicly abused by a politician or elected official in the course of their work during the COVID-19 pandemic and 14% reported having been subjected to direct censorship. This situation is even more worrying in the light of close to half of the respondents reporting politicians and elected officials as sources of disinformation.

But there is some hope. Numerous studies have documented the significant role that South Africa's news media – mostly in collaboration with scientists and civil society – played in forcing the Mbeki government to make evidence-based treatment available in the public sector (Malan, 2005). 'Journalists took on an advocacy role, which I feel was appropriate, and formed exceptionally strong relationships with scientists and activists to fight for the implementation of policies based on sound science,' stated Ida Jooste, the global health journalism advisor of the media development organisation, Internews Network. 'And [mostly health] journalists are now benefiting from those relationships when reporting on COVID-19, because South Africa's HIV scientists have also become the country's COVID experts' (Jooste, 2020, personal communication, 3 December 2020).

6.6   WHAT ARE THE ETHICAL ISSUES JOURNALISTS SHOULD CONSIDER WHEN REPORTING ON PANDEMICS?

How journalists frame stories and the words they use to tell them directly impact on news consumers' understanding of a pandemic, the levels of panic they experience and how people with a disease are perceived and treated (Jooste, 2020, personal communication, 3 December 2020). 'Journalists therefore need to select the terms they use to report on a pandemic very carefully.'

Stigma and blame, Jooste stated, are two of the most common consequences of scientifically inaccurate and badly thought-through language use. 'Patient 0 or Patient 1 are two such examples. These terms create the impression that it's scientifically possible to determine the day on which a virus travelled to a country, when that person is really only the first diagnosed case. And the consequence of such "labels" often is that people blame Patient 0 or 1 for bringing the virus into their country and stigmatise them and their families.'

For instance, after the first case of COVID-19 in the South African township, Khayelitsha in Cape Town, was diagnosed, the person was rejected by her community. A family spokesperson told the *Cape Times*: 'Her pictures are all over social media as if she had done something wrong' (Siyo, 2020).

Jooste said, 'although not ideal [because the terminology still results in the labelling of people], terms such as "the first identified patient" or "the first diagnosed patient" would be better to use and would also be more scientifically accurate'.

How much alarm to sound is another rather complex ethical issue that journalists grapple with during outbreaks. 'How do we warn Americans about the full range of potential [COVID-19] risks in the world without ringing alarm bells so constantly that they'll tune us out?' the Washington, DC-based *Vox* media rightly asks.

Studies have shown that scare-mongering people can harm public health responses because fear and panic can stigmatise a disease to such an extent that people become too afraid to get tested or to seek care and remain in the community undetected (Person, 2004). Messages such as 'Ebola kills' or adjectives like 'deadly, horrific or catastrophic' are also subjective and can lead to unnecessary panic if used out of context. 'It is true that some people die [of Ebola or COVID-19].

But we don't call the traffic jams every day in every city "deadly traffic jams" even though somebody will die every day in traffic' (Tompkins, 2020).

Brian Stelter, *CNN's* media correspondent, told *Vox* that the solution to this issue comes down to balancing 'the need to not scare … [news consumers] prematurely with the need to scare them into action' (Kafka, 2020).

Whether to name patients or not can get equally tricky. On the one hand, experts argue, not naming patients makes journalists 'tacitly complicit in perpetuating the sense that to die of the virus [in this case SARS-CoV-2] is shameful and should be kept secret' (Davis, 2020). On the other hand, naming patients could result in them being harassed and stigmatised.

One possible solution to this, the South African Press Council points out in its COVID-19 guidelines, is to only release the names of patients if their families are in agreement or if the public interest overrides someone's right to privacy (Davis, 2020).

Lastly, news organisations need to be aware of the consequences of words that carry judgment. 'Referring to people living with HIV as innocent victims, which has often been used to describe HIV-positive children or people who have acquired HIV medically, wrongly implies that people infected in other ways are somehow deserving of a punishment' (UNAIDS, 2007). It is therefore preferable, according to the Joint United Nations Programme on HIV/AIDS, to consistently talk of 'people living with HIV' or 'children living with HIV'.

6.7   THE TRAINING, MENTAL HEALTH SUPPORT AND OTHER RESOURCE NEEDS OF JOURNALISTS DURING PANDEMICS

In the ICFJ's survey, media professionals identified the mental health impact of reporting on COVID-19 as the most common difficulty that they had to deal with, and needed support for. One in every seven respondents reported that they sought psychological support to help them deal with increased anxiety, exhaustion, burn-out and sleeping difficulties, but only a quarter of the total number of respondents said their employers offered them help with counselling (Posetti, Bell and Brown, 2020).

A Reuters Institute survey (Selva, 2020) produced similar results and found that the mental health impact on reporters was so severe, that about a quarter of respondents in countries such as South Africa, Kenya, Nigeria and Botswana had clinically significant anxiety compatible with the diagnosis of generalised anxiety disorder, and 11% reported prominent symptoms of post-traumatic stress disorder. The authors of the study concluded: 'There is a strong case to be made for making sure all journalists can access support of some sort of counselling, either through their newsrooms or through external organisations such as the DART Centre for Journalism and Trauma in New York.'

Another common need that editors and journalists identified in the ICFJ survey was training for journalists in advanced verification and fact-checking techniques, as well as medical reporting, to enable them 'to accomplish better quality journalism that also more effectively responds to the threat of disinformation'.

One innovative solution during COVID-19 was two 'Epidemiology 101' courses that the epidemiologist Madhu Pai offered to African and Indian journalists. Pai, who heads up the International TB Centre in Montreal, hosted the modules in collaboration with media organisations in India, Kenya and South Africa and the courses have also been made available online for free (Makou, 2020; Pai, 2020).

But Miguel Castro, a strategy lead at the Bill & Melinda Gates Foundation's Global Media Partnerships stated the solution to the lack of health reporting skills and decrease in the number of journalists the media industry can afford, might lie in increasingly outsourcing such reporting. Media organisations will have to find ways to report on complex health matters that don't involve hiring specialist journalists. So niche media-start-ups, in the form of centres of excellence that specialise in health reporting that provide the mainstream media with well-researched stories, might become the norm rather than the exception.

'For philanthropists to fund the salaries of health reporters at media houses, is simply not scalable or sustainable: how do you choose which ones to fund among the hundreds of thousands of news media organisations? Rather, donors such as us will continue to fund specialist health reporting units that can provide mainstream media houses with evidence-based stories, consistently and at scale. We will also continue to invest funds into fact-checking organisations that can increase the news media's capacity to counter health-related disinformation and set the record straight' (Castro, 2020, personal communication, 7 December 2020).

6.8   CONCLUSION

The politics of both news and pandemics, as well as the under-resourced environment that the media currently finds itself in, make reporting on pandemics complex and challenging. The result is therefore often a combination of clear, science-based reports and misinformation.

The fact that trust in the news media is at an all-time low globally further complicates the situation.

But pandemics also bring opportunities. For one, they speed up processes, and in the case of the news media, that means partnerships between scientists and journalists, as well as among media organisations themselves, have, at least during the COVID pandemic, moved considerably faster. Scientists have become faces as frequent as politicians on television and health journalists from specialist media start-ups are increasingly being used to augment the reporting of non-specialist journalists at mainstream news outlets.

How such partnerships are nurtured and maintained will, to a large extent, determine how prepared the media is to report on future pandemics, and what kind of role they'll play in subsequent health emergencies.

6.9 SELF-ASSESSMENT QUESTIONS

1. What does the public think of the news media's reporting on COVID-19?
2. Has the news media helped scientists to identify gaps in pandemic responses?

6.10 REFERENCES

Davis, R. 2020. Should SA media name those who die of Covid-19? *Daily Maverick*, 7 April. Available at: https://www.dailymaverick.co.za/article/2020-04-07-should-sa-media-name-those-who-die-of-covid-19/.

Food and Drug Administration (2020). FDA cautions against use of hydroxy-chloroquine or chloroquine for COVID-19 outside of the hospital setting or a clinical trial due to risk of heart rhythm problems. 1 July. Available at: https://www.fda.gov/drugs/drug-safety-and-availability/fda-cautions-against-use-hydroxychloroquine-or-chloroquine-covid-19-outside-hospital-setting-or.

Elizabeth, J. 2016. 7 characteristics of effective accountability journalists. *American Press Institute*, 20 December. Available at: https://www.americanpressinstitute.org/publications/reports/white-papers/characteristics-effective-accountability-journalists/.

Gunther, A.C. 1998. The persuasive press influence: effects of mass media on perceived public opinion. *Communication Research* 25(5), pp. 486–504. Available at: https://journals.sagepub.com/doi/10.1177/009365098025005002.

Haffajee, F. 2020. Journalism in the time of COVID. *16th African Investigative Journalism Conference*, University of the Witwatersrand, Johannesburg, 6–30 October. Available at: https://www.youtube.com/watch?feature=youtu.be&v=yu_BDm9IwmA&app=desktop.

Haelle, T. 2020. Man dead from taking chloroquine product after Trump touts drug for coronavirus. *Forbes*, 23 March. Available at: https://www.forbes.com/sites/tarahaelle/2020/03/23/man-dead-from-taking-chloroquine-after-trump-touts-drug-for-coronavirus/?sh=6c4ac71572e9.

Kafka, P. 2020. What went wrong with the media's coronavirus coverage? *Vox*, 13 April. Available at: https://www.vox.com/recode/2020/4/13/21214114/media-coronavirus-pandemic-coverage-cdc-should-you-wear-masks.

Leask, J., Hooker, C. and King, C. 2010. Media coverage of health issues and how to work more effectively with journalists: a qualitative study. *BMC Public Health*, 8 September. Available at: https://bmcpublichealth.biomedcentral.com/articles/10.1186/1471-2458-10-535.

Kalogeropoulos, A. and Fletcher, R. 2019. What do people think about the news media? *Reuters Institute for the Study of Journalism*. Available at: https://www.digitalnewsreport.org/survey/2019/what-do-people-think-about-the-news-media/#fn-9857-1.

Mail & Guardian. 2000. A prayer for the living, 3–9 November, p. 30.

Makou, G. 2020. Want to do a crash course in epidemiology? Here you go. *Bhekisisa Centre for Health Journalism*, 1 August. Available at: https://bhekisisa.org/resources-for-journalists/2020-08-01-want-to-do-a-crash-course-in-epidemiology-here-you-go/.

Malan, M. 2003. The scientific politics of HIV/AIDS: a media perspective. M.Phil dissertation, University of Stellenbosch, March. Available at: https://scholar.sun.ac.za/handle/10019.1/53684.

Malan, M. 2005. Quid pro quo: a journalistic look at NGO-media interaction in Africa. *The Brown Journal of World Affairs* 11(2). Available at: http://bjwa.brown.edu/11-2/quid-pro-quo-a-journalistic-look-at-ngo-media-interaction-in-africa/.

Malan, M. 2006. Exposing AIDS. Media's impact in South Africa. *Georgetown Journal of International Affairs*, Winter/Spring. Available at: https://www.jstor.org/stable/43133659?seq=1.

Mawarire, T. 2020. Things will never be the same again: COVID-19 effects on freedom of expression in Southern Africa. *Internews*, 2 December. Available at: https://internews.org/sites/default/files/2020-12/Internews_Effects_COVID-19_Freedom_of_Expression_Southern_Africa_2020-12.pdf.

McCombs, M. and Shaw, D. 1972. The agenda-setting function of mass media. *Public Opinion Quarterly* 36(2), pp. 176–187. Available at: https://academic.oup.com/poq/article-abstract/36/2/176/1853310?redirectedFrom=fulltext.

Mitchell, A. and Oliphant, J. 2020. Americans immersed in COVID-19 news; most think media are doing fairly well covering it. *Pew Research Centre*, 18 March. Available at: https://www.journalism.org/2020/03/18/americans-immersed-in-covid-19-news-most-think-media-are-doing-fairly-well-covering-it/.

Morosoli, S., Humprecht, E., Staender, A., Van Aelst, P. and Edder, F. 2020. Perceptions of disinformation, media coverage and government policy related to the coronavirus — survey findings from six western countries. *University of Zurich and University of Antwerp*, June. Available at: https://files.designer.hoststar.ch/62/5f/625fb1a1-868d-4ff3-a809-697b654426af.pdf.

Newman, N., Fletcher, R., Kalogeropoulos, A. and Nielsen, R. 2019. Reuters Institute Digital News Report 2019. *Reuters Institute for the Study of Journalism*, June. Available at: https://reutersinstitute.politics.ox.ac.uk/sites/default/files/inline-files/DNR_2019_FINAL.pdf.

Nielsen, R., Cherubini, F. and Angi, S. 2020. Few winners, many losers: The COVID-19 pandemic's dramatic and unequal impact on independent news media. *The Reuters Institute for the Study of Journalism*. Available at: https://reutersinstitute.politics.ox.ac.uk/sites/default/files/2020-11/Nielsen_et_al_COVID-19_Pandemics_Impact_on_Independent_News_Media_FINAL.pdf.

Nielsen, R., Fletcher, R., Newman, N., Brennan, J.S. and Howard, P.N. 2020. Navigating the "infodemic": how people in six countries access and rate news and information about coronavirus. *Reuters Institute for the Study of Journalism*, 15 April. Available at: https://reutersinstitute.politics.ox.ac.uk/infodemic-how-people-six-countries-access-and-rate-news-and-information-about-coronavirus.

Nielsen, R., Kalogeropoulos, A. and Fletcher, R. 2020. Most in the UK say news media have helped them respond to COVID-19, but a third say news coverage has made the crisis worse. *Reuters*, 25 August. Available at: https://reutersinstitute.politics.ox.ac.uk/most-uk-say-news-media-have-helped-them-respond-covid-19-third-say-news-coverage-has-made-crisis.

Pai, M. 2020. 'Journalists need to get it right: epidemiology training can help'. *Forbes*, 9 August. Available at: https://www.forbes.com/sites/madhukarpai/2020/08/09/journalists-need-to-get-it-right-epidemiology-training-can-help/?sh=3eabb5f466a2.

Person, B., Sy, F., Holton, K., Govert, B. and Liang, A. 2004. Fear and stigma: the epidemic within the SARS outbreak. *Journal of Emerging Infectious Diseases* 10(2), February. Available at: https://www.ncbi.nlm.nih.gov/pmc/articles/PMC3322940/.

Pew Research Centre. 2020. American news pathways project, 24 January. Available at: https://www.journalism.org/2020/01/24/election-news-pathways-project-frequently-asked-questions/.

Posetti, P. and Matthews, A. 2020. #CoveringCOVID: six recommendations for disinformation combat. *International Center for Journalists, Washington, DC*, 27 March. Available at: https://www.icfj.org/news/coveringcovid-six-recommendations-disinformation-combat.

Posetti, P., Bell, E. and Brown, P. 2020. Journalism and the Pandemic: a global snapshot of impacts. *International Center for Journalists*. Available at: https://www.icfj.org/sites/default/files/2020-10/Journalism%20and%20the%20Pandemic%20Project%20Report%201%202020_FINAL.pdf.

Selva, M. 2020. COVID-19 is hurting journalists' mental health. News outlets should help them now. *Reuters Institute for the Study of Journalism*, 17 July. Available at: https://reutersinstitute.politics.ox.ac.uk/risj-review/covid-19-hurting-journalists-mental-health-news-outlets-should-help-them-now.

Siyo, A. 2020. Khayelitsha COVID-19 patient, family "rejected by community". *IOL, Cape Times*, 31 March. Available at: https://www.iol.co.za/capetimes/news/khayelitsha-covid-19-patient-family-rejected-by-community-45812610.

Sulcas, A. 2020. HIV and Ebola's influence on science journalism in the age of COVID-19. *Internews*, 1 December. Available at: https://internews.org/story/hiv-and-ebolas-influence-science-journalism-age-covid-19.

Swartzberg, J. 2020. COVID-19 and the media: The role of journalism in a global pandemic. *Berkeley Conversations*, University of California, Berkeley. Available at: https://m.youtube.com/watch?feature=emb_logo&time_continue=5&v=H--oW2RXuXA.

Tomkins, A. 2020. How newsrooms can tone down their coronavirus coverage while still reporting responsibly. *Poynter*, 4 March. Available at: https://www.poynter.org/reporting-editing/2020/how-newsrooms-can-tone-down-their-coronavirus-coverage-while-still-reporting-responsibly/.

UNAIDS. 2007. Words are not neutral against HIV. 3 January. Available at: https://www.unaids.org/en/resources/presscentre/featurestories/2007/january/20070103featurestorywords.

University of Washington. 2020. News: Fake news, misinformation and disinformation. *Campus Library, UW Bothell and Cascadia College*, 26 October. Available at: https://guides.lib.uw.edu/c.php?g=345925&p=7772376.

Wasserman, E. 2020. COVID-19 and the media: The role of journalism in a global pandemic. *Berkeley Conversations*, University of California, Berkeley, 6 May. Available at: https://m.youtube.com/watch?feature=emb_logo&time_continue=5&v=H--oW2RXuXA.

World Health Organization. 2020a. Novel Coronavirus (2019-nCoV) Situation Report – 13. 2 February. Available at: https://www.who.int/docs/default-source/coronaviruse/situation-reports/20200202-sitrep-13-ncov-v3.pdf.

World Health Organization. 2020b. Managing the COVID-19 infodemic: promoting health behaviours and mitigating the harm from misinformation and disinformation. 23 September. Available at: https://www.who.int/news/item/23-09-2020-managing-the-covid-19-infodemic-promoting-healthy-behaviours-and-mitigating-the-harm-from-misinformation-and-disinformation.

CHAPTER 7

CORRUPTION, LEADERSHIP AND THE CORROSION OF THE PUBLIC HEALTH SYSTEM CAPABILITIES IN SOUTH AFRICA

Prof Alex van den Heever

7.1 INTRODUCTION

The available evidence strongly indicates that the South African health system is characterised by combinations of both stagnation and deterioration, with performance levels suggestive of significant capability weaknesses relative to peer countries (van den Heever, 2019). This chapter offers a review of the factors that potentially explain why this is so and attempts to identify where reforms are required to place the overall health system onto an improving trajectory. A central theme of this chapter is that the principal drivers of dysfunction are systemic and principally driven by how leadership within the system is compromised by conflicts of interest which give rise to corruption. Under these conditions, it is argued, it is not possible for the health system to institutionalise processes of continuous improvement.

7.2 OBJECTIVES

The objectives of this chapter are:
- First, to understand the features of organisational capability relevant to continuous improvement in the public health system in South Africa.
- Second, to review the capabilities of the South African public health system.
- Third, to examine corruption in the South African state and the public health system together with its influence on health system capabilities through its influence on leadership.
- Fourth, to identify strategic governance reforms necessary to set the public health system on a continuous improvement pathway.

7.3   IMPROVING HEALTH SYSTEMS

Complex problems faced by society benefit from well-functioning public systems supported by effective leadership and technical expertise. Public systems, which are goal-oriented interconnected networks of people and organisations, are best suited to the achievement of weighty goals that require ongoing attention. A failure to achieve these goals, while potentially attributable to individual performance failures of various forms, when widespread would suggest weaknesses at the level of the system. The capabilities of a health system can be tested both by how it responds to rapidly developing health crises as well as by long-standing health needs.

All pandemics severely test health systems, but not all pandemics are the same; they may therefore test the system in different ways. Fast-moving pandemics resulting from airborne transmission require rapid responses, where even well-functioning health systems may lack the capabilities for a swift and efficient response.

However, slow-moving pandemics, such as AIDS and tuberculosis, are complicated by socioeconomic determinants of health compounded by extremely complex networks of human behaviour driving ongoing transmission. Whether faced with acute and novel crises or long-standing healthcare needs, resource allocation decisions need to be made across a wide range of prevention and treatment options. When facing a fast-moving pandemic, certain prevention options may, however, be off the table for quite some time – such as test and trace vaccines – placing an immediate strain on treatment options, which may also be unprepared in the case of a new disease. Regardless of how ineffective treatments may be, acute clinical settings may be severely impacted until such time as a successful combination of prevention and treatment can be institutionalised. While a well-functioning health system may initially fail to respond effectively to a complex health crisis, it will be able to address relatively straightforward long-standing and predictable health needs. This is achieved through incremental improvements in allocative efficiencies, where interventions are efficiently distributed between prevention and treatment over time through effective decision-making. In this way, more cost-effective interventions should replace less cost-effective interventions, constantly improving the performance of the health system (Chandra and Staiger, 2020; Paulden, McCabe and Karnon, 2014).

By way of contrast, poorly-functioning systems will not cope well with either complex or straightforward health needs. In such a system, cost-ineffective interventions are not progressively replaced, leading to poor outcomes for the resources allocated.

Given the budget constraints in all health systems, ensuring that effective interventions prevail over ineffective ones relies on processes of strategic decision-making that can make these technical distinctions and successfully execute processes to operationalise them. For this to occur, four features of a health system must be in place. First, it must be in a position to measure performance effectively. Second, competent processes of deliberation need to be in place to interrogate performance measures technically and through processes of engagement and consultation. Third, strategic management must be able to make informed decisions arising from the processes of deliberation. Fourth, the execution of decisions throughout a health system must occur allowing for flexibility, feedback and learning. Without these four elements operating effectively, even if not perfectly, complex health systems will not possess the dynamic capabilities to adapt to health needs on an ongoing basis.

7.4   UNDERSTANDING ORGANISATIONAL CAPABILITIES

In recent years, references to the 'capable state' have emerged in South Africa, largely flowing from official reports which placed a high priority on its achievement (National Planning Commission, 2011). Understanding capability regarding both the state generally and those aspects of the state that address the health system is self-evidently necessary for its achievement. Despite its prominence, at least in name, within the National Development Plan 2030, very little has happened to understand the concept in practical terms and to initiate strategies for its achievement.

The strategic management literature for both the public and the private sectors is increasingly adopting a dynamic capability approach to ensure organisational responsiveness to fast-changing conditions (Piening, 2013). Within the private sector, dynamic capabilities are used to maintain competitive advantages central to firm survival. While public sectors arguably face greater complexity in achieving public value in uncertain conditions, the public sector organisations are not necessarily threatened with extinction by competitors. The pressure to adapt is thus diminished relative to the private sector, despite facing a greater need for adaptability and innovation. When applied to public sector organisations, the dynamic capabilities approach is not focused on expanded markets or higher profits but on organisational performance in the achievement of public value (Pablo, Reay, Dewald and Casebeer, 2007).

Dynamic capabilities are usefully defined as an organisation's 'ability to integrate, build, and reconfigure internal and external competencies to address a rapidly changing environment' (Teece, Pisano and Shuen, 1997 p. 516). A related definition suggests that dynamic capabilities 'can be described as bundles of interrelated routines, which, shaped by path dependency, enable an organization to renew its operational capabilities in pursuit of improved performance' (Piening, 2013 p. 216).

The ability to hone in on those features that need to change revolves around accelerated organisational learning and institutionalised systems of feedback to management sufficient to enable revisions to strategy and execution. Learning is understood as a non-linear dynamic process which results from a combination of experimentation and repetition fully endorsed by the organisation (Pablo et al, 2007).

However, as restructuring is costly, organisations need to minimise low-value and maximise high-value change. This requires that organisations are able to timeously evaluate and execute needed and useful change to continuously improve value.

As organisational capabilities are embedded in the resources, assets, routines, values and associated cultural orientations, change is not straightforward. However, whereas for-profit private sector organisations invest in dynamic capabilities with specialised personnel with full-time commitments to their role changes, public organisations often use ad hoc project teams with part-time teams to adopt externally- rather than internally-developed innovations (Piening, 2013). Therefore, public sector organisations are generally less likely to effectively invest in the development of dynamic capabilities.

Central to capability acquisition and retention is the role of leadership in strategic management. Within a public sector, this occurs both at the level of the authorising framework, which references the executive of government or the political office bearers, and at the top management structures responsible for executing organisational strategies and therefore important to an organisation's operational capacity (Bryson, Crosby and Bloomberg, 2014). Traditional models of leadership based on power and authority are now regarded as a poor fit for modern governance in public sector settings, with a strong shift away from the inefficiencies and innovation-eroding top-down hierarchical approaches (Denhardt and Denhardt, 2011).

Instead, official authority is used strategically to decentralise processes of strategy development and execution to fully engage the technical knowledge of an entire organisation and to unlock innovation that would otherwise be ignored or discouraged (Crosby, Hart and Torfing, 2017).

The leadership role emphasises process management and focuses on the organisation's public value mission and mandate. The authority available to leadership is central to maintaining and adapting the strategic structures of an organisation, such as its managerial organisation, control processes and systems (reporting, performance review, budgets) as well as motivating arrangements to ensure organisational innovation, learning and adaptability (Ayres, 2017, 2019; Bryson et al, 2014; Crosby et al, 2017).

A central feature of dynamic capability is the availability within the organisation of highly-skilled personnel (Crespi, Fernández-Arias and Stein, 2014). This includes staff with specialised knowledge relevant to the organisation's mandate as well as professional staff central to the development, maintenance and continuous adaptation of routine processes of management and control. The retention of these skills for long periods within an organisation is also important to capture the undocumented institutional learnings and capabilities that can only emerge over time. Highly-skilled leaders are also necessary for enhancing the integrity of managerial processes and building relationships of trust at decentralised levels (needed for innovation and learning) within an organisation (Ayres, 2017).

The political executive, or the authorising environment, also has a central role to play in addressing the political aspects of engaging across government. Leadership weaknesses at this level compromise an organisation's ability to resolve standard problems associated with overlapping missions and mandates within public sectors. Without this capability, operational managers will be unable to establish the multi-agency processes necessary for holistic problem-solving, strategising and strategy execution (Crespi et al, 2014).

Avoiding capture is vital to the integrity of all aspects of any public agency's public value mandate and mission. An agency can be captured by the executive and/or the political parties and patronage networks that influence political parties and bureaucratic structures directly responsible for the administration of an agency and programme beneficiaries. A vital measure to mitigate the risk of capture and to institutionalise good appointments at the top management level involves the implementation of corporate governance in executing agencies of government (Crespi et al, 2014).

It is through such structures that it is possible to minimise all forms of capture, through the careful design of a corporate governance regime which will be different depending on the agency's context. The board would include directors that reflect a mix of technical skills (scientists, lawyers, accountants), stakeholder participation and beneficiary participation which would diminish informational asymmetries, ensure close supervision of senior managers and aggregate societal interests. Corporate governance arrangements also avoid the potential for capture through strategic appointments into the agency or organisation. The diversity of board appointments helps avoid the potential for malicious forms of coordinated conduct.

To avoid the capture of the board itself, the processes of nomination, appointment and removal should be diversified, with only a minority of appointments ever permissible by members of the executive of government.

The directors also require an accountability framework which can address material failures in performance (including inadequate commitment), misconduct and failures to meet and retain their fit and proper status. Diversifying who can remove board members (for instance, by expressly stating parties who can be regarded as aggrieved) on objective grounds is also important.

Limiting the removal of either board members or senior executives to political processes, such as through legislatures or the executive, reduces the likelihood that such decisions will be based on objective criteria and enhances the opportunities for agency capture. Instead, partisan political motivations driven by patronage will be given the space to operate and grow over time (this is indicated in the Public Protector's report into state capture: Public Protector, 2016).

Overall, therefore, dynamic organisational capabilities that enable adaption to rapidly-changing complex contexts are achieved through institutionalising skilled leadership, well-governed corporate governance arrangements, a decentralised approach to strategy development and execution, and the employment and effective deployment of highly-skilled staff. Decentralisation involves a dispersion of the traditional command and control authorities (strategies and execution) of senior management to a wider range of managers to enable innovation through organisational experimentation and learning. By way of contrast, the retention of traditional command and control approaches to public sector strategy development and implementation reduces their capacity for innovation through learning and exposes them to capture by a variety of interests detrimental to public value discovery and achievement.

7.5   CAPABILITIES IN THE SOUTH AFRICAN PUBLIC HEALTH SYSTEM

A review of the South African public health system in 2019 examined its preparedness for epidemics (van den Heever, 2019). Due to the absence of more specific performance information, three proxy indicators were applied by province.

- The first involved comparing provincial performance using facility-based maternal mortality ratios as an indicator of clinical governance.
- The second examined public domain information on Office of Health Standards Compliance (OHSC) quality assurance assessments for hospitals. Beds-in-use information by hospital was used to generate a composite provincial indicator.
- The third examined Auditor-General of South Africa (AGSA) information on irregular expenditure at a provincial level as a proxy measure for provincial health system capabilities. This was assumed reasonable given that health departments are generally the largest provincial department and

that province-wide performance is a general indicator of the performance of all provincial departments. It was however also noted by the AGSA that health departments were the worst-performing of all provincial departments in general (AGSA, 2018).

Using the maternal mortality ratio (MMR) as an indicator, the following was suggested:

- First, South Africa has a poorly-performing public sector, which cannot be explained purely by the resources allocated to it as countries at a similar level of development significantly outperform South Africa and all the provinces.
- Second, the consistent differences in performance between the Western Cape and other provinces suggest that outcomes are the result of systemic factors that influence how the services are managed.
- Third, when the two provinces of Gauteng and Western Cape were compared, both of which face near-identical social, economic and demographic challenges, the structural differences in performance can only be explained by other factors – such as management capabilities.

Using the OHSC reviews, the following was found:

- The OHSC appears to be a valid indicator of managerial capability within the provincial hospital services. However, it demonstrates a weakness in some provinces where they may have sufficient managerial capacity to achieve better scores on the OHSC indicator while still not being able to achieve the more difficult objective of better health outcomes (indicated by the MMR).

Using the AGSA's reports, the following was found:

- The AGSA's findings with respect to both provincial governments as a whole and health expenditure are consistent with the view that the public health system is in crisis.
- Consistent with the MMR and OHSC indicators, the Western Cape stands out as a relatively well-performing outlier, with the other provinces all performing poorly.

The analysis finds therefore that all three sets of indicators support a finding that the public health system is generally poorly managed and operating below its potential. In the form of facility-based MMRs, the health outcome indicator directly implicates the health services rather than wider socio-economic factors as the source of higher-than-normal mortality. Countries of a similar level of development to South Africa and with comparable or lower levels of fiscal support for public health services achieve better MMR results (also see (Development Bank of South Africa, 2008 pp. 16–17)). There is no evidence to suggest that South Africa's public health services are systematically improving. Furthermore, there are publicly-expressed concerns that the health system is in crisis and calls for serious intervention from both a governance and finance perspective (van den Heever, 2019).

Of relevance to the provincial health system, the AGSA notes specifically that '[t]he financial health of provincial departments of health and education needs urgent intervention to prevent the collapse of these key service delivery departments. In comparison with the other departments, these sectors (particularly the health sector) are in a bad state' (AGSA, 2018 p. 76).

These findings point to performance failures that are systematic in nature, as eight out of nine provinces demonstrate broadly similar capability findings, with the Western Cape a clear outlier. This suggests that there are common features driving capability weaknesses in eight provinces.

7.6   CORRUPTION IN THE PUBLIC HEALTH SYSTEM

Corruption could be regarded as a particularly pernicious form of performance failure, as it involves a fundamental deviation from the mission of public sector organisations, which is to consistently strive to achieve public value. The prevalence of corruption both in the state as a whole and within the public health system is substantial (Davis, 2021) and is now increasingly raised as relevant to an understanding of overall performance weaknesses (Rispel, De Jager and Fonn, 2015; South African Lancet Commission, 2018).

Irregular expenditure levels and the failure to follow up findings made by the AGSA are suggestive of systemic corruption. All provinces except the Western Cape have extraordinary levels of irregular expenditure: Gauteng R6.4 billion (5.9% of the budget), Mpumalanga R2.2 billion (5.3% of the budget), Northern Cape R1 billion (6.7% of the budget), Eastern Cape R0.86 billion (1.2% of the budget), Free State R3.9 billion (11.9% of the budget), KwaZulu-Natal R9.9 billion (9.0% of the budget), North West R3 billion (8.2% of the budget), and Limpopo R2.5 billion (4.1% of the budget) and the Western Cape R44 million (0.1% of the budget) (AGSA, 2018).

In the most recent AGSA report, the Gauteng Department of Health (GDOH) is identified as having the second-largest accumulated balance of irregular expenditure of R13.6 billion as identified in 2018/19, none of which (0%) was addressed in 2019/20. This is a remarkable finding, and suggests that either the GDOH lacks the capability to follow up irregular expenditure or it does not wish to do so (and does not fear the consequences).

The extensive corruption noted in the COVID-19 relief efforts (Muvunyi, 2020) clearly demonstrates that corruption is widespread and reflected in the culture of provincial and national government. Despite extensive reporting of corruption within the health sector and more broadly within the state, no members of the executive have to date been prosecuted, with the principal political party (the African National Congress or ANC) implicated in the corruption reluctant to take any substantive action against the growing number of senior politicians involved. The relationship between performance failures, levels of corruption and the failure to hold senior members of the executive to account is self-evident.

7.7   CORRUPTION CAUSES AND THE IMPLICATIONS FOR PERFORMANCE

As corruption is manifest, widespread and apparently deeply rooted in South Africa's state structures at all levels of government, there is a need to understand the conditions that have led to this situation. This section therefore offers a reasoned narrative of the probable structural causes of corruption and performance failures in the public health system. As corruption is widespread, the causes lie outside of the health system and are reflected in all the organs of state.

First, the form of corruption dominating South Africa's public sector and public health system needs to be identified. In this regard, two basic forms of corruption should be distinguished. The first takes the form of petty corruption that expressly deviates from the rules and norms of an organisation and its senior management and authorising environment, which is referred to here as 'bottom-up corruption'. The second and far more pernicious form arises from complete organisational capture and involves corruption permitted by those in a position to exercise state authority – or 'top-down corruption'.

This latter form has been labelled 'state capture' following the 2016 report of the Public Protector (Public Protector, 2016). Based on financial estimates flowing from the Judicial Commission of Inquiry into Allegations of State Capture, approximately R49.2 billion can be related just to the activities they are investigating (Davis, 2021).

This Commission, which to date has not issued a report, together with the Nugent Commission (Nugent, 2018), which identified the strategic capture of the South African Revenue Service (SARS) through the powers exercised by the President of South Africa, reflects what appears to be a general modus operandi in relation to the capture of all public sector organisations, including those within the health sector. This involves the coordinated deployment of people into the leadership teams of organs of state. Once in place, they replace the full executive team from within. At this point, all strategic aspects of the organisation, including procurement and further employment within the organisation, are under the total control of the corrupt leadership team.

Second, organisational capture within the public sector is enabled through the considerable discretion that members of the executive have at all levels of government to appoint the leadership team into agencies, administrations and public services, such as public health services. This includes all regulators responsible for private sector regulation, including, for instance, the OHSC which must evaluate public services for quality and is earmarked to license all private health facilities that will be permitted to contract with the National Health Insurance Fund (National Department of Health, 2017).

The present governing party, the ANC, has also been found to determine appointments for all parts of government through a deployment committee – generally referred to as 'cadre deployment' (Paton, 2021). In this way, a private organisation, a political party, is able to coordinate strategic appointments into all parts of the state while excluding appropriate candidates based on merit.

When appointments by the executive are combined with the process of political deployment, substantial discretion is provided to hidden actors to strategically capture organisations and thereby to bypass the accountability processes of government. All processes of procurement, licensing as well as public and private sector regulation, police investigation and associated law enforcement, and public prosecution can then be aligned with a malign strategic goal by a relatively small and invisible group of actors. The resulting impunity from prosecution emboldens continued and escalating corruption, resulting in the rapid hollowing out of state organisations.

Third, South Africa's version of democratic governance provides for a legislative branch that is intended to be independent of the executive and judicial branches of government. While the judicial branch appears to be independent for now, the legislative and executive branches are connected via structures of political party control.

Coordination of both branches effectively occurs through party structures which can discipline any member of Parliament who chooses to properly execute their constitutional role of supervision over the executive. Where membership is removed by the party, members of the legislature must resign. While it is technically possible to challenge the lawfulness of such a removal in the courts, it is unlikely that many will risk an expensive court entanglement.

The conflict of interest established by the current proportional representation system, as presently practised in South Africa, therefore successfully eliminates the legislative branch as an independent supervisor of the executive branch and strengthens the strategic coordination potential of unaccountable political party structures.

Fourth, it can be argued that electoral politics offers final arbitration on the misconduct of political parties. Elections are, however, a relatively blunt instrument of accountability where misconduct and poor performance can be obfuscated in political contests, with much riding on the maintenance of independent institutions of civil society and the media.

State capture, however, offers the opportunity to interfere with the independence of election administrations and vote-counting. While this may take some time, once the other organisations of government accountability have been captured, there is little to protect the integrity of elections or the independent voices of civil society. While South Africa may not yet be at this point, it remains a contingent risk that is very much alive.

An interaction between electoral politics and corruption also occurs where election funds are raised through, inter alia, tenders allocated to coincide with elections. This can involve in-party elections and access to party lists as well as general elections. It is possible that the increased service delivery just prior to elections has more to do with party fundraising and patronage (e.g. payoffs to access party lists) than with attracting popular support.

Fifth, once state organisations have been captured, their public mandates become secondary and performance in the public interest is no longer pursued as a strategic objective. When combined with the highly-centralised top-down hierarchies of public sector administrations and agencies, the potential for the achievement of dynamic capabilities disappears. Under these conditions, the organisations also cease to solve basic public value problems as their capabilities are eroded.

It is probable under these circumstances that innovation is penalised rather than rewarded, and highly-skilled staff depart the public sector as senior management becomes exclusively populated by political appointments lacking in the incentives to pursue public value. The skilled staff that remain will largely carry the burden of the substantive operational responsibilities while lacking the authority to influence and execute innovative strategies.

Sixth, the mismatch between the resulting weakened capabilities and the context-related complexity of health systems exacerbates the failures of health systems. As the fragility of the health system increases, the frequency of systems failures increases. With each increase, highly-skilled personnel exit, driving a new cycle of fragility. Within the South African context, it is not unreasonable to conclude that a cycle of ever-increasing fragility is in play that cannot be addressed adequately with additional resourcing, as the capability to efficiently deploy resources is compromised.

Seventh, while it could be argued that the capability failures of the state that plague the health system are artefacts of a single administration of the governing party, this is not supported by the evidence. The weaknesses in the state that opened the door to top-down (or state) capture were established in 1994 and have apparently gathered momentum over time.

The rapidity with which corruption in COVID-19 procurement occurred, as reflected in the report of the Special Investigate Unit (SIU) (Special Investigative Unit, 2021), demonstrates a state that is primed for corruption. While it could be argued that the activation of the SIU to tackle this corruption is indicative of a change, it is too early to tell whether this is merely addressing some bottom-up corruption carried out by an out-of-favour faction of the governing party, or authentic action to counter top-down corruption. The retention of the structural features that enable top-down corruption therefore remains a contingent risk that can be exploited at any moment in time.

7.8   ARRESTING THE NEGATIVE CYCLE

It is not clear that the capabilities of the health system can be addressed separately from the wider issues of top-down capture prevalent throughout the state. This section nevertheless highlights the features of the health system that need to be considered to address corruption and thereby the capabilities of the health system.

First, a clear separation needs to be institutionalised between the public health administrations and the executive of government. This should apply to all agencies of the health system.

Second, the corporate governance arrangements of key agencies, regulators and health service functions should be modified to establish independent supervisory boards and councils. These boards and councils should appoint and remove the senior executives of the organisations they oversee, approve their strategies and oversee the execution of their strategies. The boards should not be appointed by any part of the executive and their membership should include appropriate skills and aggregate the interests of the served population and relevant stakeholders.

Third, health service delivery should be decentralised, with autonomy allocated to the executive management to carry out their operations in accordance with strategic parameters drawn up by provincial departments or regional authorities and supervised by the relevant boards. This is required to institutionalise the emergence of dynamic capabilities within public health services.

Fourth, the authority to plan and execute regional strategies should be allocated to autonomous regional authorities in order to facilitate the emergence of dynamic capabilities in strategy formation and execution at the level of the region.

Finally, this framework can be established through a combination of legislative reforms at the national level of government, thereby ensuring a degree of national uniformity, and at the provincial level where local experimentation and innovation can inform context-specific strategies.

In this approach, the top-down institutional interventions that establish the governance superstructure of the health system should lock out opportunities for top-down corruption through structurally separating the executive of government from public administrations and agencies. This framework also allows for the localised or bottom-up development of institutional arrangements that encourage leadership and dynamic capabilities in pursuit of clear public sector missions (or public value).

7.9 CONCLUSION

This chapter evaluated the state of corruption in both the South African state and the public health system, its structural roots and its implications for strategic leadership as well as organisational and systems capability. It did this by examining the central elements needed for the achievement of dynamic capabilities in public sector organisations and public health systems.

The analysis suggests that the public health system reflects significant capability weakness and is at risk of increasing cycles of fragility which could see even current capabilities deteriorate further. This fragility is caused principally by the failure of the state to separate party and state, combined with a top-down hierarchical approach to public administration.

The party-political conflicts of interest contaminate the integrity of leadership in all public sector organisations, corrupting their strategy formation and execution, while the centralisation smothers innovation as well as organisational and systems learning.

Turning around the performance of the public health system will require inverting many of the current institutional arrangements.

First, the executive (and, by association, party-political structures) must be separated from public administrations, agencies and services.

Second, independent supervisory corporate governance arrangements must be introduced for key agencies, services and regional authorities. Supervisory boards and councils must have the powers to appoint and remove the relevant key executives at the management level.

Third, substantial autonomy must be allocated to key agencies, services and regional authorities to formulate and execute strategies subject to national and provincial strategic direction. This would be consistent with a general approach to decentralise decision-making as far as possible.

Fourth, the overriding governance framework should be established in national legislation, which would, inter alia, lock out opportunities for top-down capture throughout the health system.

As a strategic approach, this framework would enable bottom-up innovation through decentralisation while removing the risk of top-down capture by separating the executive from operational decision-making together with a corporate governance framework that allows for localised and more immediate supervision of decentralised functions.

7.10 SELF-ASSESSMENT QUESTIONS

1. What role does leadership play in the achievement of dynamic capabilities in the public health system?
2. What features of the dynamic capabilities approach generate continuous improvement in public sector organisations?

7.11 REFERENCES

Auditor-General of South Africa. 2018. *Consolidated general report on national and provincial audit outcomes: PFMA 2017–18*. Pretoria: Auditor-General of South Africa.

Ayres, S. 2017. Assessing the impact of informal governance on political innovation. *Public Management Review* 19(1), pp. 90–107. doi:10.1080/14719037.2016.1200665.

Ayres, S. 2019. How can network leaders promote public value through soft metagovernance? *Public Administration* 97(2), pp. 279–295. doi:https://doi.org/10.1111/padm.12555.

Bryson, J.M., Crosby, B.C. and Bloomberg, L. 2014. Public Value Governance: Moving beyond traditional public administration and the new public management. *Public Administration Review* 74(4), pp. 445–456.

Chandra, A. and Staiger, D.O. 2020. Identifying sources of inefficiency in healthcare. *The Quarterly Journal of Economics* 135(2), pp. 785–843. doi:10.1093/qje/qjz040.

Crespi, G., Fernández-Arias, E. and Stein, E. 2014. The Hard Part: Building public sector capabilities. In G. Crespi, E. Fernández-Arias and E. Stein (Eds) *Rethinking Productive Development: Sound Policies and Institutions for Economic Transformation*. New York: Palgrave Macmillan US, pp. 321–358.

Crosby, B.C., Hart, P. and Torfing, J. 2017. Public value creation through collaborative innovation. *Public Management Review* 19(5), pp. 655–669. doi:10.1080/14719037.2016.1192165.

Davis, R. 2021. The total(ish) cost of the Guptas' State Capture: R49,157,323,233.68, Analysis. *Daily Maverick*, 24 May. Available at: https://www.dailymaverick.co.za/article/2021-05-24-the-totalish-cost-of-the-guptas-state-capture-r49157323233-68/?utm_source=top_reads_widget.

Denhardt, J.V. and Denhardt, R.B. 2011. Leadership. In M Bevir (Ed) *The Sage Handbook of Governance*. Los Angeles/London/New Delhi/Singapore/Washington DC: Sage, pp. 419-435.

Muvunyi, F. 2020. South Africa's double blow: Corruption and the coronavirus. *Deutsche Welle*. Available at: https://www.dw.com/en/south-africas-double-blow-corruption-and-the-coronavirus/a-54423065.

National Department of Health. 2017. White Paper: Towards a national health insurance policy. Pretoria: Government Gazette.

National Planning Commission. 2011. National Development Plan 2030, our future, make it work (978-0-621-41180-5).

Nugent, R. 2018. Commission of Inquiry into Tax Administration and Governance by SARS.

Pablo, A.L., Reay, T., Dewald, J.R. and Casebeer, A.L. 2007. Identifying, enabling and managing dynamic capabilities in the public sector. *Journal of Management Studies*, 44(5), pp. 687–708. doi:https://doi.org/10.1111/j.1467-6486.2006.00675.x.

Paton, C. 2021. Cyril Ramaphosa defends ANC cadre deployment. *Business Day*, 28 April. Available at: https://www.businesslive.co.za/bd/national/2021-04-28-cyril-ramaphosa-defends-anc-cadre-deployment/.

Paulden, M., McCabe, C. and Karnon, J. 2014. Achieving allocative efficiency in healthcare: Nice in theory, not so nice in practice? *PharmacoEconomics* 32(4), pp. 315–318. doi:10.1007/s40273-014-0146-x.

Piening, E.P. 2013. Dynamic capabilities in public organizations. *Public Management Review* 15(2), pp. 209–245. doi:10.1080/14719037.2012.708358.

Public Protector. 2016. State of Capture. Report of the Public Protector.

Rispel, L.C., De Jager, P. and Fonn, S. 2015. Exploring corruption in the South African health sector. *Health Policy and Planning* 31(2), pp. 239–249. doi:10.1093/heapol/czv047.

South African Lancet Commission. 2018. *Confronting the Right to Ethical and Accountable Quality Health Care in South Africa: Synopsis of the Findings and Recommendations of the Consensus Report of the South African Lancet National Commission*. Pretoria.

Special Investigative Unit. 2021. Finalised matters in respect of the: Investigation into the procurement of, or contracting for goods, works and services, including the construction, refurbishment, leasing, occupation and use of immovable property, during, or in respect of the National State of Disaster, as declared by the Government Notice No 313 of 15 March 2020, by or on behalf of the State Institutions Proclamations No R23 of 2020 23 July 2020 to 25 November 2020. Online.

Teece, D.J., Pisano, G. and Shuen, A. 1997. Dynamic capabilities and strategic management. *Strategic Management Journal* 18(7), pp. 509–533. doi:https://doi.org/10.1002/(SICI)1097-0266(199708)18:7<509::AID-SMJ882>3.0.CO;2-Z.

Van den Heever, A.M. 2019. Preparedness for epidemics in South Africa: The health system and proposals for National Health Insurance. In Z. Mazibuko (Ed) *Epidemics and Healthcare Systems in Africa*. Johannesburg: Mapungubwe Institute for Strategic Reflection, pp. 413.

AN UNDERSTANDING OF THE SUPPLY, DISTRIBUTION AND USE OF PERSONAL PROTECTIVE EQUIPMENT DURING PANDEMICS

Stavros Nicolaou

Yahya E. Choonara

8.1 INTRODUCTION

In the twentieth century, pandemics occurred in 1918, 1957, and 1968 with the highest mortality recorded in the 1918 influenza outbreak that resulted in more than 50 million deaths globally (Johnson and Mueller, 2002; Morens and Fauci, 2007). At the turn of the twenty-first century, the Severe Acute Respiratory Syndrome-Coronavirus-1 (SARS-CoV-1) struck in 2003 with Healthcare Professionals (HCPs) among the most vulnerable due to poor compliance with using Personal Protective Equipment (PPE) as a component of infection control (CDC, 2003). In 2009, the H1N1 virus was detected in Mexico and the United States (US) Strategic National Stockpile allocated nearly 39 million pieces of PPE to protect people (Patel, 2017). In 2012, the Middle East Respiratory Syndrome-Coronavirus (MERS-CoV) emerged with PPE again instituted to reduce viral transmission (Rothan et al, 2020). In March 2020, Coronavirus Disease-2019 (COVID-19) was declared a pandemic and is currently the largest outbreak of the twenty-first century that has overwhelmed even the most developed healthcare systems with an estimated mortality rate of 2.92% by July 2020 (Carty and DiNicolantonio, 2020). The number of reported cases worldwide had reached over 18 million, with more than 600 000 deaths recorded at the time of writing this Chapter (Roser et al, 2020).

Lessons learnt from previous pandemics reflect that PPE plays a fundamental role in the hierarchy of infection control and 'Flattening the Curve', especially when parameters of viral transmission are uncertain during the initial stages. In the absence of a vaccine, governments enforce national lockdowns and activate quiescent Disaster Management Acts that regulate the use of PPE to protect people, reduce mortality and shield economies from collapsing. PPE protects individuals from cross-infection based on contact, droplet and airborne viral transmission and includes visible control items such as gloves, masks, visors, gowns, respirators and aprons. However, PPE should not be relied on as a primary prevention strategy as its effectiveness depends on the sustainability of supply, adequate staff training and use as well as appropriate remodelling of human behaviour towards compliance. In the absence of effective administrative, environmental and engineering controls, the benefits of PPE among measures adopted to protect people during pandemics is limited.

The virulence and spread of a novel virus is largely unknown during the early stages. This confounds decision-making in terms of PPE supply, distribution and use. The global demand for PPE is driven by the number of cases and misinformation, panic buying and stockpiling which results in PPE shortages. In addition, the capacity for developing countries to expand PPE production is limited, and the demand cannot be met. Policies that do not protect against the unsystematic use of PPE also negatively impact the supply and distribution chain.

Ubiquitous PPE items that are routinely used in hospitals to care for infectious patients rapidly become a scarce commodity during pandemics. Mitchell and co-workers (2012) have reported stochastic simulation data on PPE quantities needed (and the rate of use) during pandemics which limits forecasting and adequate planning. Data by the World Health Organization (WHO) reflects that nearly 20–25 PPE sets are required per patient with variable compliance by HCPs wearing PPE. National stockpiles are likely inadequate during pandemics and progressive strategies are required for countries to be adequately prepared in making PPE supply and demand projections more certain. National lockdowns also disrupt global supply chains by reducing economic activity, loss of labour and limitations on raw material inputs. This has impelled countries to impose restrictions on the export of PPE and even material precursors.

Lessons are continually being learnt to ensure the effective use, supply and distribution of PPE during pandemics. It is important that countries build on past experiences to not only address current concerns, but also strategise for the future. Coordinated effort is needed between government, business, professional associations and communities to address PPE matters through standards-setting (quality and training), emergency response readiness, overseeing pricing and ensuring the optimal supply, distribution and use of PPE during pandemics.

8.2 OBJECTIVES

The objectives of this chapter are:

- To provide a concise incursion into the role of PPE during pandemics and highlight the nuances and challenges of its supply, distribution and use with reference to the COVID-19 pandemic.

- To outline the best practices to reduce the risk of viral transmission and the sustainable supply of high-quality PPE via complementary sourcing, supplier vetting, stockpiling and establishing a PPE Procurement Platform.

- To discuss research related to the design, innovation, effectiveness, and reuse of PPE.
- To reflect on lessons learnt that could potentially be incorporated into prospective PPE policies, standards-setting, regulatory guidelines and training manuals for countries to be better prepared for future pandemics.

8.3 THE ROLE OF PPE IN THE HIERARCHY OF INFECTION CONTROLS DURING PANDEMICS

Based on available evidence, SAR-CoV-2 is transmitted through close contact, droplet spread and by airborne transmission (Liu et al, 2020). People most at risk are those who have close contact with a positive patient or who care for COVID-19 patients. Figure 8.1 outlines effective preventive measures to physically prevent viral transmission and the overall role of PPE use among HCPs.

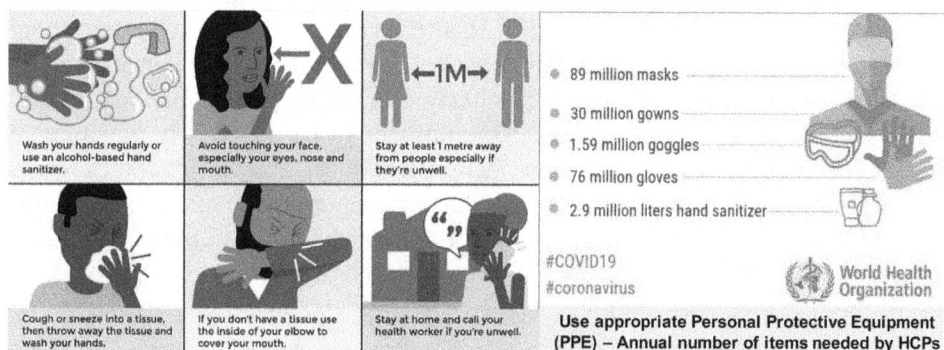

Figure 8.1: Outline of the measures used to prevent viral transmission highlighting the role of PPE, especially among Healthcare Professionals (HCPs)

The role of PPE is complementary within a suite of measures that also comprise administrative, environmental and engineering controls such as appropriate healthcare infrastructure, the development of infection prevention and control policies, access to laboratory testing, appropriate triage, adequate staff-to-patient ratios, staff training, decontaminating surfaces and adequate space to allow for social distancing. Implementing a PPE usage programme requires monitoring with the aim of continuous improvement, adopting accountability and best practices. In addition, the environmental impact (i.e. emerging trace pollutants) throughout the life cycle of non-degradable PPE will be magnified by the scale at which PPE is typically used during pandemics.

In addition, the misuse of PPE can equally contribute to individuals becoming infected and results in its wastage. Hence, the WHO published a guideline on conserving PPE that focuses on appropriate use, preventing misuse and sustaining supply chains (WHO, 2020). Overall, there is a lack of high-quality evidence on what type of PPE (particularly masks) is required in various settings contributing to much confusion. The allocation of PPE to those considered frontline or essential workers provided significant debate and has become an important (and emotive) component of healthcare systems. Therefore, it is essential to understand the role of PPE as part of a system to reduce viral transmission during pandemics.

8.4   ELEMENTS THAT IMPACT THE EFFICIENT USE OF PPE

Understanding the elements that impact the use of PPE is crucial to ensure compliance. The use of PPE should be aligned to the mode of viral transmission. This has led to much debate for example, on the type of mask to be used in various settings and who should be considered as frontline workers (FDA, 2020b). PPE elements relevant to HCPs are also applicable to essential workers and communities. The US Centres for Disease Control and Prevention (CDC) has published a tiered approach to transmission-based precautions (Siegel et al, 2007). Tier 1 refers to standard precautions applicable to HCPs caring for all patients and Tier 2 refers to precautions where patients have infections that could be transmitted to HCPs. Viral transmission routes include direct and indirect contact, droplet spray, and aerosol routes (Li et al, 2020).

In addition, several experts have questioned whether the SARS-CoV-2 virus can spread via airborne transmission and therefore makes transmission difficult to interpret (Van Doremalen et al, 2020; Bourouiba, 2020). The WHO provided some consensus recommending precautions for aerosol-generating settings that require the use of high-performance FFP2/FFP3 or N95 masks (WHO, 2020). Using a different or higher level of PPE than is required can be considered misuse and may affect PPE supplies.

8.4.1   Patterns of PPE use in the workplace

While much of the world remains at home during pandemics, essential workers (other than HCPs) need to report to work to ensure continuity in providing essential goods and services. PPE is a central component of infection prevention programmes in the workplace. At minimum, employees should consider the provision of PPE aligned to the employee's task and the organisational context. Although there are gaps in knowledge based on PPE usage, existing knowledge is sufficient to recommend deliberate planning and preparation at organisational level, provide staff training on the use of PPE and ensure the availability as well as accountability of appropriate PPE.

8.4.1.1 PPE for essential workers

It should be acknowledged that PPE use is fundamental to provide a safe environment for essential workers. PPE use should be functional, convenient, affordable and factored into decisions involving work activities and staffing. Employee input should be used for planning and maximising compliance. Administrative controls should ensure the sustainable equitable supply and distribution of PPE to workers. This includes establishing policies, standards, procedures, and practices which will limit staff exposure and improve worker safety. The responsibilities for Occupational Health and Safety (OHS) measures fall within the purview of governments under the Ministries of Health and Labour with OHS Acts that speak to employee health and safety during pandemics. These Acts must speak to the role of standards-setting for PPE and developing guidelines and assisting organisations with PPE-related matters.

Professional associations, regulatory bodies and standards development bureaus also play significant roles to ensure PPE is effective at the workplace. Work environments with the potential for infection risk such as cleaning and catering services are considered part of the healthcare workforce. During pandemics, non-HCPs may also become caregivers, such as family members who also require access to PPE.

8.4.1.2 PPE for Healthcare Professionals (HCPs)

HCPs may be defined broadly as workers in direct patient care and support services who are employed by health facilities, those working in emergency medical services or who are self-employed as well as health sciences students who work under supervision in health facilities or as trained healthcare volunteers during a pandemic. For HCPs, the nature of work provides challenges for the design and wearing of PPE. These include interaction with patients (and family members) that make communication important and pose challenges in exposure monitoring. Figure 8.2 illustrates the relevant concerns faced by HCPs regarding the use of PPE.

RELEVANT CONCERNS TO THE USE OF PPE BY HCPs

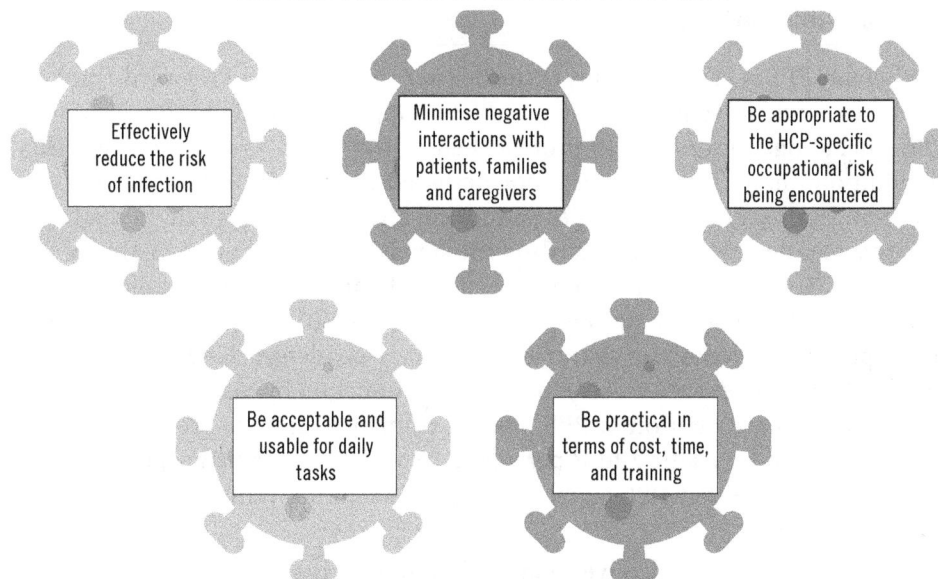

Effectively reduce the risk of infection

Minimise negative interactions with patients, families and caregivers

Be appropriate to the HCP-specific occupational risk being encountered

Be acceptable and usable for daily tasks

Be practical in terms of cost, time, and training

Figure 8.2: Illustration of the relevant concerns to the use of PPE by Healthcare Professionals (HCPs) as a starting point for selecting appropriate PPE

Various organisations have published guidelines on PPE related to HCPs which is broadly consistent (WHO, 2020; ECDC, 2020; PHE, 2020). Such efforts support the rationale use of PPE by restricting the movement of personnel, instituting stringent facility decontamination, minimising unnecessary patient contact, ensuring best practice in donning, doffing and disposal of PPE. Consensus among the guidelines states that airborne precautions comprise Filtering Facepiece (FFP2/FFP3) masks, visors, long-sleeved fluid-repellent gowns and gloves as core PPE for HCPs.

Lessons learnt from the SARS epidemic in Canada where a high rate of infection was recorded among HCPs indicated that complex PPE increased the risk of contamination removal. The 'buddy system' is quite effective with an observer using a checklist to ensure donning and doffing is performed correctly. Training on PPE use before patient management is essential for staff and patient safety. In addition, the classification of procedures as aerosol-generating is also not rooted in clear science. Some studies report low rates of HCP infection associated with tracheal intubation when PPE was appropriately used (Nicolle, 2003; Alhazzani et al, 2020; Meng et al, 2020).

8.5 MAPPING THE GLOBAL SUPPLY AND DISTRIBUTION OF PPE DURING PANDEMICS

Predictably PPE is in short supply at the height of a pandemic as forward-thinking countries work fervently to safeguard the supply and distribution chains of PPE (including stockpiling) to protect their self-interests and reduce mortality. In addition, many PPE items are not designed for re-use or reprocessing and common sterilisation technologies cannot effectively reprocess PPE in a safe and effective manner. Hence, safeguarding the supply and distribution chains of PPE is crucial. Given the global magnitude of pandemics, scaling up supply chains to meet the PPE demand surge in an equitable and sustainable manner among developed and developing countries remains a challenge. Governments have developed incentives for industry to ramp up production by easing restrictions on the export and distribution of PPE. Hence, countries resort to creating strategic national stockpiles leading to a perceived lack of inventory transparency with reports suggesting that PPE supplies are distributed unevenly or insufficient to meet the demand.

Furthermore, many unconventional solutions have been suggested, for example the use of cloth masks and recruiting commercial launderers under lockdown that normally service hotels. Cloth masks are best used by communities despite the uncertainty on their effectiveness but are still better than wearing no mask. The use of snorkel masks and tubes have also been suggested since they can be easily reused. In addition, high-grade filters used in N95 masks also exist in air-conditioning filters with a Minimum Efficiency Reporting Value (MERV) rating that can be effective against transmitting viral particles <0.2µm.

Although countries place much effort on ramping up the local production of PPE to keep pace with the demand, bottlenecks are encountered in the upstream supply chain from which speciality PPE raw materials are sourced. Many countries therefore explore repurposing sectors of their economies to boost PPE manufacturing capacity. These include the acquisition of PPE from suppliers in non-healthcare industries such as construction, research laboratories, salons, dentists, veterinarians, and farms, and reclaim stocks purchased through government treasury, solidarity funds, charity campaigns or community organisations.

During pandemics there is a significant disruption to the global supply of PPE caused by rising demand, panic buying, stockpiling and misuse. Without secure supply chains, the risk to people (especially HCPs) is real and governments need to act quickly and work with supply chain networks to improve supply, ease export restrictions and put measures in place in collaboration with industry to stop speculation and stockpiling as well as increase manufacturing capacity to meet the global demand for PPE. Hospital administrators and governments have a critical role to partner with manufacturers and develop a reliable supply system.

Linked to the sustainable supply of PPE there are guidelines published to optimise the responsible use of PPE at various levels of operation, i.e. Conventional, Contingency or Crisis mode.

Since the COVID-19 outbreak was reported, PPE prices have surged in many countries with supplies delayed and market manipulation rampant. Based on WHO modelling a global estimate of 89 million medical masks are required monthly by HCPs for the COVID-19 response. This has led to WHO guidelines demanding the rational and appropriate use of PPE and effective supply chain management.

One of the challenges highlighted by the US Food and Drug Administration (FDA) is that PPE distribution to health facilities is based on historical rather than projected usage data, resulting in shortages. Hence, conservation strategies developed by healthcare facilities have been recommended by the FDA. The FDA had also provided Emergency Use Authorization (EUA) for importing non-National Institute of Occupational Safety and Health (NIOSH)-approved N95 and FFP2 masks to mitigate shortages based on accepted standards from countries who have similar standards to the NIOSH. In addition, the FDA had adjusted its import screening to expedite imports of PPE to prevent and mitigate any supply issues and to help alleviate supply pressures by expediting review of manufacturing site changes or premarket submissions for manufacturers to increase PPE availability. The FDA also reviews PPE before they can be legally sold in the US where manufacturers must show they meet specific criteria for performance, labelling, and intended use (FDA, 2020).

In South Africa (SA), the SA Medical Technology Industry Association (SAMED) had called for an increase in local production of PPE. A large majority of PPE is manufactured and procured internationally. Africa has been outbid by developed countries and has lagged in the global race for PPE during the COVID-19 pandemic with calls for a more equitable approach to help developing nations with PPE. The African Union (AU) has stepped in to create a pooled purchasing platform to improve negotiating power. The WHO and UN also provide PPE donations across Africa sourced from philanthropists. SA has worked with economic allies to obtain PPE from China but with the pandemic arriving later in Africa the supply chain has been highly constrained.

Further investigation is needed on PPE supply chains into decision-making under epistemic and stochastic uncertainty, optimising supply chain planning considering agility, resilience and sustainability, understanding conflicts of interest among suppliers in global value chains, determining the life-cycle sustainability of PPE items and developing PPE allocation strategies under resource or supply constraints. Figure 8.3 lists broad strategies for the supply, management and conservation of PPE.

SUPPLY	MANAGEMENT	CONSERVATION
International imports from markets with manufacturing skill, experience and a decline in cases	Limit non-essential healthcare services by cancelling elective procedures	Reclaim PPE via construction and aerospace industries, universities, dentists and farmers
Partner with business to manage procurement, supply and distribution chains	Employ 'immune' workers who have recovered from clinical illness or with demonstrated immunity	Reuse of PPE via sterilisation, disinfecting and rotating over 72-hour cycles where applicable
Use government policy to regionalise supply, ration supply and loosen import regulations	Reduce patient contact by utilising telemedicine and batching chronic medication supply	Repurpose supply via prefabricated masks (3D printed masks, welding/scuba masks)
Create supply by producing unconventional PPE (fabric masks)	Stratify the use of PPE items by patient risk in healthcare facilities	Extend supply via improvisation of PPE items

Figure 8.3: List of broad strategies employed for the supply, management and conservation of PPE

8.6   ESTABLISHMENT OF A PPE PROCUREMENT PLATFORM TO OPTIMISE SUPPLY AND DISTRIBUTION DURING PANDEMICS: LESSONS FROM THE BUSINESS 4 SOUTH AFRICA (B4SA) HEALTH STREAM CASE STUDY

Pandemics create the need to source large quantities of PPE. In SA, at the onset of the COVID-19 pandemic (in March 2020), steps were taken to source PPE not only to protect people but also to avert strike action by HCPs and essential workers. The challenge was confounded by the global scarcity of PPE, escalating prices and limited local manufacturing capability. In response to this public health emergency, the SA Government mobilised social partners at the National Economic Development and Labour Council (NEDLAC) to consolidate resources and build a coordinated response to tackle COVID-19. Business for South Africa (B4SA) was born as an independent and broad coalition of volunteers to accelerate and support the country's response to the pandemic.

The B4SA team included over 450 professionals from across academia, healthcare, business and industry, volunteering to support the country in three fundamental areas, i.e. Health, Labour and the Economy. In a relatively short period of time, the B4SA Health Stream established an independent, efficient and scalable PPE Procurement Platform with a Supplier Portal to source, validate and contract with PPE suppliers. The demand for PPE was also ascertained via the Platform and from the SA National Department of Health (NDoH).

The Platform enabled PPE buyers, suppliers and donors to timely access bulk orders which met the required specifications on a cost-effective basis. The end-to-end logistics to ensure the delivery of PPE sourced by B4SA was undertaken by a vetted logistics company, Imperial Health Sciences (IHS), on a cost-recovery basis. The fundamental criteria that underscored the PPE Procurement Platform were price, quality, availability and where possible support for SME's, empowerment and local manufacturers. All suppliers were vetted through the B4SA Supplier Portal via a three-stage process 1) supply company vetting, 2) product certificate authentication and 3) product quality inspection.

A key focus of the Platform was to institute a framework to screen the quality of PPE items using the National Regulator for Compulsory Specifications (NRSC) standards and the South African Bureau of Standards (SABS) approval to avoid the risk of sub-standard PPE reaching the market and leading to infection among HCPs. PPE items used in healthcare facilities are considered medical devices and are regulated. All PPE importers and manufacturers were asked to obtain a license from the South African Health Products Regulatory Authority (SAHPRA) for the company to be listed on the Supplier Portal. Manufacturers/importers were required to demonstrate to SAHPRA that the items have been tested to meet specified consensus standards. The regulations were designed to control the manufacture and sale of PPE.

The COVID-19 pandemic has also exposed the global risk of an over-reliance on single markets for the supply of PPE. At the onset of the pandemic, PPE represented <2% of the overall medical equipment sales in SA, with surgical gloves making up the vast majority. To compound this, SA (like much of the world) had limited internal manufacturing and supply capacity to deliver the vast quantities of PPE that was needed. While B4SA's PPE Procurement Platform initially focused on urgently securing bulk quantities of PPE from constrained global markets its focus morphed to identify, capacitate and source PPE from local manufacturers, black-owned suppliers and small and medium-sized enterprises (SMEs) in partnership with Government, Labour and Donors. This strategy did not only provide opportunities for local manufacturing, but also contributed to the country's economic recovery plan and the preservation of jobs where 97% of all PPE items ordered were from local Broad-Based Black Economic Empowerment (B-BBEE) Level 1 manufacturing companies.

8.6.1   The Six Tenets of the B4SA PPE Procurement Platform

Since the COVID-19 pandemic impacts on both the public and private sectors in SA, it was imperative to coordinate the management of the national state of disaster. Initially, the B4SA Procurement Platform focused on purchasing PPE from suppliers who met the criteria of quality, volume of supply and timing of delivery. Later, suppliers were validated and had to register on the Supplier Portal.

As the Platform evolved, the procurement system was formalised to include PPE for essential workers in addition to HCPs as the lockdown eased and employees returned to work. The development of the platform was built on six tenets.

8.6.1.1   Tenet 1: The relationship between B4SA and donors

B4SA was not a juristic person but an initiative of Business Unity South Africa (BUSA). Therefore, volunteers who provided services as part of the B4SA PPE procurement platform acted on BUSA's behalf as the entity that entered into contracts, acquired rights, and incurred obligations relating to the platform. In the case of medical-grade PPE, B4SA instituted a process of vetting and approving suppliers that were recommended to donors before a contract of sale between the supplier, donor and the Lead Logistics Provider (LLP) was finalised. The PPE was then distributed to provinces or sold to designated private wholesalers. In the case of non-medical PPE, the vetting and approval of suppliers resulted in a recommendation to the relevant business and, if approved, a contract of sale between the supplier and the business was instituted.

8.6.1.2   Tenet 2: Sourcing and validation of PPE suppliers

B4SA established an online Supplier Portal (https://covid19manager.co.za) using the Tencent Platform and developed the PPE Procurement Platform with consultants. The Fraxses platform was also used to establish a PPE Dashboard to reflect information on supplier stock availability, healthcare provider stock information and records of purchase orders, donations and distributions. A call for submissions from prospective suppliers was made, followed by the establishment of the portal that received more than 7 000 applications. Three components were used to validate suppliers via the Portal.

First, the supplier's submission was confirmed complete and those validated needed to complete exclusions of liability to be eligible for contracting in respect of orders.

Secondly, suppliers were vetted through 'know-your-customer' criteria. including proof of company registration, industry affiliations and tax status. A vetted supplier was conditionally approved and notified to submit documentation for PPE items via the Portal.

Thirdly, technical vetting of the supplier and product occurred by an independent technical team that reviewed the submissions by supplier against regulatory standards approved by the SABS, NRCS, NDoH and SAHPRA. Figure 8.4 outlines the technical criteria that were considered.

1. Provision of manufacturers export licence for medical grade PPE from country of origin

2. Refer suppliers to obtain SAHPRA approval licence for any unlicensed PPE items

3. Review of SAHPRA medical device licence to ensure relevant product to be imported or manufactured

4. Review ISO13485 certificate of manufacturing site and certificate authenticity for PPE item and its specification

5. Review the product test report to ensure specifications within WHO standards

6. Review product certification and conformity to standards (EN, SANAS, SABS, NRCS or ISO)

7. Review product label to ensure that it did not include claims beyond its registered specification

Figure 8.4 Outline of technical vetting criteria used for the PPE supplier and product by the B4SA team

To ensure that SMEs met the supplier qualification criteria, B4SA aided SMEs in fulfilling the technical criteria. The technical vetting process was undertaken by a team of SABS inspectors, who operate independently and objectively. In addition, the SABS and NRCS inspectors conducted an inspection of the imported PPE products either on arrival at the airport or at the LLP warehouse. To enhance the independence of the validation process, each inspector in the vetting process was required to complete a non-disclosure agreement and declare any conflicts of interest. The supply of PPE by black-empowered and local suppliers with a high B-BBEE score were prioritised in the verification process. If an aspirant supplier failed the vetting process, the supplier was informed of this outcome and the reasons thereof. Suspected invalid certificates were handed over to SAHPRA, and the NDoH.

8.6.1.3 Tenet 3: Ascertaining the demand specifically for medical-grade PPE

The primary focus was to procure PPE for use in the public and private healthcare sectors. The demand for PPE was aligned to the NDoH's demand forecast via a dashboard managed by an audit firm (Deloitte Touche Tohmatsu Limited) that produced a weekly demand gap analysis by comparing the demand forecasts with the PPE orders that were placed. This data was used to prepare estimated projections of the total demand and extrapolated the portion of the demand that the B4SA PPE Procurement Platform sourced.

8.6.1.4 Tenet 4: Preparation and approval of purchase orders and contracting with suppliers

There were two scenarios in which procurement occurred through the B4SA PPE Procurement Platform. In Scenario 1 (the normal scenario), procurement was considered relatively urgent and a comparison was undertaken between validated suppliers on price with the lowest price approved. If prices were close, preference was given to majority black-owned suppliers and thereafter a supplier with the best B-BBEE score. In Scenario 2 (the emergency scenario), where there was an urgent need to purchase PPE (either because of a sudden spike in demand or a threatened shortage in the PPE markets), offers already received from validated suppliers were assessed by an approval panel and immediately approved.

The purchase order included a clause in which the supplier indemnified BUSA, B4SA, the donor and personnel involved in the procurement process in respect of any loss from their involvement in the process, including defects in the PPE to be supplied. The approval panel constituted five persons who were required to approve an order before it could proceed. To enhance its independence, the panel comprised one BUSA appointee, one Black Business Council (BBC) appointee and three B4SA Steering Committee appointees. The mandate of the approval panel was to consider purchase orders as follows:

1. Whether the price conformed to (or was below) the relevant benchmarks;
2. The immediate availability of the stock;
3. Confirm that the supplier was vetted;
4. Ensure that due diligence was done on airfreight costs and the route for consignment of goods; and
5. Preference given to black-owned/local manufacturers to promote localisation and transformation.

Once the purchase order was approved it was submitted to the donor or, in the case of non-medical PPE, the third party purchaser for approval, and, if approved by the donor/purchaser a purchase contract was concluded with the supplier.

8.6.1.5 Tenet 5: Distribution of PPE in the public and private sectors

Once the B4SA PPE procurement platform was established, the team recognised the benefit of having a competitive end-to-end logistics provider. Pursuant to this process, B4SA had appointed IHS on a medium-term basis. Through the B4SA procurement platform the requisite PPE items were distributed by the LLP to provincial depots (as determined by the SA Government Procurement Team). Thereafter the NDoH distributed the donated items at the provincial level. The distribution for PPE in the private healthcare sector was served through private wholesalers who placed orders via the LLP.

8.6.1.6 Tenet 6: Relationship between the LLP and wholesalers

B4SA appointed IHS to provide end-to-end logistics for all PPE procured through the B4SA PPE Procurement Platform on a cost-recovery basis, considering the six criteria below:

1. Provide end-to-end logistics including uplifting of stock in foreign primary markets (e.g. China);
2. Preparedness to operate on a cost-recovery basis;
3. Compliance with regulatory and statutory requirements;
4. A track record of supply to the state;
5. Quality assurance and integrity; and
6. Have international billing items and codes.

8.7 OVERCOMING SHORTAGES THROUGH PPE LIFETIME EXTENSION

Extending the lifetime of PPE items for multiple uses may help to alleviate shortages. There is a paucity of scientific literature reporting on the reprocessing of PPE since most PPE items are manufactured for single use only. In addition, limited knowledge dissemination due to Intellectual Property (IP) protection makes this area unclear. However, leading manufacturers have published findings that also assist in shaping International Organization for Standardization (ISO) standards, guidelines and regulations with a focus on reuse of PPE (McEvoy and Rowan, 2019). Fisher and Shaffer (2011) advocated physical or chemical decontamination of N95 masks. However, the decontamination treatment must maintain mask fit and filtration performance without leaving harmful residues. The process may also not comply with low cost and high throughput as a factor for PPE decontamination. The greatest challenge to reprocessing PPE is ensuring material functionality post-treatment. Many researchers have acknowledged the uncertainty of sterilising PPE, and there is some evidence that the fibres in masks and respirators that filter viral particles can degrade and lose their efficacy with PPE reprocessing.

Some Original Equipment Manufacturers (OEMs) of single-use PPE have made available methods for reprocessing items given the global need to consider contingency plans arising from PPE shortages during pandemics. In addition, the US FDA has published an enforcement policy for sterilising masks that informs reprocessing of PPE (FDA, 2020b). Lessons on the reprocessing of PPE can also be learnt from best practices exploited in the food industry.

8.8 RESEARCH LANDSCAPE INTO PPE: DESIGN, INNOVATION, EFFECTIVENESS AND POLICY

Research into improving PPE needs to be strengthened at all levels. There are many opportunities for current PPE research to build on past experiences on the design, innovation, effectiveness, regulatory and policy fronts. Lessons learnt from previous pandemics should drive research into PPE cost-effectiveness as well as innovation into the reuse of PPE. Policy research and implementation mechanisms for PPE use, supply and distribution are critical during pandemics to support infection control plans established by HCPs as well as all professional and government stakeholders.

The design and innovation arm should focus on engineering PPE that is effective, ongoing and aligned to policy, regulatory, standards setting and certification. Such research needs to extend to identifying and translating evidence-based requirements and realistic assessments of PPE performance. Research into the reuse of PPE focus on various sterilisation methods of used PPE. Novel proposals also include mask-fibre impregnation with copper or sodium chloride and rendering PPE greener where feasible through multidisciplinary research. An interesting focus is the use of positive pressure airflow helmets that can be cleaned and reused as no filters are used. Where possible, bespoke production of PPE using medical grade materials to provide additional options during shortages should be considered. For example, using crowdfunding to develop simple and affordable masks and three-dimensional (3D)-printed visors.

Research and innovation into PPE should be continually supported to keep the momentum between pandemics. The focus of many researchers largely detracts to other areas, and countries remain critically underprepared. The exploration of smart software, mobile tracking apps and networking between supply and distribution channels is also needed to meet the gaps in PPE supply and demand.

8.9 CONCLUSIONS

The world changes after and between pandemics and brings with it a high degree of nationalism to ensure citizens are well equipped and effectively protected. Taking the opportunities that are born out of a crisis, pandemics have triggered the drive for localisation and transformation among developing countries with a determined focus on manufacturing PPE to secure supplies locally. During pandemics, developing countries need to compete for PPE supplies with more industrialised nations. It is therefore crucial to maintain a system-wide perspective on PPE use, supply and distribution to ensure the broader availability of PPE and intensely scrutinise the quality of items that are made available to the market, especially for frontline HCPs. Important lessons can also be learnt from establishing PPE Procurement Platforms that add significant value to optimise the supply and distribution of PPE. It is imperative that countries learn from such informed best evidence and practice to be better prepared. In addition, digitalised technologies such as artificial intelligence (AI) tools capable of tracking global suppliers/consumers are required to assist with more accurate forecasting of PPE demand and supply. The *status quo* revealed from the current COVID-19 pandemic highlight that despite the astounding advancements made within the 4th Industrial Revolution (4IR) our world remains vulnerable in terms of the equitable and sustainable supply, distribution and use PPE during pandemics.

8.10 SELF-ASSESSMENT QUESTIONS

1. What advances to PPE are needed to enhance effectiveness?
2. What are the key areas of PPE research that should be strengthened?

8.11 REFERENCES

Alhazzani, W., Hylander, M.M. and Arabi, Y.M., et al. 2019. Surviving Sepsis Campaign: Guidelines on the management of critically ill adults with coronavirus disease 2019 (COVID-19). *Intensive Care Medicine* 46, pp. 854–887.

Bourouiba, L. 2020. Turbulent gas clouds and respiratory pathogen emissions: potential implications for reducing transmission of COVID-19. *Journal of the American Medical Association* 323(18), pp. 1837–1838.

British Standard Institute. 2009. Respiratory protective devices. Filtering half masks to protect against particles. Requirements, testing, marking, BS EN 149:2001+A1:2009. Available at: https://www.bsigroup.com/en-GB/topics/novel-coronavirus-covid-19/medical-devices-ppe/.

Carty, M.F. and DiNicolantonio, J.J. 2020. Nutraceuticals have potential for boosting the type 1 interferon response to RNA viruses including influenza and coronavirus. *Progress in Cardiovascular Diseases* 63(3), pp. 383–385.

Centres for Disease Control and Prevention (CDC), US Department of Health and Human Services, GA, Atlanta, USA. 2003. Guidelines for environmental infection control in health-care facilities. Recommendations of CDC and Healthcare Infection Control Practices Advisory Committee (HICPAC). Available at: https://stacks.cdc.gov/view/cdc/45796.

European Centre for Disease Prevention and Control (ECDC). 2020. Infection prevention and control for COVID-19 in healthcare settings. Available at: https://www.ecdc.europa.eu/en/publications-data/infection-prevention-and-control-covid-19-healthcare-settings.

Fisher, E.M. and Shaffer, R.E. 2011. A method to determine the available UV-C dose for the decontamination of filtering face piece respirators. *Journal of Applied Microbiology* 110(910), pp. 287–295.

Food and Drug Administration (FDA), USA. 2020a. Personal protective equipment for infection control. Available at: https://www.fda.gov/medical-devices/general-hospital-devices-and-supplies/personal-protective-equipment-infection-control.

Food and Drug Administration (FDA), USA. 2020b. Enforcement policy for face masks and respirators during the coronavirus disease (COVID19) public health emergency (Revised). Available at: https://www.fda.gov/regulatory-information/search-fda-guidance-documents/enforcement-policy-face-masks-and-respirators-during-coronavirus-disease-covid-19-public-health.

Johnson, N.P.A.S. and Mueller, J. 2002. Updating the accounts: Global mortality of the 1918–1920 "Spanish" Influenza Pandemic. *Bulletin of the History of Medicine* 76(1), pp. 105–115.

Li, Q., Guan, X., Wu, P., Wang, X., Zhou, L. and Tong, Y., et al. 2020. Early transmission dynamics in Wuhan, China, of novel coronavirus-infected pneumonia. *New England Journal of Medicine* 382(13), pp. 1199–1207.

Liu, J., Liao, X. and Qian, S., et al. 2020. Community transmission of severe acute respiratory syndrome coronavirus 2, Shenzhen, China. *Emerging Infectious Diseases* 26(6), pp. 1320–1323.

McEvoy, B. and Rowan, N.J. 2019. Terminal sterilization of medical devices using vaporized hydrogen peroxide: A review of current methods and emerging opportunities. *Journal of Applied Microbiology* 127(5), pp. 1403–1420.

Meng, L., Qiu, H. and Wan, L., et al. 2020. Intubation and ventilation amid the COVID-19 outbreak: Wuhan's experience. Anaesthesiology 132, pp. 1317–1332.

Mitchell, R., Ogunreai, T., Astratianakis, S., Bryce, E., Gervais, R. and Gravel, D., et al. 2012. Impact of the 2009 influenza A (H1N1) pandemic on Canadian health care workers: a survey on vaccination, illness, absenteeism, and personal protective equipment. *American Journal of Infection Control* 40(7), pp. 611–616.

Morens, D.M. and Fauci, A.S. 2007. The 1918 influenza pandemic: Insights for the 21st century. *Journal of Infectious Diseases* 195(7), pp. 1018–1028.

Nicolle, L. 2003. SARS safety and science. *Canadian Journal of Anesthesia* 50, pp. 983–988.

Patel, A., D'Alessandro, M.M., Ireland, K.J., Burel, W.G., Wencil, E.B. and Rasmussen, S.A. 2017. Personal protective equipment supply chain: Lessons learned from recent public health emergency responses. *Health Security* 15(3), pp. 244–252.

Public Health England (PHE). 2020. COVID-19: infection prevention and control guidance. [online] Available at: https://www.gov.uk/government/publications/wuhan-novel-coronavirus-infection-prevention-and-control/wuhan-novel-coronavirus-wn-cov-infection-prevention-and-control-guidance#mobile-healthcare-equipment.

Public Health England. 2020. When to use a surgical face mask or FFP3 respirator. Available at: https://www.fbu.org.uk/circular/2020hoc0204ad/official-guidance-when-use-surgical-face-mask-or-ffp3-respirator.

Roser, M., Ritchie, H., Ortiz-Ospina, E. and Hasell, J. 2020. Coronavirus Pandemic (COVID-19). OurWorldInData.org. Official Website. Available at: https://ourworldindata.org/coronavirus.

Rothan, H.A. and Byrareddy, S.N. 2020. The epidemiology and pathogenesis of coronavirus disease (COVID-19) outbreak. *Journal of Autoimmunity* 109, pp. 102433. Available at: https://doi.org/10.1016/j.jaut.2020.102433.

Siegel, J., E. Rhinehart, M. Jackson, L. Chiarello, and the Healthcare Infection Control Practices Advisory Committee. 2007. 2007 guideline for isolation precautions: Preventing transmission of infectious agents in healthcare settings. Available at: https://www.cdc.gov/infectioncontrol/guidelines/isolation/index.html.

Van Doremalen, N., Bushmaker, T. and Morris, D.H., et al. 2020. Aerosol and surface stability of HCoV-19 (SARS-CoV-2) compared to SARS-CoV-1. *New England Journal of Medicine* 382, pp. 1564–1567.

World Health Organization (WHO). 2020a. Rational use of personal protective equipment (PPE) for coronavirus disease (COVID-19). Available at: https://apps.who.int/iris/bitstream/handle/10665/331498/WHO-2019-nCoV-IPCPPE_use-2020.2-eng.pdf?sequence=1&isAllowed=y.

World Health Organization (WHO). 2020b. Transmission of SARS-CoV-2: implications for infection prevention precautions. Available at: https://www.who.int/news-room/commentaries/detail/transmission-of-sars-cov-2-implications-for-infection-prevention-precautions.

World Health Organization (WHO). 2020c. Clinical management of severe acute respiratory infection when novel coronavirus (nCoV) infection is suspected. Available at: https://www.who.int/publications-detail/clinical-management-of-severe-acute-respiratory-infection-when-novel-coronavirus-(ncov)-infection-is-suspected.

CHAPTER 9

PANDEMICS, HEALTH INEQUITIES AND THE SOCIAL DETERMINANTS OF HEALTH

Laetitia Rispel

David Chiriboga

9.1 INTRODUCTION

Notwithstanding the evidence and warnings of the global risk of high-impact, potentially fast-spreading outbreaks of complex infectious diseases (Global Preparedness Monitoring Board 2019), the novel coronavirus disease 2019 (COVID-19) took the world by surprise. By 5 October 2021, around 235 million COVID-19 cases and more than 4.8 million deaths were reported to the World Health Organization (WHO) (https://covid19.who.int/). Table 9.1 shows the number of confirmed COVID-19 cases for the different WHO regions.

Table 9.1: COVID-19 situation by WHO region, 5 October 2021

Region	Number of confirmed cases	Percentage
Americas	90,479,144	38.5
Europe	70,896,282	30.1
South-East Asia	43,189,962	18.4
Eastern Mediterranean	15,871,955	6.7
Africa	6,056,076	2.6
Western Pacific	8,680,923	3.7

Source: World Health Organization. Available at: https://covid19.who.int/ [Accessed 6 October 2021].

Very few countries have been prepared for the impact of the COVID-19 pandemic on health systems and the shocks to economic and social systems (Paintsil, 2020; WHO Europe, 2020). In most affected countries of the world, COVID-19 has caused untold hardship, suffering and devastation, laying bare and amplifying the pre-existing social injustices both within and among countries and regions (Abrams and Szefler, 2020; Chiriboga et al, 2020).

This chapter explores pandemics and their intersection with the social determinants of health (SDH), highlighting that pandemics are both biological and social phenomena that magnify pre-existing socioeconomic inequities.

9.2   OBJECTIVES

The specific objectives of the chapter are to:
- Define the concept of SDH and its relationship to health equity.
- Distinguish between the notions of health [in]equality and health [in]equity.
- Explain the relationship and intersection between pandemics, the SDH and health inequities.
- Provide evidence on the amplified impact of the SDH and the COVID-19 pandemic on pre-existing inequities in South Africa.
- Outline the possible actions of health sciences educational institutions and civil society organisations in addressing the SDH and health inequities.

9.3   EVOLUTION AND DEFINITION OF THE SOCIAL DETERMINANTS OF HEALTH

The concept of the SDH, or the socioeconomic conditions that influence individual and/or group differences in health status, has its roots in ancient civilisations (Tountas, 2009). Hippocrates often referred to as the 'father of modern medicine', defined health as an equilibrium between environmental 'forces' and individual 'habits' (Tountas, 2009).

In the inter-war period, Latin America scholars played a major role in defining and enhancing the discourse on social medicine (Carter, 2019). They emphasised the social, economic, and political causes of ill-health, and they advocated for a strong role for the state in healthcare delivery, and universal health systems to meet the needs of populations (Carter, 2019). Importantly, these scholars expanded the boundaries of the study and practice of medicine to include the political, economic and social structures that influence and shape life (Carter, 2019). They also underscored the social determinants of illness and death; the impact of social policies on health and health care; and the relationships between work, reproduction, and the environment (Iriart et al, 2002; Waitzkin et al, 2001). Many of the Latin American countries played a central role in the establishment of the WHO, based on principles of universal social and health rights (Cueto and Palmer, 2014).

The original 1948 WHO Constitution defines health as 'a state of complete physical, mental and social well-being and not merely the absence of disease or infirmity' (WHO, 2006 p. 1). Article 2(i) of the WHO Constitution underscores the importance of the SDH, and notes that WHO will collaborate with other agencies to promote 'the improvement of nutrition, housing, sanitation, recreation, economic or working conditions and other aspects of environmental hygiene' (WHO, 2006 p. 1). Despite this broader definition of health, the 1950s and 60s witnessed the emergence of technology-driven, vertical health programmes and campaigns with little acknowledgement of the social and/or political contexts (Solar and Irwin. 2007).

The 1978 international conference on primary healthcare (PHC) was a significant global development to change the discourse in favour of the critical role of the SDH (Solar and Irwin, 2007). The final Alma Ata Declaration on PHC reiterates the WHO's definition of health and underscores health as a fundamental human right (WHO, 1978). The first clause of the PHC Declaration highlights the relationship between the 'attainment of the highest possible level of health' and action by 'other social and economic sectors in addition to the health sector' (WHO, 1978). The Declaration also highlights the social injustice because of the health inequities between and within countries (WHO, 1978).

However, the emphasis on the SDH in achieving health for all, created by the Alma-Ata PHC Declaration, was short lived. During the 1980s and 1990s, a combination of powerful vested interests, neoliberal economic models and structural adjustment programmes imposed on many countries in sub-Saharan Africa, Latin America and the Caribbean resulted in a reduction in social spending which affected the ability of policymakers to address the SDH and address inequities (Hartmann, 2016; Solar and Irwin, 2007). Furthermore, Hall and Taylor argued that many politicians and donor agencies were unwilling to support community participation, another central element of PHC, because of its transformative potential in challenging the status quo (Hall and Taylor, 2003).

In the 2000s, a series of developments created a window of opportunity to revitalise the global discourse on the SDH and strategies to address health inequities. In 2003, the late Dr Lee Jong-Wook assumed the position of Director-General of WHO and stated publicly his commitment to health equity and social justice (Jong-Wook, 2005). An additional impetus for a discourse and/or action on the SDH, was increasing evidence of the worsening health inequities among and within countries, exacerbated by the failure of health and social policies to reduce these disparities (Blas and Kurup, 2010; Commission on Social Determinants of Health, 2008; Graham, 2004; Irwin and Scali, 2007).

In 2005, Lee established the Commission on Social Determinants of Health (CSDH), with a mandate of generating and consolidating knowledge on SDH that could be turned into policy action to promote health equity, especially in low- and middle-income countries (LMICs) (Solar and Irwin 2007). The CSDH was mandated to release its report in 2008, to coincide with the 30-year anniversary of the Alma-Ata conference on PHC and 60 years after the enactment of the WHO Constitution (Commission on Social Determinants of Health, 2008; Solar and Irwin, 2007).

The WHO's definition of the SDH is shown in Box 1 (Commission on Social Determinants of Health 2008). In its final report, the Commission presented evidence to demonstrate that although diseases have biological causes, the SDH explain the distribution of disease and health inequities within and between regions, countries and populations (Commission on Social Determinants of Health, 2008).

Definition of SDH

The social determinants of health are the conditions in which people are born, grow, live, work and age. These circumstances are shaped by the distribution of money, power and resources at global, national and local levels. The social determinants of health are mostly responsible for health inequities – the unfair and avoidable differences in health status seen within and between countries.

Source: https://www.who.int/social_determinants/sdh_definition/en/

The CSDH defined health equity as 'the absence of unfair and avoidable or remediable differences in health among population groups defined socially, economically, demographically or geographically' (Solar and Irwin, 2007 p. 7).

Although there are different theories and models on the SDH (Solar and Irwin, 2007), the CSDH developed a conceptual framework which includes the socioeconomic and political context, structural determinants, and intermediary determinants to explain health outcomes at individual and group levels, and the relationship between health equity and the SDH (Commission on Social Determinants of Health, 2008). The CSDH framework includes structural drivers, including socioeconomic, cultural, the natural environment, and climate change, the legacy of colonialism and systemic racism and discrimination, which in turn influence the conditions of daily life (Commission on Social Determinants of Health, 2008). These conditions include the educational system, neighbourhood and physical environment, employment, social support networks and healthcare systems (Commission on Social Determinants of Health, 2008). All these factors combined comprise the conditions for a dignified life which determine the level of health equity within a population (Commission on Social Determinants of Health, 2008). In 2019, the Pan American Health Organization updated and simplified the framework (Figure 9.1) (Pan American Health Organization, 2019).

INTERSECTIONALITY: SOCIAL AND ECONOMIC INEQUITIES, GENDER, SEXUALITY, ETHNICITY, DISABILITY, MIGRATION

STRUCTURAL DRIVERS

Political, Social Cultural and Economic Structures

Natural Environment, Land and Climate Change

History and Legacy, Ongoing Colonialism, Structural Racism

CONDITIONS OF DAILY LIFE

Early Life and Education

Working Life

Older People

Income and Social Protection

Violence

Environment and Housing

Heath Systems

HEALTH EQUITY AND DIGNIFIED LIFE

TAKING ACTION

Governance
Human Rights

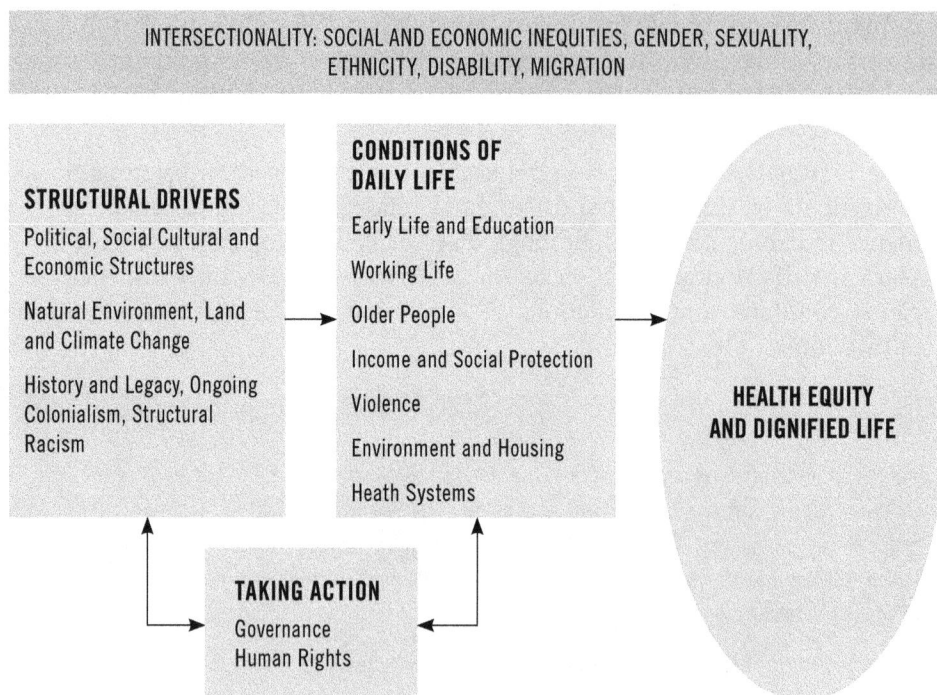

Figure 9.1: Conceptual framework on social determinants of health
Source: Pan American Health Organization, 2019 p. 5

The 2008 Commission proposed a new global agenda for health equity, and three overarching recommendations: improve daily living conditions; tackle the inequitable distribution of power, money, and resources; and measure and understand the problem and assess the impact of action (Commission on Social Determinants of Health, 2008).

Three years after the release of the CSDH report in 2011, the Rio Political Declaration on Social Determinants of Health reaffirmed the global commitment to health equity, through addressing the SDH (WHO, 2011). The key commitments or resolutions include governance for health and development, people's participation in policy-making and implementation, reorientation of the health sector towards reducing health inequities, monitoring of progress on SDH, and enhanced accountability (WHO, 2011).

In 2015, the United Nations adopted Agenda 2030, with 17 Sustainable Development Goals (SDGs) that provide for a global vision towards sustainable development (United Nations, 2015). The SDGs aim to achieve a balance across the economic, social and environmental dimensions of sustainable development (United Nations, 2015). The list below shows these 17 sustainable developments goals. Although Goal 3 focuses specifically on health and well-being, the other 16 SDGs deal with the SDH, and are linked inextricably to SDG 3. However, there are several challenges associated with the SDGs, including fragmentation, lack of binding mechanisms and international financial strategies, and weak metrics to hold governments accountable (United Nations, 2019).

The 17 SDGs to transform our world:

Goal 1: No Poverty

Goal 2: Zero Hunger

Goal 3: Good Health and Well-Being

Goal 4: Quality Education

Goal 5: Gender Equality

Goal 6: Clean Water and Sanitation

Goal 7: Affordable and Clean Energy

Goal 8: Decent Work and Economic Growth

Goal 9: Industry, Innovation and Infrastructure

Goal 10: Reduced Inequality

Goal 11: Sustainable Cities and Communities

Goal 12: Responsible Consumption and Production

Goal 13: Climate Action

Goal 14: Life below Water

Goal 15: Life on Land

Goal 16: Peace and Justice Strong Institutions

Goal 17: Partnerships to Achieve the Goals

Source: United Nations, 2015.

9.4 HEALTH EQUALITY VS HEALTH EQUITY

Many authors, including the final report of the CSDH, use the terms [in]equality and [in]equity interchangeably (Commission on Social Determinants of Health, 2008). However, these concepts are not the same, often influenced by different disciplinary perspectives and ideology.

Therborn argues that inequality is a social construct, and makes a distinction between difference and inequality (Therborn, 2012). Therborn describes vital, existential and resource inequality (Therborn, 2012). Vital inequality refers to socially determined distributions of health and ill-health and of lifespan (Therborn, 2012). Existential inequality is the unequal social treatment of persons, including denial of recognition, autonomy, existential security, dignity and respect, and structured and processed by categories and lenses of othering, e.g. race, ethnicity, and/or gender (Therborn, 2012).

Resource inequality refers to the unequal allocation of means among human actors, often measured through distributions of income and wealth. Therborn highlights the intersectionality and contextual influences of these types of inequalities, both globally and nationally (Therborn, 2012).

The well-known illustration by the Interaction Institute for Social Change shows the difference between the two concepts of equality and equity.

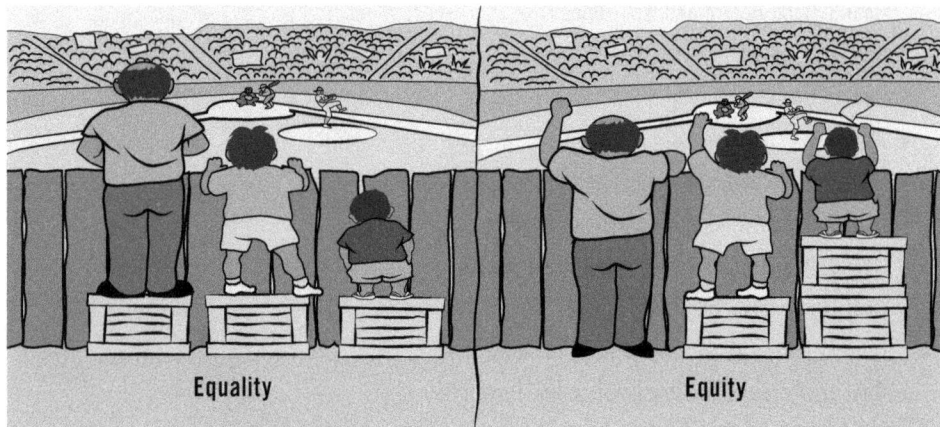

Figure 9.2: Difference between equality and equity (Levine, n.d.)

Source: Peter Levine. Available at: https://peterlevine.ws/?p=20430. [Accessed 16 October 2020].

In 2017, Garay and Chiriboga outlined the difference between health inequality and health inequity (Table 9.2) in order to achieve socioeconomic justice and health for all (Garay and Chiriboga, 2017). An inequality is any difference, whereas an inequity is a socially and ethically unfair difference. They pointed out that one of the risks of the SDH approach is the dependence on ratios of inequalities between sub-populations and the myriad categories leading to fragmentation and dilution of efforts to combat such inequalities (Garay and Chiriboga, 2017). These differences do not happen in a vacuum, but rather are a consequence of the socioeconomic conditions, which in turn are determined by the prevailing national and international political and socioeconomic models (Graham, 2004; Hartmann, 2016; Iriart et al, 2002; Pan American Health Organization, 2019). Garay and Chiriboga proposed a systematic, root-cause analysis approach to analysing inequities (Garay and Chiriboga, 2017).

Table 9.2: Health inequalities vs health inequities

Domain	Inequality	Inequity
Concept	Differences	Unfair differences
Measurement	Differences or ratios between subpopulations	Gap from best feasible and sustainable standards: burden of inequity
Conclusions	Arbitrary conclusions	Measurable objective, inter and intra national, intra and intergenerational
Strategy	Approach to disadvantaged groups: poverty alleviation	Approach to minimum threshold: social cohesion (address both extremes), levels of dignity, and universal rights
Effect	Mitigation	Transformation

Source: Garay and Chiriboga, 2017 p. 151.

In the next section, we use the term inequity, unless inequality or inequalities are used in the specific publications referenced.

9.5   PANDEMICS, THE SDH AND HEALTH INEQUITIES

Perhaps no observation during the great influenza epidemic of 1918-1919 was more common than the familiar comment that **"the flu hit the rich and the poor alike"**. Apparently, there was ample ground for a belief in the impartiality of the disease. Like many conclusions based on general impressions, this observation was true only in part. Epidemic influenza undoubtedly was very prevalent among all classes of persons and its mortality toll was levied from the wealthy as well as from the poor. But when the generalization was subjected to the closer analysis afforded by actual records of influenza incidence in 1918 in enumerated populations, the interesting indication appeared that there were marked and consistent differences in its incidence-with respect both to morbidity and to mortality-among persons of different economic status.

Source: Sydenstricker, 1931 pp. 154–155.

The quote by Edgar Sydenstricker, the then statistician of the United States (US) Public Health Service, illustrates the intersection between pandemics, the SDH and health inequities. In a seminal analysis of the 1918–1919 influenza pandemic records, Sydenstricker demonstrated marked and consistent differences in both morbidity and mortality rates among persons of different socioeconomic status in the US (Sydenstricker, 1931). The study found that the influenza attack rate was higher among lower socioeconomic groups, even after adjusting for age, sex and certain other conditions (Sydenstricker, 1931).

Earlier in 2020, Bambra and colleagues summarised evidence from different studies which confirmed the inequalities in the 1918 influenza pandemic prevalence and mortality rates between high-income and low-income countries, more and less affluent neighbourhoods, higher and lower socioeconomic groups, and urban and rural areas (Bambra et al, 2020). For example, India had an influenza mortality rate 40 times higher than Denmark and the mortality rate was 20 times higher in some South American countries compared to Europe (Bambra et al, 2020).

South Africa was among the worst-hit countries in the world, with estimates of around 300 000 deaths because of the 1918 influenza pandemic (Phillips, 1984). Given the country's history of colonisation and apartheid, the white authorities used the influenza pandemic as an opportunity to implement oppressive, discriminatory legislation, such as residential segregation, that benefited the white population at the expense of the black majority (Finn and Kobayashi, 2020). Finn and Kobayashi have pointed out that the 1918–19 influenza pandemic has shaped, and continues to shape, South Africa's urban, spatial, and social landscapes (Finn and Kobayashi, 2020).

Definition of a syndemic

A syndemic is a set of intertwined and mutually enhancing epidemics involving disease interactions at the biological level that develop and are sustained in a community or population because of harmful social conditions and injurious social connections.

Source: Singer and Clair, 2003 p. 434.

In 2003, Singer and Clair coined the term 'syndemic' to refer to the intersection and interactions between epidemics, the SDH, and health inequities (Singer and Clair, 2003). They defined a syndemic as 'a set of intertwined and mutually enhancing epidemics involving disease interactions at the biological level that develop and are sustained in a community or population because of harmful social conditions and injurious social connections' (Singer and Clair, 2003 p. 434). Using the findings from a study among HIV-positive injecting drug users in the US, the authors argued that the 'recognition of the existence of syndemics suggests the need for a biosocial re-conception of disease', requiring a holistic approach that would address 'the structural violence of social inequality' (Singer and Clair, 2003 p. 434).

In the US, Pellowski et al demonstrated that the HIV epidemic is concentrated in socially marginalised and disenfranchised communities, such as communities of colour and sexual minorities (Pellowski et al, 2013). The inequities are driven by disparities in the structural and economic conditions faced by these groups, including environmental resource constraints, access to care, and psychosocial influences (Pellowski et al, 2013).

The 2020 Global AIDS update underscores the 'enormous, unfinished business of the HIV pandemic' (UNAIDS, 2020). Notwithstanding tremendous progress in managing HIV&AIDS, sub-Saharan Africa remains the worst-affected region (UNAIDS, 2020). The drivers of the HIV pandemic continue to be gender inequalities, gender-based violence and other SDH, with the report noting that 'the HIV epidemic continues to run along the fault lines of inequalities' (UNAIDS, 2020 p. 7). These inequities account for the gaps in HIV responses and resulting HIV infections and AIDS-related deaths (UNAIDS, 2020).

Figure 9.3 illustrates the relationship between HIV prevalence and income disparity in 46 sub-Saharan African countries (UNAIDS, 2020). The study found that after controlling for education, gender inequality and income per capita, a one-point increase in a country's 20:20 ratio (i.e. the ratio of average income of the wealthiest 20% to the poorest 20% of the population) corresponds to a two-point increase in HIV prevalence (UNAIDS, 2020).

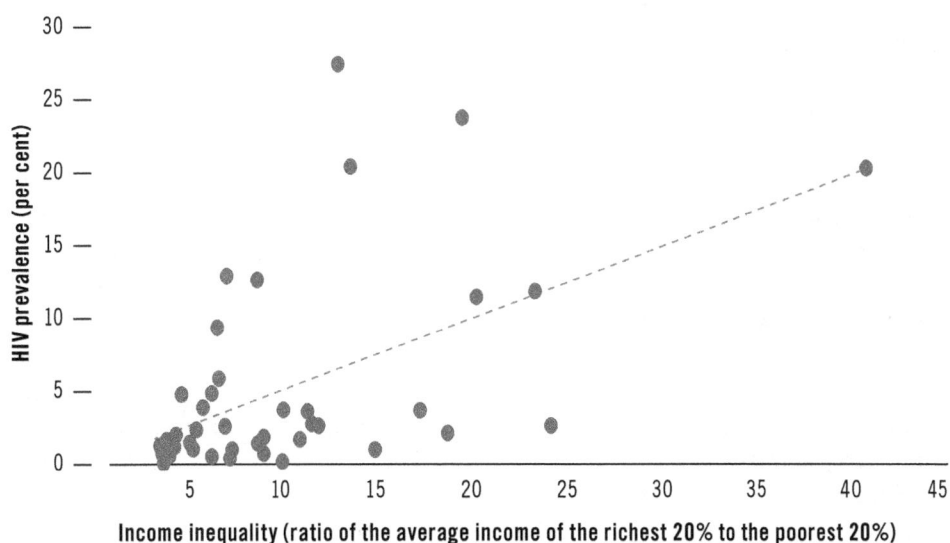

Figure 9.3: HIV prevalence and income inequality, sub-Saharan African countries, 2019

Source: UNAIDS, 2020 p. 17.

In 2012, Lowcock and colleagues examined the effects of the SDH on the 2009 H1N1 influenza severity and the role of clinical risk factors in mediating such associations in Ontario, Canada (Lowcock et al, 2012). The study found that the main clinical risk factors for severe H1N1 pandemic illness explained only a portion of the associations observed between the SDH and hospitalisation (Lowcock et al, 2012).

A 2019 case study on epidemics in Africa illustrated the inter-relatedness of disease outbreaks and the wider socioeconomic context, including health policy, infrastructure, staffing, funding, and governance models (Mazibuko, 2019).

The COVID-19 pandemic has amplified the pre-existing health inequities, with some calling for the pandemic to be recognised as a syndemic (Bambra et al, 2020; Horton, 2020). The disparities in the SDH result in differential exposure to the virus, differential vulnerability to infection and differential consequences of the disease (Bambra et al, 2020; Burström and Tao, 2020). Several scholars have pointed out that COVID-19 vulnerability is inequitably distributed, and is concentrated among communities that experience limited education, low socioeconomic status, unemployment, discrimination and structural racism (Bambra et al, 2020; Burström and Tao, 2020; Chiriboga et al, 2020; Gray et al, 2020; Rollston and Galea, 2020). In a country-level analysis of 50 countries with the highest number of cases, Chaudry et al found that a higher per cent unemployment rate was associated with an increased number of COVID-19 critical cases per million for any given country (Chaudhry et al, 2020). These SDH contribute to downstream adverse health outcomes, which are exacerbated by poor access to a high-quality healthcare system, itself an SDH. The healthcare system as an SDH is illustrated in a study by Khan et al that examined the association between healthcare capacity and COVID-19 case fatality rates (Khan et al, 2020). After adjusting for demographic, health expenditure, population density, and prior burden of non-communicable disease, the study found that greater healthcare capacity was related to lesser case fatality, with every additional unit increase in the healthcare capacity index associated with a 42% decrease in the case fatality (Khan et al, 2020).

The Global Network against Food Crises has highlighted that COVID-19 has placed an additional burden on fragile political and social systems, compounding existing risks, including conflict, economic crises, natural disasters, climate extremes/variability, serving as additional stresses on agri-food systems and exacerbating acute food insecurity (Global Network Against Food Crises, 2020). Although the impacts of COVID-19 on livelihoods and acute food insecurity are highly context-specific, a general worsening of acute food insecurity is being observed across several countries compared with the situation reported in 2019.

9.6   THE SDH AND THE COVID-19 PANDEMIC: A CASE STUDY OF SOUTH AFRICA

South Africa's rights-based Constitution provides the platform for the transformation efforts since the first democratic elections in 1994 (Republic of South Africa, 1996). Despite significant progress towards the vision of a 'free, non-racial and equal society', the 25-year review by the South African Presidency highlights the 'lingering challenges of social inequality, the enduring connection between race and poverty, gender and class disparities, unequal economic opportunities, and spatial exclusion' (The Presidency, 2019 p. 6).

South Africa remains one of the most unequal countries in the world, with a Gini coefficient of 0.68 (The Presidency, 2019). The table below highlights key aspects of the SDH in South Africa, found in a 2018 study that predates the COVID-19 pandemic.

Table 9.3: Pre-existing socioeconomic inequities in South Africa, 2018

1. Since 1994, South Africa has sought to address poverty and inequality with a wide range of initiatives, including the use of fiscal policy to support redistributive measures.

2. Consumption expenditure shows that South Africa is one of the most unequal countries in the world.

3. Although there is strong correlation between levels of inequality in consumption and wealth, wealth inequality is also high and has been growing over time.

4. High unemployment remains the key challenge for South Africa. The labour market is split into two extreme job types: a small number of people with highly paid jobs in largely formal sectors and larger enterprise, and, the majority of the population, who work in informal, poorly paid jobs.

5. Inequality of opportunity is high, measured by the influence of race, gender, parents' education, parents' occupation and place of birth.

6. South Africa has high levels of chronic poverty (almost half of the population) and a relatively small middle class.

7. Labour market incomes, education, gender and race are important drivers of inequality in South Africa

8. Food security has a clear spatial dimension; with rural areas recording the highest level of food insecurity compared to urban and farm areas.

Source: World Bank, 2018.

The National Income Dynamics Study (NIDS) – Coronavirus Rapid Mobile Survey (CRAM) conducted during 2020 has demonstrated that the impact of the measures used to combat the COVID-19 pandemic (e.g. the lockdown) has been uneven, exacerbating socioeconomic inequities by race, gender and geography (Spaull et al, 2020). The NIDS-CRAM study found that vulnerable populations in informal and precarious employment have been most affected by job losses and the resulting income loss, thus worsening the income inequalities (Spaull et al, 2020). Furthermore, 3 million jobs were lost between February and April 2020, or put differently, the percentage of reported unemployment increased from 43% to 53% (Spaull et al, 2020). The situation remained largely unchanged when measured again in June 2020 (Spaull et al, 2020). Black Africans and people with less than matric (completion of high or secondary school) reported the lowest employment recovery rates (Spaull et al, 2020). Similarly, rural areas have been more affected by job losses than urban areas (Spaull et al, 2020).

Women experienced greater job losses during the pandemic (Spaull et al, 2020). Between February and April, employment declined by 23% for women, compared to a decline of 10% for men (Spaull et al, 2020). The study found that childcare has had a disproportionate influence on women's labour market outcomes, compared to those of men (Spaull et al, 2020). In the second wave of the NIDS-CRAM study, 3.4 million women compared to 1.7 million men reported that difficulties in childcare prevented them from going to work or made work very difficult (Spaull et al, 2020). Importantly, wage inequality between men and women in the poorest 40% of the earning distribution (or category) has increased by a factor of up to five between February and June 2020 (Spaull et al, 2020).

The NIDS-CRAM study found that income had a much stronger relationship with health during the COVID-19 crisis than before (Nwosu and Oyenubi, 2020). Income-related health inequality in the COVID-19 period was six times higher compared to that obtained in the 2017 NIDS (Nwosu and Oyenubi, 2020). The key factors that predicted the observed income-related health inequalities in the COVID-19 era were race, hunger, and income (Nwosu and Oyenubi, 2020).

There was also increasing educational inequality during lockdown, with wealthy children twice as likely to attend school despite their grade being 'closed' (because of the lockdown regulations) compared to children in no-fee schools (Spaull et al, 2020).

In summary, the South African case study shows how the COVID-19 pandemic has worsened, and laid bare the pre-existing socioeconomic inequities.

9.7   ADDRESSING SDH AND HEALTH INEQUITIES DURING PANDEMICS

As shown in this chapter, pandemics are syndemics, often exposing the social injustice and deep social and economic inequities at both global and national levels (Chiriboga et al, 2020; Gray et al, 2020; Institute for Economic Justice, 350Africa. org and Climate Justice Coalition, 2020; Martin-Howard and Farmbry, 2020). At the same time, civil society organisations have pointed out that the extraordinary responses of government have demonstrated 'the realms of possibility when there is the appropriate political will' (Institute for Economic Justice, 350Africa.org and Climate Justice Coalition, 2020 p. 5). Furthermore, many have pointed out that the COVID-19 pandemic provides an opportunity to address the SDH and health inequities, through a people-centred approach and just economic recovery (Burström and Tao, 2020; Chiriboga et al, 2020; Gray et al, 2020; Institute for Economic Justice, 350Africa.org and Climate Justice Coalition, 2020; Martin-Howard and Farmbry, 2020; Rollston and Galea, 2020; UNAIDS, 2020).

The literature is replete with evidence and recommendations on the actions needed to address the SDH and health inequities (Commission on Social Determinants of Health, 2008; Global Preparedness Monitoring Board, 2019; United Nations, 2015; WHO, 2011). Instead of repeating these recommendations, we conclude this section with a call to action by health sciences educational institutions and civil society organisations to contribute to a transformative vision for society.

Although the CSDH, recommended that the SDH should be incorporated into the pre-service education and training of all health professionals, this is seen as a 'nice-to-have', rather than an essential component of the curriculum (Commission on Social Determinants of Health, 2008). Health sciences education institutions are in a unique position, as they are responsible for the production of the future generation of the health workforce. The COVID-19 pandemic requires rethinking educational systems and curricula to include the SDH, championed by senior faculty and powerful clinicians. We call on health sciences education institutions to provide strong ethical and accountable leadership to achieve these curriculum changes that have the SDH and health equity at the core.

We advocate for collective and individual action to address the social, economic and political factors that drive health inequities, because these factors are shaped by policies, which make them amenable to change or intervention. Civil society should develop structures and processes that support health equity and that confront structural and systemic racism, and other SDH. To this end, the launch of the Sustainable Health Equity Movement in July 2020 is an important initiative to highlight the role and importance of sustainable health equity in response to the pandemic and beyond (https://www.sustainablehealthequity.org/).

As highlighted, the COVID-19 pandemic amplifies pre-existing socio-economic and health inequities, hence the response to the *syndemic* needs to be comprehensive and equity-focused, prioritising interventions in resource-poor settings, and among poor communities. However, action is unlikely to happen unless there is strong advocacy from civil society. Such advocacy efforts should focus on populations or communities at high risk of exposure, and high risk of severe morbidity and mortality, and include universal mask use and social distancing policies, economic relief packages, universal labour laws to protect employment and to protect essential workers, and universal access to testing and vaccination, and appropriate care and treatment.

COVID-19 also provides the opportunity to reorient and revitalise information systems to collect data, broken down by SDH and to highlight and monitor health inequities. Civil society has a critical role to play in advocating for vaccines, testing, medicines and health technologies to be recognised as global public goods. This implies the abolition of pandemic-related patents, transparency and accountability frameworks for initiatives such as the Act tool Accelerator.

9.8   CONCLUSION

This chapter reviewed pandemics and their intersection with the SDH. We highlighted how the concept of SDH has its roots in antiquity, advanced by the Social Medicine movement in Latin America during the last century, and revitalised almost 60 years after the creation of WHO, through the CSDH (Carter, 2019; Commission on Social Determinants of Health, 2008; Iriart et al, 2002; Tountas, 2009). Although the SDH were incorporated in UN 2030 Sustainable Development Agenda, the lack of a cohesive approach, lack of binding mechanisms and international financial strategies, and weak metrics to hold governments accountable adversely affect implementation and demonstrable progress on the SDGs, both nationally and globally (United Nations, 2019).

Pandemics are not the 'great equalizers' they are portrayed to be. The COVID-19 pandemic, with untold hardship, suffering and devastation, has disproportionately affected the most vulnerable and disadvantaged populations worldwide, laying bare and amplifying the pre-existing social injustices both within and among countries and regions (Abrams and Szefler, 2020; Bambra et al, 2020; Burström and Tao, 2020; Chiriboga et al, 2020; Finn and Kobayashi, 2020; Gray et al, 2020; Horton, 2020). The existing disparities in the SDH have resulted in differential exposure to the virus, differential vulnerability to infection and differential consequences of the disease. This vulnerability is exacerbated by limited or non-existent access to high-quality healthcare systems, itself an SDH, and is directly associated with COVID-19 disease outcomes (Chaudhry et al, 2020; Khan et al, 2020). COVID-19 has also placed an additional burden on fragile political and social systems, compounding existing risks, including conflict, economic crises, natural disasters, climate extremes/variability, serving as additional stresses on agricultural and food supply systems and exacerbating acute food insecurity (Chiriboga et al, 2020; Global Network Against Food Crises, 2020).

At the same time, the COVID-19 pandemic also provides an opportunity to address the SDH and health inequities, through a people-centred approach and a fairer economic recovery (Chiriboga et al, 2020; Institute for Economic Justice, 350Africa.org and Climate Justice Coalition, 2020).

This chapter is a call to action by health sciences educational institutions and civil society organisations in all fields to contribute to a transformative vision for society. We recommend the inclusion of ethical leadership, the concept and principles of equity, and the SDH in pre-service education and the continuing professional development of all practising health professionals. We advocate for collective and individual action to address the social, economic and political factors that drive health inequities, because these factors are shaped by policies, which make them amenable to change or intervention.

This is a call for an ethical, comprehensive and global response to the pandemic. Such a pandemic response should incorporate all the healthcare system components, such as universal access to tests, vaccines and medical technologies and quality healthcare. Furthermore, the response should ensure the elimination of intellectual property rights for pandemic related medicines, and a strong, global, social and economic safety net to confront the devastating impact of the pandemic (Chiriboga et al, 2020; Institute for Economic Justice, 350Africa.org and Climate Justice Coalition, 2020). We need to build back more just societies, fighting the inhumane, austerity measures that have led to the unprecedented inequities worldwide, because we have failed to place the health of all people and the planet before short-sighted, unethical economic profit for a few.

The central message of this chapter is that an appropriate response to the COVID-19 pandemic requires the recognition of the centrality of addressing the SDH and health inequities in an integrated, inclusive, and multi-disciplinary approach.

9.9 SELF-ASSESSMENT QUESTIONS

1. Why is it important to address the SDH?
2. What action is needed to address the SDH and health inequities during pandemics?
3. What are the priority research areas on SDH and health equity?

9.10 REFERENCES

Abrams, E.M. and Szefler, S.J. 2020. COVID-19 and the impact of social determinants of health. *The Lancet. Respiratory Medicine* 8(7) doi:https://doi.org/10.1016/S2213-2600(20)30234-4.

Bambra, C., Riordan, R., Ford, J. and Matthews, F. 2020. The COVID-19 pandemic and health inequalities. *J Epidemiol Community Health* doi:10.1136/jech-2020-214401.

Blas, E. and Kurup, A.S. (Eds). 2010. *Equity, social determinants and public health programmes.* Geneva: WHO.

Bridgman, G., Van der Berg S. and Patel, L. 2020. Hunger in South Africa during 2020: Results from Wave 2 of NIDS-CRAM. Stellenbosch.

Burström, B., and Tao, W. 2020. Social determinants of health and inequalities in COVID-19. *European Journal of Public Health* 30(4), pp. 617–18.

Carter, E.D. 2019. Social medicine and international expert networks in Latin America, 1930–1945. *Global Public Health* 14(6–7), pp. 791–802.

Chaudhry, R., Dranitsaris, G., Mubashir, T., Bartoszko, J. and Riazi, S. 2020. A country level analysis measuring the impact of government actions, country preparedness and socioeconomic factors on COVID-19 mortality and related health outcomes. *EClinicalMedicine* 25, p. 100464.

Chiriboga, D., Garay, J., Buss, P., Madrigal, R.S. and Rispel, L.C. 2020. Health inequity during the COVID-19 pandemic: A cry for ethical global leadership. *The Lancet.*

Commission on Social Determinants of Health. 2008. Closing the gap in a health generation: Health equity through the social determinants of health. Geneva: World Health Organization.

Cueto, M., and Palmer, S. 2014. *Medicine and public health in Latin America: A history.* Cambridge: Cambridge University Press.

Finn, B.M. and Kobayashi, L.C. 2020. Structural inequality in the time of COVID-19: Urbanization, segregation, and pandemic control in sub-Saharan Africa. *Dialogues in Human Geography* 10(2), pp. 217–20.

Garay, J.E. and Chiriboga, D.E. 2017. A paradigm shift for socioeconomic justice and health: from focusing on inequalities to aiming at sustainable equity. *Public Health* 149, pp. 149–58.

Global Network Against Food Crises. 2020. Food Crises and COVID-19: Emerging evidence and implications. An analysis of acute food insecurity and agri-food systems during COVID-19 pandemic: Technical note. Brussels: European Union, Food and Agriculture Programme of the United Nations and World Food Programme.

Global Preparedness Monitoring Board. 2019. A world at risk: annual report on global preparedness for health emergencies. Geneva: World Health Organization.

Graham, H. 2004. Social determinants and their unequal distribution: clarifying policy understandings. *The Milbank Quarterly* 82(1), pp. 101–24.

Gray, D.M., Anyane-Yeboa, A., Balzora, S., Issaka, R.B. and May, F.P. 2020. COVID-19 and the other pandemic: Populations made vulnerable by systemic inequity. *Nature Reviews Gastroenterology & Hepatology* 17(9), pp. 520–22.

Hall, J.J. and Taylor, R. 2003. Health for all beyond 2000: The demise of the Alma-Ata Declaration and primary health care in developing countries. *The Medical Journal of Australia* 178(1), pp. 17–20.

Hartmann, C. 2016. Postneoliberal public health care reforms: Neoliberalism, social medicine, and persistent health inequalities in Latin America. *American Journal of Public Health* 106(12), pp. 2145–51.

Horton, R. 2020. Offline: COVID-19 is not a pandemic [Editorial]. *The Lancet* 396(10255), p. 874.

Institute for Economic Justice, 350Africa.org and Climate Justice Coalition. 2020. No going back to normal: Imagining a Just Recovery in South Africa. Braamfontein: The Institute for Economic Justice, 350Africa.org and the Climate Justice Coalition.

Iriart, C., Waitzkin, H., Breilh, J., Estrada, A. and Merhy, E.E. 2002. Latin American social medicine: contributions and challenges. *Revista Panamericana de Salud Pública* 12(2), pp. 128–36.

Irwin, A. and Scali, E. 2007. Action on the social determinants of health: A historical perspective. *Global Public health* 2(3), pp. 235–56.

Jong-Wook, L. 2005. Public health is a social issue. *The Lancet* 365(9464), pp. 1005–06.

Khan, J.R., Awan, N., Islam, M. and Muurlink, O. 2020. Healthcare capacity, health expenditure, and civil society as predictors of COVID-19 case fatalities: a global analysis. *Frontiers in Public Health* 8, p. 347: doi: 10.3389/fpubh.2020.00347.

Levine, P. N.d. Available at: https://peterlevine.ws/?p=20430.

Lowcock, E.C., Rosella, L.C., Foisy, J., McGeer, A. and Crowcroft, N. 2012. The social determinants of health and pandemic H1N1 2009 influenza severity. *American Journal of Public Health* 102(8), pp. e51–e58.

Martin-Howard, S. and Farmbry, K. 2020. Framing a needed discourse on health disparities and social inequities: Drawing lessons from a pandemic. *Public administration review* 80(5), pp. 839–44.

Mazibuko, Z. (Ed). 2019. *Epidemics and the health of African nations.* Johannesburg: Mapungubwe Institute for Strategic Reflection (MISTRA).

Nwosu, C. and Oyenubi, A. 2020. COVID-19: How the lockdown has affected the health of the poor in South Africa. in *The Conversation*. Johannesburg. Available at: https://theconversation.com/covid-19-how-the-lockdown-has-affected-the-health-of-the-poor-in-south-africa-144374?utm_medium=email&utm_ca%E2%80%A6.

Paintsil, E. 2020. COVID-19 threatens health systems in sub-Saharan Africa: The eye of the crocodile. *Journal of Clinical Investigation* 130(6).

Pan American Health Organization. 2019. Just Societies: Health Equity and Dignified Lives. Executive Summary of the Report of the Commission of the Pan American Health Organization on Equity and Health Inequalities in the Americas. Revised edition. Washington, D.C.: Pan American Health Organization (PAHO).

Pellowski, J.A., Kalichman, S.C., Matthews, K.A. and Adler, N. 2013. A pandemic of the poor: Social disadvantage and the US HIV epidemic. *American Psychologist* 68(4), pp. 197–209. doi:10.1037/a0032694.

Phillips, H. 1984. Black October: The impact of the Spanish influenza epidemic of 1918 on South Africa. In *Historical Studies*. Cape Town: University of Cape Town.

Republic of South Africa. 1996. Constitution of the Republic of South Africa 1996, Act 108 of 1996.

Rollston, R. and Galea, S. 2020. COVID-19 and the social determinants of health. *American Journal of Health Promotion* 34(6), pp. 687–89.

Singer, M. and Clair, S. 2003. Syndemics and Public Health: Reconceptualizing disease in bio-social context. *Medical Anthropology Quarterly* 17(4), pp. 423–41.

Solar, O. and Irwin, A. 2007. A conceptual framework for action on the social determinants of health: Discussion paper for the Commission on Social Determinants of Health. Geneva: World Health Organization, Commission on Social Determinants of Health.

Spaull, N., Oyenubi, A., Kerr, A., Maughan-Brown, B., Ardington, C., Christian, C., Shepherd, D., Casale, D., Espi, G., Wills, G., Bridgman, G., Bhorat, H., Turok, I., Bassier, I., Kika-Mistry, J., Kotze, J., Budlender, J., Visagie, J., Ingle, K., Rossouw, L., Patel, L., Benhura, M., Leibbrandt, M., Mohohlwane, N., Magejo, P., English, R., Daniels, R.C., Hill, R., Zizzamia, R., Jain, R. and Burger, R. 2020. National Income Dynamics Study (NIDS) – Coronavirus Rapid Mobile Survey (CRAM): Wave 2 Synthesis Report. Stellenbosch.

Sydenstricker, E. 1931. The incidence of influenza among persons of different economic status during the epidemic of 1918. *Public Health Reports (1896-1970)*, pp. 154–70.

The Presidency, South Africa. 2019. *Towards a 25 year review: 1994–2019.* Pretoria: Government Printing Works.

Therborn, G. 2012. The killing fields of inequality. *International Journal of Health Services* 42(4), pp. 579–89.

Tountas, Y. 2009. The historical origins of the basic concepts of health promotion and education: the role of ancient Greek philosophy and medicine. *Health Promotion International* 24(2), pp. 185–92.

UNAIDS. 2020. Seizing the moment global AIDS update | 2020. Tackling entrenched inequalities to end epidemics. New York: United Nations, Joint United Nations AIDS Programme (UNAIDS).

United Nations. 2015. Transforming our world: the 2030 Agenda for Sustainable Development. New York: United Nations.

United Nations. 2019. Report of the Secretary-General on SDG Progress 2019: Special Edition. New York: United Nations.

Waitzkin, H., Iriart, C., Estrada, A. and Lamadrid, S. 2001. Social medicine then and now: lessons from Latin America. *American Journal of Public Health* 91(10), pp. 1592–601.

WHO. 1978. Alma-Ata 1978: Primary health care. Geneva: World Health Organization.

WHO. 2011. Rio Political Declaration on Social Determinants of Health, World Conference on Social Determinants of Health, Rio de Janeiro, Brazil, 21 October 2011.

WHO. 2006. Constitution of the World Health Organization, Basic Documents, Forty-fifth edition, Supplement. Geneva: World Health Organization.

WHO Europe. 2020. Strengthening the health system response to COVID-19 Maintaining the delivery of essential health care services while mobilizing the health workforce for the COVID-19 response. Copenhagen: World Health Organization Regional Office for Europe.

World Bank. 2018. Overcoming poverty and inequality in South Africa: An assessment of drivers, opportunities and constraints. Washington D.C.: The World Bank.

CHAPTER 10

PANDEMICS: MANAGING PSYCHOSOCIAL DIMENSIONS FOR THE PUBLIC GOOD

Garth Stevens[1]

10.1   INTRODUCTION

The psychosocial dimensions of pandemics have historically been poorly researched and even less understood by those tasked with the responsibility of care and authoritative leadership during disease outbreaks, epidemics, and pandemics. Understandably, this is because pandemics are global events that do not present with high frequency during the normal human lifespan, while epidemics are often localised geographically, and the extant knowledge bases related to their management are therefore not as rapidly evolving as with more habitually encountered diseases.

Often featuring as a secondary consideration to the immediate and sometimes catastrophic health, social and economic consequences, there is perhaps much less attention directed towards the centrality of psychosocial dimensions (i.e. the intersecting psychological, behavioural and social factors) in the transmission, spread and potential containment of infectious diseases and contagions. This chapter engages with this apparent paradox, in order to foreground the importance of a more holistic approach to pandemic management.

It also highlights the most common psychological effects of pandemics, including increased health awareness and help-seeking behaviours, amplified levels of anxiety and depression, compassion fatigue, burnout, substance abuse, interpersonal violence, stigma, etc., in order to adequately consider how mental health services may require additional injections of resources, at the level of both upskilling and upscaling.

The chapter then unpacks some of the key mechanisms for enhancing broader prosocial behaviour in times of pandemics, which is often scaffolded on population confidence in governance and science, and the generation of a consensus of common plight, ultimately yielding increased levels of empathy, altruism, social compliance with any restrictive social regulations, and actions in the service of the broader public good.

---

[1]   All correspondence should be directed to the author at Garth.Stevens@wits.ac.za

However, it also highlights the limitations of this level of adherence and points to the need to anticipate and mitigate the inevitability of behavioural non-adherence and vaccine hesitancy as populations transcend the fear threshold for morbidity and mortality. This is especially the case when initial social compacts in times of pandemics are undermined by pre-existing levels of inequality and social fault lines, that ultimately result in differentiated experiences of pandemics and their consequences across heterogeneous populations.

Finally, the chapter explores the relationship between scientific knowledge and political governance in managing pandemics across large populations. It recognises the critical role of science in guiding this process, but also acknowledges its limitations, and suggests that it must be combined with savvy and compassionate political governance, communication strategies, and advocacy, to optimise prosociality within populations in times of pandemics.

10.2 OBJECTIVES

The objectives of this chapter are therefore:
- To comprehend the centrality of the psychosocial dimensions of managing pandemics in the service of the public good.
- To understand the common psychological consequences of pandemics, in order to develop more responsive healthcare and mental healthcare management systems.
- To examine the processes and factors underpinning prosocial behavioural adherence during times of pandemics, in order to maximise population volition in the creation of widespread health and well-being, oriented towards the collective good.
- To anticipate non-adherence to prosocial behaviours in times of pandemics, and to consider how to mitigate the underlying drivers that compromise collective prosocial responses.
- To suggest ways in which we can develop an awareness of the relationships between scientific knowledge, political governance, and the psychosocial management of pandemics.

10.3 A PSYCHOSOCIAL APPROACH

In the context of most pandemics, the immediate responses (and correctly so) are initially focused on the provision of primary interventions (e.g. vaccine delivery), secondary interventions (e.g. containment strategies for patients in health facilities), and tertiary interventions (e.g. health interventions to attenuate the long-term effects of disease) to minimise the health impacts on populations. The psychosocial elements of pandemics are often relegated to a set of ancillary interventions, but herein lies a paradox. Where health systems are fragile or underdeveloped, when services are still being ramped up, or where the health science of pandemics is still evolving, we require an understanding of the psychosocial dimensions of pandemics, as they are crucial to helping contain the psychological effects and physical transmission of the disease through an awareness of the social and psychological context of contagion control and suppression. In the context of the COVID-19 pandemic, for example, social distancing, mask-wearing, and frequent hand-washing are some basic examples of the non-pharmacological interventions that have played an important role in flattening the curve of infections. But understanding why these are taken up or disavowed by populations requires an intimate understanding of the drivers of behaviour, from both a psychological and social perspective.

Frosh (2010) offers some insights into the idea of a psychosocial framework, when he speaks of the psychosocial as being concerned with the interplay between what is typically understood as external social reality and the psychological elements of human interaction, thereby problematising the simplistic division of inner and outer realities. As Saville-Young (2011) notes, a psychosocial framework questions the traditional division of the personal and the social, arguing instead for a psychosocial zone where the social and the psychological are both involved in the simultaneous and ongoing co-construction of one another. This approach helps us to understand the interface between socio-structural and psychological constituents in the production of effects and responses to pandemics today, and how they are intertwined with other aspects of social life such as race, gender, class, inequality, spatial geographies, etc. Stated differently, this framework allows us to contemplate how psychological elements such as emotions, affective responses, and behavioural repertoires are mutually and reciprocally influenced by social conditions such as the prevailing political, economic, and cultural domains of social life (Stevens, Duncan and Hook, 2013).

10.4   PSYCHOLOGICAL SEQUELAE OF PANDEMICS

There are a plethora of psychological sequelae that often accompany pandemics, but these sometimes only surface as the pandemic becomes embedded in the collective consciousness of a society, as a significant threat to health and well-being. There is thus often a temporal lag, and health and mental health systems can be caught unprepared for their impact.

For example, levels of health and bodily awareness, information-seeking, and help-seeking behaviours can commonly spike in the context of epidemics and pandemics. Randle, Nelder, Sider and Hohenadel (2018) found significantly increased levels of web-searches, telemedicine calls, doctor visitations, and laboratory testing amongst Canadians in the immediate aftermath of the 2016 Zika virus outbreak in Brazil, revealing a level of awareness, but also anxiety about the potential transmission of the virus. Similar findings have also been described in the context of the Ebola virus outbreak in 2014 (Blakey, Reuman, Jacoby and Abramowitz, 2015), with the exacerbation of transmission risk fears after public awareness of the disease outbreak.

Related to this form of health anxiety, the fear of death (or death anxiety) has also been shown to increase in mortality salient situations such as pandemics, where death rates appear, or are reported, to be higher than usual or in excess of the general mortality rates in a given context. Arrowood, Cox, Kersten, Routledge, Shelton and Hood (2017) have suggested that this anxiety increases individuals' access to death-related thoughts and defensive behaviours, manifesting in cognitive distortions and the possibility for compulsivity in behavioural repertoires. More generally, contamination fears can escalate obsessional thoughts related to death, which are then temporarily offset by compulsive behaviours (Aardema, 2020), such as excessive hand-washing and overuse of sanitisers in the context of the COVID-19 pandemic.

In South Africa, parallel findings have been recorded during the COVID-19 pandemic, with higher self-reported rates of anxiety and depression associated with self-isolation, quarantine, social isolation and limited social contact with others during restrictive social conditions such as 'lockdown' (SADAG, 2020). In a survey conducted by the American Psychological Association (APA, 2020), most psychologists who treated anxiety and depressive disorders reported an increase in patients seeking treatment, again highlighting the relationship between pandemic conditions and neurotic symptoms, and disproportionately affecting monitories who are more marginalised within society.

Several studies have also shown higher rates of drug and alcohol abuse during the COVID-19 pandemic, for example, and even though all of these increases may not be attributable to the pandemic, resilience-promoting activities such as physical exercise have not always been deemed safe; there has thus been an increase in dysfunctional behaviours to help people cope under stressful conditions (APA, 2020).

Recent studies of frontline healthcare workers have also revealed significantly higher levels of burnout and fatigue in managing high patient loads in health facilities caring for COVID-19 patients (Lasalvia et al, 2021), but also higher levels of compassion fatigue when de-sensitisation to death occurs and frontline healthcare workers are expected to make daily decisions about resource rationing and utilisation in the context of critical care (Alharbi, Jackson and Usher, 2020). This of course is all the more challenging under conditions of fiscal austerity in countries with struggling economies, where health systems are often threatened by under-resourcing.

Interpersonal violence, and violence against women in particular, tends to increase in most social emergencies or crises, including epidemics and pandemics.

Stress, disruption of socially protective schemes and networks, economic distress and decreased access to services can exacerbate the risk for gender-based violence. Escalated emotional tension can occur under these 'lockdown' conditions where troubled family members spend more time together, resulting in greater risks for domestic violence (WHO, 2021).

In its comparison of the challenge of stigma in the context of both the AIDS and COVID-19 pandemics, UNAIDS (2020a) notes that stigma and discrimination can rapidly follow after the initial fear and uncertainty associated with pandemics. This can expose people to violence, harassment and isolation, and hamper disclosure of health statuses, the uptake of essential health services, and the rollout of public health measures. Stigma can then also take on a socially inflected form by victim-blaming of marginal groups along social cleavages of race, socioeconomic status, occupation, gender, immigration status, social geographies and sexual orientation. Similar experiences in other epidemics such as those associated with Tuberculosis and Polio outbreaks have also been found historically, reducing health-seeking behaviours as disclosure was curtailed by elements of contagion-fear, shunning and social shaming.

All of the above are predictors of generally poorer mental health outcomes for populations, but in the context of frontline healthcare workers, they also increase the likelihood of increased errors and the potential for a lower quality of care (Alharbi, Jackson and Usher, 2020).

Clearly, responses to mitigate and remediate these psychosocial sequelae are required right at the outset of any pandemic, and not as an ancillary set of interventions. Some of these interventions may include developing an awareness of the differential vulnerabilities across populations; developing appropriate psychosocial referral networks; upskilling practitioners in appropriate therapeutic modalities; building social cohesion through community interventions to offset the effects of stigmatisation; providing sound and timely information through communication strategies to dispel myths and reduce anxiety and uncertainty; ramping up health and mental health systems to avoid burnout and compassion fatigue; and implementing policy measures proactively to ensure adequate funding/resourcing of appropriate psychosocial and health services.

10.5   FOSTERING A CULTURE IN THE SERVICE OF THE PUBLIC GOOD

One of the key questions that will face decision-makers within the context of a national or global emergency such as a pandemic, is how to ensure that the population at large acts in the service of a collective good rather than simply in the direction of individual self-interest. This is key to any contagion containment and suppression strategy, as population buy-in is essential to rupturing disease transmission cycles within communities and other spaces of daily living, especially where state enforcement is simply not possible, or where the reach of various arms of government can be weak or unevenly developed in parts of countries, and where behavioural interventions can inhibit further disease transmission. While some enforcement strategies will invariably be necessary for most national and global emergencies, decision-makers ultimately need to strive for population volition, and a sense of empowerment and ownership, if individuals are to act in the service of the public good.

The concept of the public good is generally understood to be any service or product, that is equally available to all in a given society, in ways that are both non-rivalrous and non-exclusionary. In other words, the use of the service or product by some should not exclude others from obtaining that service, nor should the service or product be so scarce that only some can enjoy it on a competitive basis and at the expense of others. In the context of global pandemics, services and products that are central to population health and well-being are a key public good, and decision-makers must consider how to promote population-level actions that act to maintain that public good for all.

Such a culture of acting in the service of the public good is scaffolded upon several features. Population confidence in structures of governance and those in authoritative positions to make decisions that are equitable across a heterogeneous society is crucial, scientific information and outcomes need to be rationally and fairly deployed for all, resources need to be as evenly distributed as possible, and where social constraints are necessary, they must be equally endured across variable populations. The extent to which this is successful will determine the degree to which a society is able to engender a consensus of common plight, generate increased levels of empathy, a sense of collective altruism based on a shared future, and ultimately, actions in the service of the public good.

But all of this pivots on how decision-makers address the question of heterogeneous populations, especially in the context of high levels of inequality. During the early phases of the COVID-19 'lockdown' in South Africa, the sale of alcohol was banned. While the actual merits of that decision will continue to be debated into the future, the central driver of this decision appeared to be an attempt to minimise hospital admissions related to violence and injuries that are frequently associated with alcohol consumption. It would have been untenable to decide to close taverns and bars in working-class communities, while allowing high-end restaurants with more affluent patrons to continue sipping on Chardonnay! Simply put, this social constraint or impingement needed to be evenly endured by all. Similarly, with the resumption of teaching and learning through emergency remote modalities in the education sector after the initial period of 'lockdown', this entitlement or right needed to be evenly distributed. More affluent students with access to data, computing devices and high-speed fibre connectivity had to be matched with the provision of computing devices, data, and connectivity for those less privileged. Again, irrespective of the merits of these decisions, the crucial lesson to be learnt here is that distributional regimes for both social constraints or impingements as well as entitlements or rights must be as evenly deployed as possible, especially in contexts of inequality within social formations. Failure to adopt such a position is likely to increase existing experiences of inequality and foster resistance to any sense of a collective good.

10.6   FURTHER IMPEDIMENTS TO POPULATION VOLITION IN PROSOCIAL BEHAVIOUR

Population non-adherence to prosocial and health-promoting behaviours such as non-pharmacological interventions, ultimately occurs when the fear threshold for morbidity and mortality of self and others, is transcended. Stated differently, when cohorts within populations start to experience the adherence to prosocial behaviour as more 'costly' to them or others than the threat of death or disease, these behaviours will diminish in favour of non-adherence. But inherent cost-benefit analyses are not the only factors that allow for the transcending of the fear threshold; several psychological, socioeconomic, and knowledge-related factors may impede population volition in prosocial and health-promoting behaviours.

Recently, for example, behavioural non-adherence has been increasingly evident and witnessed during the protracted COVID-19 pandemic. Non-pharmacological interventions that include mask-wearing, social-distancing, hand-sanitising, deep-cleaning, health status disclosure, self-isolation, self-quarantine, etc. have all waxed and waned over the course of several months (see for example, Haischer et al, 2020). Part of this variable uptake is related to the science of the pandemic constantly evolving, revealing which of these interventions have greater levels of efficacy. In other instances, it surfaces a very real reduction in the traction that these interventions have amongst populations. Even technological advancements such as tracking and tracing apps that can promote prosocial behaviour have not always been taken up. For example, whilst there are some 25 million mobile phone users across South Africa's population of approximately 60 million (Statista, 2021), the government-sponsored tracking and tracing app has been downloaded by only a fraction of users. In addition, we also ironically see increasing levels of vaccine hesitancy, even as the dominant narrative of how we return to a sense of normalcy is being constructed through vaccine adherence. How do we then understand the apparently declining levels of traction for what is broadly considered health-promoting and prosocial behaviour in times of pandemics?

At a psychological level, one of the most widespread mechanisms to cope with the traumatic possibilities of death and disease, is through the denial of personal risk and vulnerability. This mode of response is not uncommon, of course, as we have seen similar trajectories in health research on HIV and AIDS, as well as in sexually transmitted infections (UNAIDS, 2000b). Alongside this is the concept of pandemic fatigue, which is perhaps best described as the everyday burnout experienced from the perpetual pressures of pandemics that come to constitute every aspect of our lives. The psychological burden associated with pandemics can thus result in a compensatory response to avoid and deny risk, resulting in complacency and declining investments in health-promoting and prosocial behaviour. Regarding vaccine hesitancy – the delay in acceptance, or refusal of vaccines when available – several cultural, religious, and psychological motives are often drawn upon, and may not only reflect a knowledge deficit (Shen and Dubey, 2019; Robertson et al, 2021). Certainly, one of the key features in the psychological construction of contemporary human subjects is that we are encouraged to take individual control of our own healthcare in many respects – tracking our heart rates and blood pressure, our activity levels, our sleep patterns, our weight, and seeking health information and knowledge independently of practitioners. Under these circumstances, there is an increasing devolution of expertise to individual citizens themselves, making population-level compliance with expert directives less likely in some instances. In thinking about how to address these challenges, several possibilities arise. While we may be tempted to simply suggest the provision of more accurate information and knowledge, and to persuade those non-adherent members of a population to act in the interest of a collective good, the risk of alienation is greater if such an approach is adopted. Fundamentally, the social crisis of the pandemic has been devolved to the realm of individual and personal self-management, and this level of burden means that many simply opt to disengage publicly or to retreat into their individual self-interest as they manage their own fears and anxieties. What is perhaps required under these circumstances are interventions that provide accurate information on updated knowledge for informed debate and decision-making, foregrounding the pandemic as a public crisis and not one for individual self-management, and fostering intercommunal spaces for dialogue that also implicitly stimulate social cohesion and solidarity. In this way, the public crisis is managed by multiple publics, and is not left to the domain of self-management for individuals who are retreating from public life.

In the social and economic terrains, many within a population will make the decision that the costs to livelihoods are simply too great, and that riskier behaviours must inevitably be engaged in, while health-promoting prosocial behaviour needs to be placed on the backburner (see for example, Staunton, Swanepoel and Labuschaigne, 2020). Livelihoods can of course also include social dimensions that are compromised when there are expectations of populations to act in the direction of the public good (e.g. being isolated from family, friends and loved ones). Pull factors towards maintaining livelihoods may reduce the investment in prosocial and health-promoting behaviours. While this is particularly the case for those in unequal and precarious economic positions within a society, it is even more the case when the broader economic climate is also ailing. Inequality, under these circumstances, drives a differential experience of pandemics and their consequences across heterogeneous populations. For the marginal, there may be an expectation of a foreshortened future in which death is inevitable, and where the pursuit of living in the moment is thus elevated. Adherence to non-pharmacological interventions may therefore be negatively impacted upon. For others, the adage that *only a life worth living is a life worth saving*, will have strong resonance, and so cultivating a sense of protecting human life during pandemics must include the protection of *all* human life, especially in unequal societies. Examples of bailout packages to prevent economic catastrophe in business and higher rates of consequent unemployment, sustained social security safety nets and protections, and pandemic-related grants, are all examples of interventions that have the capacity to reduce population-level disparities, maintain livelihoods, and buttress prosocial behaviours if they are appropriately implemented.

Access to limited information and knowledge, poor information and knowledge, or an over exposure to too much information and knowledge, can also hamper a population's behavioural adherence in times of pandemics by creating increased levels of confusion. For example, as the science of pandemics evolves, questions about incubation, transmission, mitigation, and so forth, are constantly changing in the early days of scientific inquiry. Poor communication of accurate information and knowledge compromises sound decision-making in many instances. Communication, right from the outset, should stress that the information and knowledge will change rapidly as more becomes known, so that populations expect and are prepared for a degree of contradictory information as the science evolves. Information and knowledge should also be communicated timeously and with a degree of regularity to ensure that this becomes routinised within the social sphere. Importantly, populations need to understand the rationale behind decision-making and how information and knowledge contribute to that process. Poorly rationalised decisions by those in authority are likely to be rejected and resisted. It requires the translation of complex forms of scientific rationality into the most accessible forms of understanding, for heterogenous populations who will have different knowledge bases from which they are departing. These are all likely to foster a baseline of commonly shared information within a society at a given point in time within a pandemic, creating the potential basis for common prosocial action.

10.7   SCIENCE, POLITICS AND GOVERNANCE IN PANDEMICS

The COVID-19 pandemic has provided us with some insights into the complex but vital relationship between science, politics and governance during health emergencies of this magnitude. In reflecting on the development of this relationship, a broad sequencing of events could be identified in many parts of the world as countries attempted to manage the global pandemic. Initially, governments took a wait-and-see approach, but when the nature and scale of the challenge became apparent, they rapidly turned to scientists for direction on immediate contagion containment and longer-term prevention and possible eradication of the virus. Health scientists, in particular, were at the forefront of many debates and guided many of the initial critical decisions. While this was important, there was less emphasis placed on the economic, socio-cultural, and psychosocial dimensions of these decisions, and this was perhaps a limitation in this developing relationship between science, politics and governance. In many countries, some immediate decisions were met with a degree of public resistance (e.g. cigarette and alcohol bans, closure of industries, etc.). Political leaders soon became mindful of the range of political and related consequences to decision-making, and in some instances, overtly political decisions were then made through cherry-picking selective elements of the evolving health science. Again, this was a limitation, as decisions were sometimes being made primarily from a political vantage point and at the expense of other considerations. At this point, perhaps belatedly, many political leaders started to incorporate larger advisory teams into the decision-making process, as it was clear that there would be cascading effects into every aspect of society. Instructive for us is the important role that science can play in guiding decision-making, but this should include multiple forms of science right from the outset (i.e. health, economic, social, etc.). While forms of governance do have to consider the prevailing political conditions, savvy governance is compassionate and sensitive to the human and political dimensions, but should also be acting by mobilising the full range of intellectual, industrial and civil resources of a country to the maximum.

As indicated earlier, sound governance must also include the communication of accurate information, knowledge, decisions and their underlying rationales, in ways that are clear, and consistent for populations to apprehend. The importance of communicating scientific knowledge is central to any large-scale emergency, and the crisis management that is required in its immediate wake – especially when levels of education and literacy are variable across populations.

Similarly, savvy governance involves the balancing of lives and livelihoods in contexts of pandemics, but it again must draw on the resources of those in various sectors to be at the leading edge of predicting future consequential developments. Good governance not only attends to the immediacy of the crisis but must anticipate the effects thereof in the aftermath. Some examples, in recent times, have included fundamental impacts on the ways in which we think about the nature and future of work, remote forms of work, education and remote access, and technological leaps that were catalysed by the COVID-19 pandemic. Planning for the distal consequences in the aftermath of a pandemic is as critical as attenuating its proximal effects.

Sound political governance must also rely on a range of resources in society to guide its own advocacy drives inside a global geopolitical terrain that is uneven. In relation to advocacy within the COVID-19 pandemic, vaccine development, production, procurement, equitable distribution, and rollout are all excellent examples of where some political leaders were either exemplary, or simply failed to act expeditiously. The nature of advocacy of course also requires the harnessing of the resources of a society as it contends with global inequality across countries, variable purchase power capacities, international law, requests for cost caps and skills transfers, and must contend with elements such as vaccine nationalism and pandemic profiteering, amongst others. Governments have to act decisively in managing the crisis locally, on the one hand, but also have to proactively advocate for the population's interests globally, on the other hand.

For far too long, the relationship between science, politics and governance has either been denied, or deliberately obfuscated. For the political establishment, this has also meant a declining relationship to its constituencies as a political base, as populations increasingly second-guess the rationality of political decision-making. What is apparent from our recent experiences is that the success of the overall management of pandemics will require a deliberate and new social contract between those tasked with political governance, knowledge workers, industries, and the citizenry more broadly. In this way, a more holistic approach to managing pandemics may be possible when we are next confronted with one.

10.8 CONCLUSION

This chapter has outlined the centrality of incorporating the psychosocial dimensions of disease outbreaks, epidemics, and pandemics into a more inclusive strategy for their management. In arguing for a psychosocial approach, it stresses the importance of a layered, cross-disciplinary, intersectoral, and contextual process to understanding population effects and responses in times of large-scale emergencies of this nature. By exploring some of the common psychological sequelae of pandemics; the factors underpinning prosocial behavioural adherence or behavioural non-adherence during such crises; and the relationships between scientific knowledge and political governance; it suggests that comprehensive strategies to address the health, psychological, behavioural and social components of pandemics are best considered from the very outset of any outbreak, to ensure optimal responsiveness to overall population health and well-being.

10.9 SELF-ASSESSMENT QUESTIONS

1. What are some of the psychological effects that are experienced within populations during pandemics?

2. What are some of the interventions and strategies that can be employed to mitigate the psychological sequelae of pandemics for populations?

10.10 REFERENCES

Aardema, F. 2020. COVID-19, obsessive-compulsive disorder and invisible life forms that threaten the self. *Journal of Obsessive-Compulsive and Related Disorders* 26, p. 100558. https://doi.org/10.1016/j.jocrd.2020.100558.

Alharbi, J., Jackson, D. and Usher, K. 2020. The potential for COVID-19 to contribute to compassion fatigue in critical care nurses. *Journal of Clinical Nursing* 29 (15–16), pp. 2762–2764. https://doi.org/10.1111/jocn.15314.

APA. 2020. *Stress in America 2020*. Washington, D.C.: APA.

Arrowood, R.B., Cox, C., Kersten, M., Routledge, C., Shelton, J.T. and Hood, R.W. 2017. Ebola salience, death-thought accessibility, and worldview defense: A terror management theory perspective. *Death Studies* 41(9), pp. 585–591. https://doi.org/10.1080/07481187.2017.1322644.

Blakey, S.M., Reuman, L., Jacoby, R.J. and Abramowitz, J.S. 2015. Tracing "fearbola": Psychological predictors of anxious responding to the threat of Ebola. *Cognitive Therapy and Research* 39(6), pp. 816–825. https://doi.org/10.1007/s10608-015-9701-9.

Frosh, S. 2010. *Psychoanalysis outside the clinic: Interventions in psychosocial studies.* London & New York: Palgrave.

Haischer, M.H., Beilfuss, R., Hart, M.R., Opielinski, L., Wrucke, D., Zirgaitis, G., Uhrich, T.D. and Hunter, S.K. 2020. Who is wearing a mask? Gender-, age-, and location-related differences during the COVID-19 pandemic. *PloS one* 15(10), p. e0240785. https://doi.org/10.1371/journal.pone.0240785.

Lasalvia, A., Amaddeo, F., Porru, S., Carta, A., Tardivo, S., Bovo, C., Ruggeri, M. and Bonetto, C. 2021. Levels of burn-out among healthcare workers during the COVID-19 pandemic and their associated factors: A cross-sectional study in a tertiary hospital of a highly burdened area of north-east Italy. *BMJ Open* 11, p. e0455127. https://doi.org/10.1136/bmjopen-2020-045127.

Randle, J., Nelder, M., Sider, D. and Hohenadel, K. 2018. Characterizing the health and information-seeking behaviours of Ontarians in response to the Zika virus outbreak. *Canadian Journal of Public Health/Revue Canadienne de Sante Publique* 109(1), pp. 99–107. https://doi.org/10.17269/s41997-018-0026-9.

Robertson, E., Reeve, K.S., Niedzwiedz, C.L., Moore, J., Blake, M., Green, M., Katikireddi, S.V. and Benzeval, M. 2021. Predictors of COVID-19 vaccine hesitancy in the UK household longitudinal study. *Brain, Behaviour and Immunity* 94(2021), pp. 41–50. https://doi.org/10.1016/j.bbi.2021.03.008.

SADAG. 2020. SADAG online survey on COVID-19 and mental health. Available at: https://www.sadag.org/index.php?option=com_content&view=article&id=3092: sadag-s-online-survey-findings-on-covid-19-and-mental-health-21-april-2020&catid=149&Itemid=132.

Saville-Young, L. 2011. Research entanglements, race and recognisability: A psychosocial reading of interview encounters in (post-)colonial, (post-) apartheid South Africa. *Qualitative Inquiry* 17(1), pp. 45–55.

Shen, S.C. and Dubey, V. 2019. Addressing vaccine hesitancy: Clinical guidance for primary care physicians working with parents. *Canadian Family Physician/ Medecin de Famille Canadien* 65(3), pp. 175–181.

Statista. 2021. Number of smartphone users in South Africa from 2014 to 2023. Available at: https://www.statista.com/statistics/488376/forecast-of-smartphone-users-in-south-africa/.

Staunton, C., Swanepoel, C. and Labuschaigne, M. 2020. Between a rock and a hard place: COVID-19 and South Africa's response, *Journal of Law and the Biosciences* 7(1), lsaa052. https://doi.org/10.1093/jlb/lsaa052.

Stevens, G., Duncan, N. and Hook, D. 2013. The Apartheid Archive Project, the psychosocial and political Praxis. In G. Stevens, N. Duncan and D. Hook (Eds.). *Race, memory and the apartheid archive: Towards a transformative psychosocial praxis*. London/Johannesburg: Palgrave Macmillan/Wits University Press, pp. 1–17.

UNAIDS. 2020a. *Addressing stigma and discrimination in the COVID-19 response.* Geneva. UNAIDS.

UNAIDS. 2020b. *HIV and AIDS-related stigmatization, discrimination and denial: Forms, contexts and determinants. Research studies from Uganda and India.* Geneva: UNAIDS.

WHO. 2021. Levels of domestic violence increase globally, including in the Region, as COVID-19 pandemic escalates. WHO EMRO. Available at: http://www.emro.who.int/violence-injuries-disabilities/violence-news/levels-of-domestic-violence-increase-as-covid-19-pandemic-escalates.html.

WHY HEALTH ECONOMICS INPUT AND OTHER ECONOMIC CONSIDERATIONS ARE NECESSARY FOR MANAGING PANDEMICS

David Francis

Imraan Valodia

11.1 INTRODUCTION

The COVID-19 pandemic has highlighted the lack of integration between health policy and economic policy. In the immediate aftermath of the early spread of the SARS-CoV-2 virus, most countries, including South Africa, imposed hard lockdowns to curb the spread of the virus. The hard lockdowns had significant deleterious impacts on an economy that was already facing significant growth and public finance challenges. While there is debate about the cost to date, with estimates from 5–16% of GDP, economists agree that this has been significant. From a fiscal policy perspective, the pandemic may well have pushed South Africa's delicate fiscal situation into a crisis. What is already quite clear is the deep effect on the South African labour market.

Even before the onset of the pandemic, South Africa had one of the highest open unemployment rates in the world at just under 30% (in terms of the narrow definition). Evidence from the last 12 months suggests that the pandemic and the associated economic fallout has had a severe impact on unemployment (Statistics South Africa, 2021b). This in large part reflects the bind that faces South Africa, and other middle-income countries: they cannot afford to let the pandemic run rampant, while at the same time they are unable to afford the economic and social protections which would buffer the economy and the labour market, as has been the case in economically developed countries such as the United Kingdom.

In this chapter, we argue that, in a country like South Africa, which faces existential economic challenges, public health policy must be informed by the economic reality. Where lockdowns are necessary, they need to be accompanied by appropriate economic support which allows businesses to remain solvent, and workers to stay at home.

Many debates in the early stages of the pandemic wrongly positioned public health and the economy in a dichotomous relationship; countries either protected public health (first through lockdowns and more recently through mass vaccinations) or the economy, but the evidence has shown, perhaps unsurprisingly, that interventions in public health and the economy are mutually supporting and reinforcing.

11.2 OBJECTIVES

The objectives of the chapter are:
- Outline the macroeconomic effects of the COVID-19 pandemic in South Africa.
- Explore the employment impacts of the pandemic and responses.
- Examine the implications of the pandemic and responses for inequality.
- Suggest policy proposals for the reconstruction of a more equitable society.

11.3 THE SOUTH AFRICAN POLITICAL ECONOMY

Before we discuss the impact that the COVID pandemic and lockdowns have had on the South African economy, it is important to understand the broader political economy of the country. Pre-pandemic, in early 2020, South Africa was faced with several pressing economic challenges. These included high and rising unemployment, high inequality (indeed, among the highest in the world) in terms of income, wealth, race, gender and ownership (Francis and Webster, 2019; Webster, Valodia and Francis, 2020), growing poverty (Sulla and Zikhali, 2018), and low economic growth with declining per capita income. Furthermore, as we discuss below, the country faced a rapidly deteriorating macroeconomic position, which curtailed its fiscal space to address the pandemic.

It is South Africa's inequality that is particularly striking and has been brought into sharp relief by the current crisis. Economic data can help us construct a picture of the financial inequalities across South African households. If we divide households in the country into five groups (called quintiles), from the poorest 20% to the richest 20%, we see the depth of inequality in the country. According to research by our colleague Gabriel Espi at the Southern Centre for Inequality Studies, drawing from the National Income Dynamics Study from 2017, approximately 18 million South Africans live in the poorest 20% of households. Almost half of these poorest households are in rural areas (while there are some doubts about the reliability of population counts generated by the National Income Dynamics Study, and whether the data underestimate poverty, the household-level insights it provides are very useful).

On average, these poorest households have about five members and a total monthly household income of R2 600 (or about R567 per person in the household). Only 45% of households have an employed member. In contrast, 7 million people live in the richest 20% of households, with approximately two people per home (the average size is 1.93 people per household). The average monthly income for these households is almost R38 000 per month (or R21 000 per person). Almost 80% of these households have at least one employed member, and they work far more hours at a far higher wage than those in the poorest 20% of households.

Many of the people in the richest households can continue to earn an income by working from home. For others, in lower-paid formal employment, the pandemic and the sporadic lockdowns have exposed many to the risk that they could lose their jobs. For this group, the Unemployment Insurance Fund provides some temporary relief, but this has not been sufficient to protect jobs. While we do not yet know what the impact of the last year will be on the headline measure of inequality – the Gini coefficient of inequality in income – it is clear from the data we have already that inequality will continue to increase in the coming months.

11.4 MACROECONOMIC EFFECTS

The COVID-19 pandemic and associated economic impacts caused by lockdowns and the necessity of social distancing have had a significant impact on economic output in the country. The South African case is a revealing example of the interdependence of public health and economic imperatives, and so it is important to understand the macroeconomic picture in some detail.

While total output growth had been tepid for some time before the pandemic, the initial lockdown beginning in March 2020 had the effect of reducing output from R782 billion in the first quarter of 2020 to R652 billion for the second quarter, when the lockdown was at its most extreme level. The economy rebounded somewhat in the third and fourth quarters of 2020 as the lockdown was eased, notwithstanding the second wave of the pandemic during the fourth quarter of 2020. By the end of the first quarter of 2021, with the rebound continuing, output had reached R761 billion (Statistics South Africa, 2021a). However, this left the economy at about the same level as it was in the first quarter of 2016. In other words, the effect of the pandemic on output has been to wipe out the admittedly limited growth that has occurred over the last five years.

There was some debate in the economics literature about the nature of the post-COVID recovery. In essence, the debate was whether the recovery would take the shape of a 'V', implying an immediate rebound to pre-pandemic levels, a 'W', implying a volatile recovery but still to pre-pandemic levels, or a 'Nike swoosh', implying that the recovery would be long and not return in the short term to pre-pandemic levels (Beech, 2020; Smialek, 2020). While it is probably still too early to reach definitive conclusions about the pattern of the GDP recovery in South Africa, and further waves of the pandemic will no doubt influence matters, it is quite clear that the pandemic has had a long-term deleterious impact on economic output. As we shall see, the picture for the key issues of employment, fiscal policy and poverty and inequality confirm this.

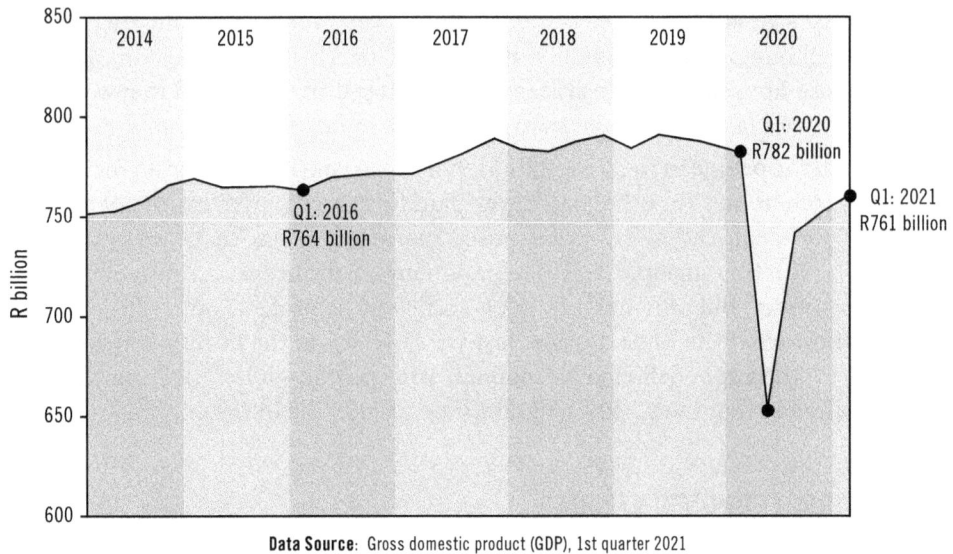

Data Source: Gross domestic product (GDP), 1st quarter 2021

Figure 11.1: Real GDP (seasonally adjusted) (Statistics South Africa, 2021a)

The pandemic plunged South Africa's already precarious fiscal situation into a full-blown crisis. Prior to the pandemic, the Minister of Finance had announced a budget that attempted to deal with a growing public debt problem with a 2020 budget that planned a containment in government consumption, with deep and sustained cuts in expenditure and a freeze, in nominal terms, in public sector remuneration (National Treasury, 2020a).

As a result of the pandemic, the Minister announced a series of measures in a Supplementary Budget, in June 2020 (National Treasury, 2020b). Key measures here included additional expenditures to deal with COVID-19 and relief measures to support additional grants, a revised estimate of revenue, a revised budget deficit estimate from -6.8% pre-pandemic to -14.6% as government revenues plunged as a result of the lockdown.

A critical element of the supplementary budget was the revised fiscal consolidation plan outlined by the finance minister, shown on the graph below. The minister argued for the active scenario below, which consolidates the debt/GDP ratio at 73.5%, arguing that the passive scenario would involve a debt spiral that would not be sustainable. However, the active scenario involved further significant reductions in government expenditure over the period, with a primary budget surplus (revenue less expenditure before debt servicing costs) in the year 2023/24.

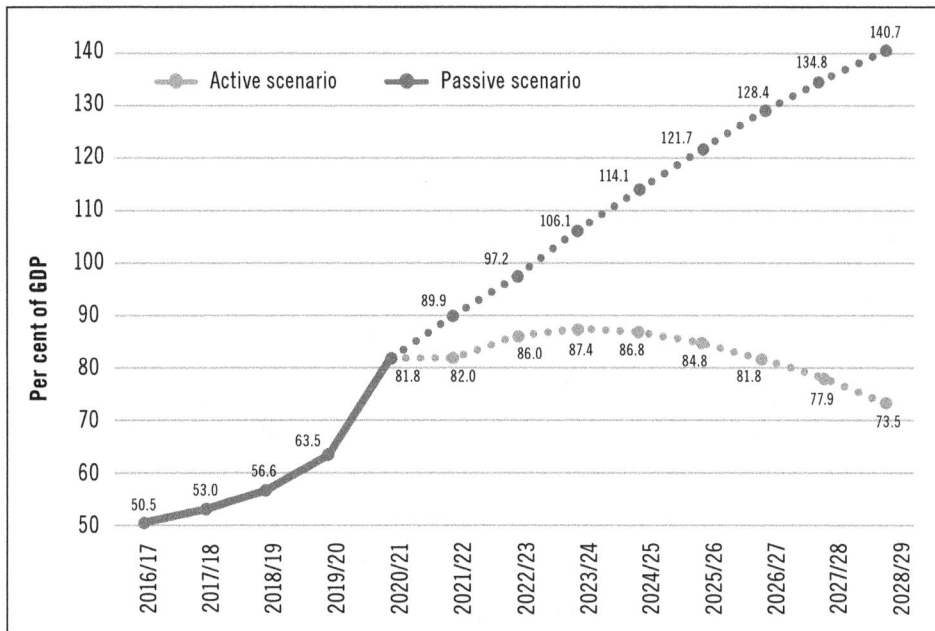

Figure 11.2 Debt outlook scenarios (National Treasury, 2020b p. 30)

We have argued before that this raises two important questions (Francis and Valodia, 2020). First, how will this surplus be achieved, and at what cost, to whom? The projections were that the budget will be balanced through significant cuts in expenditure (rather than rapid revenue growth), projected at R230 billion in 2021/22 and 2022/23, and even further in 2023/24, across all government departments but also in the key areas of education, health and higher education.

The second is why it is necessary at all to have a primary surplus in the budget so soon in the recovery cycle. The austerity measures required to balance a budget, we argued, will inflict permanent economic damage on the economy and will have significant negative impacts on the poorest and most vulnerable citizens, and deepen inequality.

This austerity plan continued into the 2021 budget plans, where the minister of finance provided further details of the fiscal consolidation plans (National Treasury, 2021). While there was some room for manoeuvre, with higher than expected revenues generated by the global recovery in commodity prices, government stuck to its plans to cut expenditure in key social areas.

Interestingly, Michael Sachs has characterised the South African fiscal position as one of austerity without consolidation. He argues that this has led to–

> a regressive deterioration in the allocation of public resources, increasing reliance on inefficiency and regressive tax handles, and a fall in the real value of public services received by poor South Africans. While austerity conditions were increasingly felt on the frontline of service delivery, the fiscal consolidation needed to stabilise the public finances never took place (Sachs, 2021 p. 17).

The macroeconomic picture, then, is bleak. The country lacks the resources to respond adequately to the pandemic, and the pandemic has further damaged the macroeconomic position. To cite but one example, the country's vaccination roll-out has been hampered by a lack of funds to administer vaccines on weekends (Sguazzin, 2021). Whether or not this is a real constraint, it is evidence of the situation outlined by Sachs above.

11.4.1   Employment, Unemployment and the South African Labour Market

When we turn from the macroeconomic picture to the labour market, the situation is equally bleak. Unemployment is the single largest economic existential threat facing South Africa. Figure 11.3, below, charts the narrow unemployment rate from 2008 to the end of 2020. Not only has unemployment risen across the period, but it has done so increasingly rapidly. Ignoring the blip in the second quarter of 2020 (a statistical phenomenon caused by the definition of unemployment – when people are locked down at home and cannot search for work, they are not counted as unemployed), there has been a marked increase in unemployment since 2018. By the end of the first quarter in 2021, the narrow unemployment rate had reached 32.6%. By the expanded definition, which includes discouraged work seekers, the unemployment rate reached 43.2% (Statistics South Africa, 2021b).

As we have argued previously, these headline figures mask significant variation within the labour market, where the pain of the pandemic has not been evenly felt (Francis, Ramburuth-Hurt and Valodia, 2020b; 2020a). Findings from early studies show that women have been disproportionately affected by job losses, as have those working in the informal economy (Casale and Shepherd, 2020; Francis, Ramburuth-Hurt and Valodia, 2020b). Early research from the NIDS-Cram survey found that women accounted for two-thirds of all job losses in the first few months of the pandemic, and data from STATS SA shows the those in the informal economy suffered twice the rate of job losses (Statistics South Africa, 2020). Secondly, what the unemployment ratios hide is the true number of people out of work in the country. There were only 558 000 new jobs created between the first quarter of 2008 and the first quarter of 2021, but there are 2.9 million more unemployed people (for a total of 7.24 million), and a further 1.9 million additional discouraged work seekers (for a total of 3.13 million) (Statistics South Africa, 2021b).

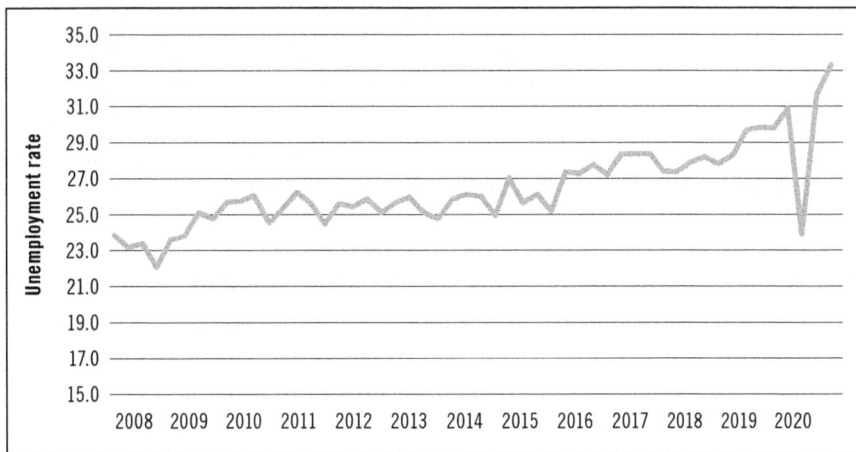

Figure 11.3 Narrow Unemployment Rate at end 2020 (Statistics South Africa, 2021c)

Figure 11.4 shows the actual level of employment in the country across the period from 2008 to the end of 2020. It is here that the precipitous decline in employment because of the pandemic and lockdowns is evident. Almost 2.5 million jobs were lost in the second quarter of 2020, and while many of these jobs have been recovered, employment is only back to levels last seen in 2013. Furthermore, it is likely that many of these recovered jobs will be more precarious and lower paid. While it is true that the government has provided temporary support to workers through the Temporary Employer/Employee Relief Scheme (TERS) and those in the informal economy through a special COVID-19 Social Relief of Distress Grant (SRD), this support has fallen far below that which would have been required to mitigate the impact of the pandemic and the lockdowns, and this is evident from the level of job destruction which is now evident.

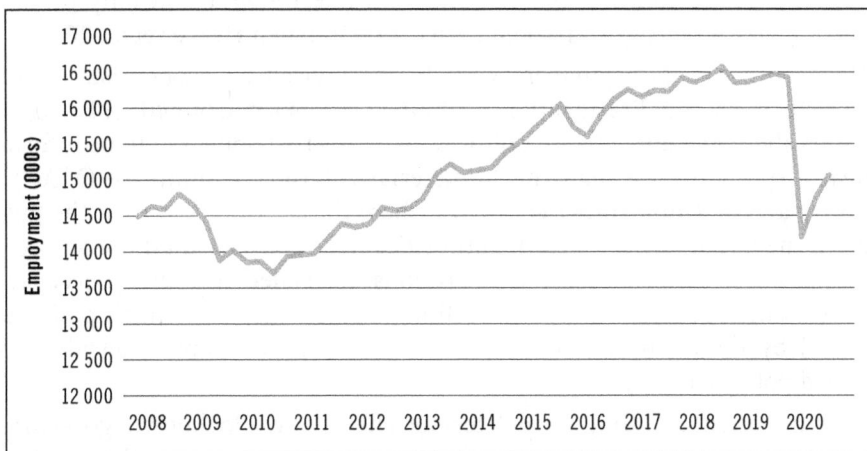

Figure 11.4 Employment in South Africa 2008–2020 (Statistics South Africa, 2021c)

Despite this dire situation, it appears that the official policy position in South Africa is that the unemployment problem will self-correct when other economic fundamentals are in place. However, there is mounting evidence in the post-apartheid period that the unemployment problem is not a technical one, nor an economic epiphenomenon, but a central characteristic of the political economy, and as such, one which requires a political as well as economic solution.

11.4.2   Making Public Health Policy – The Importance of Economics

In this third part of the chapter, we now turn to an analysis of the intersection of public health and economics that was highlighted during the pandemic. As the pandemic unfolded, we have benefitted greatly in our understanding of the health impacts of the virus by working together with a number of colleagues in a multi-disciplinary group, including economic and health experts. Our group published a number of articles on understanding the economic and health interactions in the management of COVID-19. These were published mainly in *The Conversation* (for example, see Madhi et al, 2020). From these contributions, a number of key points are worth emphasising. First, while government claimed to have its pandemic response policy informed by medical science, this itself was highly contested, with the suspension of the Medical Research Council President for publicly criticising some of the lockdown regulations as 'unscientific and nonsensical'.

Second, quite clearly, policy was being driven primarily by health considerations, with economic policy having to respond rather than being integrated into the strategy. As the pandemic evolved, and government developed its risk-assessed five-level planning framework, economic and health policy was somewhat better linked, but economic policy was still reactive. This is best demonstrated by the fact that government's vaccine programme, so critical to opening up the economy, was very much an afterthought and only began in earnest in 2021 following widespread criticism (Van den Heever et al, 2021).

Third, although policymakers were being advised by economists through forums such as the Presidential Economic Advisory Council (PEAC), key decisions about lockdowns were political decisions that appeared to be informed by health specialists through the Ministerial Advisory Committee (MAC) on the Coronavirus. Unlike other countries where the advisories were in the public domain, the South African health authorities have not placed all the advisories in the public domain, and the deliberations are veiled in secrecy because of non-disclosure agreements. It is thus difficult to be sure how much policy was informed by the scientific advice, and whether any economic considerations informed policy choices.

Fourth, notwithstanding the deleterious effects of the lockdown, government policy on the economic policy front continued to follow a path of austerity. To be fair, government did implement a number of programmes, including the

COVID-19 grant, to address the impact of the lockdown on the most vulnerable, but the austerity stance limited government's ability to implement counter-cyclical measures to boost the level of economic activity and protect households and economic infrastructure, contrary to the approach taken by many other countries around the world.

11.4.3   Toward a Conceptual Linking of Economic and Health Policies

As we have argued elsewhere (Valodia, 2020), the economic fallout from COVID-19 is, for a number of reasons, unique and takes policy into unchartered terrain. First, it has been by far the most significant decline in economic activity since the Great Depression. Second, and more complex, is the fact that during a pandemic, economic policy is unable to deal with the resultant economic crisis by employing the normal set of tools used in an economic crisis. When an economic crisis occurs, and the level of aggregate demand in the economy falls, we find ways – typically through increasing government expenditure or loosening monetary policy – to boost the level of aggregate demand. In other words, policymakers act to counteract the factors leading to a fall in demand. The uniqueness of the pandemic situation is that we are, from a health perspective, actively trying to *suppress* the level of aggregate demand.

In order to manage the spread of the pandemic, governments have been forced, through lockdowns, to ask the population to stay at home, close schools and universities, and restrict spending in restaurants and bars. In other words, our policy response has been to further reduce the level of demand. Furthermore, our health policy actions also impacted the supply side of the economy. Asking workers to stay at home negatively impacts on firms' ability to supply goods to the market, as normal distribution systems are shut down.

Even as governments get a better handle on the public health dimension of the pandemic, the economic crisis is far from over. In designing the response to the economic challenges, it is worth noting that the economic fallout has very little to do with purely economic factors, unlike many other economic crises, such as the global financial crisis in 2008. However, unless policymakers act to address the economic fallout, vast swathes of our economic system will be significantly undermined, if not destroyed. The state of the economy prior to the pandemic, and the levels of economic development, are critical for how the pandemic has to be managed from an economic and health perspective.

Under these particular and perhaps unique conditions, what is an appropriate economic policy stance to adopt? First, and critically, from a macroeconomic point of view, the policy stance has to be expansionary. Since the economic fallout of the pandemic is a temporary phenomenon and uncertainty drives the actions of economic agents, the macro stance has to be expansionary and counter-cyclical. Of course, the nature and extent of the expansionary stance will be determined by the level of economic development, and the state of the economy pre-pandemic.

Second, given the challenges in aggregate demand and the complexities with supply chains, firms, both large and small, suffer a significant fall in revenue, but not in costs (which often increase). This places temporary pressure on firms' and households' liquidity and balance sheets. Consequently, governments have to implement measures to tide firms and households over this temporary 'financial shock': many will be forced to lay off workers and cease operations (for firms), or plunge into severe stress (for households). Here, collaborative strategies with development finance institutions and the commercial banking sector are likely to have significant ameliorative impacts – policies such as temporary mortgage holidays will give firms and households the breathing space to manage the challenge. Interventions of this sort are needed for more systemic temporary relief. Mortgage holidays for owners of a property will allow them to, in turn, allow temporary rent holidays to tenants.

Third, resources have to be urgently diverted to the health sector to address the immediate health pandemic, but also to develop contingency strategies to address the high levels of uncertainty, in both the health effects of the pandemic but also in seeking solutions to ensure that the economy recovers to pre-pandemic levels.

11.5 CONCLUSION – LESSONS FROM SOUTH AFRICA'S EXPERIENCES

Throughout 2021, the COVID-19 pandemic continues to fundamentally impact on the South African economy. In July, the new Delta variant spread at an alarming rate and forced a move to level four of the lockdown with more restrictions on economic activity. While restrictions were subsequently relaxed, it is thus too soon to draw out any final lessons. However, some key conclusions can already be identified.

Strategies for dealing with the pandemic have to better integrate health considerations with economic imperatives that allow for more effective management of the immediate health crisis, and provide the necessary support to assist the economic recovery in the medium term. The lack of integration, has, we argue, led to two serious failures.

First, government's economic response was too late and, in proportion to the negative effects of the pandemic, too little. The result is that some parts of the economic infrastructure have been undermined over the long term. There is some evidence that the lockdown resulted in a large number of firms closing down. According to Statistics South Africa (2021d), the number of liquidations in 2020 was 14.2% higher than in 2020. BusinessTech (2020) reported that up to 42.7% of small firms may have closed at least temporarily as a result of the lockdown. As the GDP data outlined above demonstrates, the recovery has been incomplete.

Moreover, the social implications of not better integrating policy have been serious. The current crisis is really worsening enormous existing inequalities, in addition to creating new ones. Far more needs to be done to counter the economic destruction currently underway. South Africa cannot tackle the problem with marginal economic policy interventions. It needs immediate and drastic action informed by the best available economic evidence which is being offered by researchers across the country (Bassier et al, 2020). South African society is at risk if it does not address these economic inequalities.

Indeed, the COVID-19 pandemic makes it clear how interrelated society really is. The country can't successfully flatten the curve of infection unless all have the ability to stay at home. For many, the choice between staying at home and starving, or going out in search of work, is a reality. For many others, spatial apartheid and extremely high levels of poverty make it virtually impossible to conform to the social distancing required to contain the spread of the coronavirus.

Second, the lack of integration has also accentuated the health challenges. The only long-term strategy for managing the pandemic and returning the economy to some level of its pre-pandemic output is a comprehensive vaccination programme. South Africa's vaccine rollout started off poorly, with strategic errors in procurement, among other problems. The full extent of this is traversed in Van den Heever et al (2021). Shockingly, given the economic effects of the pandemic, South Africa's policymakers only began to seriously consider a vaccine rollout after criticism from a group of eminent scientists in January 2021 (South Africa's Eminent Scientists, 2021). Moreover, a series of poor decisions on the health front, including bureaucratic inertia to address the re-opening after a fire of key health infrastructure has forced the economy into another potential slowdown. One of the key lessons of the South African experience is the need for planning frameworks to be both integrated and also for policymakers to plan on a contingency basis. Under high levels of uncertainty, policy should be risk-assessed and flexible.

The COVID-19 pandemic has starkly highlighted the links between public health and the economy all around the world. But in South Africa – the country with the world's highest income inequality – the links are particularly pronounced. The enduring public health and economic policy failures in the country have combined to produce one of the worst COVID-19 epidemics in the world, with a shocking per capita excess death rate, and a pronounced economic shock. While there have been many policy and planning lessons from the pandemic, the one we have highlighted is how public health and economic policy are inextricably linked. Good public health policy supports the economy, and the only good economic policy is that which supports public health, protecting people and prioritising public health. South Africa has failed on both fronts – individualising public health by transferring risks onto citizens – and by failing to provide the necessary economic support to people, workers and firms.

11.6 SELF-ASSESSMENT QUESTIONS

1. How was the South African government's economic response during the COVID-19 pandemic different to that of developed countries globally?

2. What are the two serious failures of not integrating health considerations with economic imperatives in particular during a pandemic?

11.7 REFERENCES

Bassier, I., Budlender, J., Leibbrandt, M., Zizzamia, R. and Ranchhod, V. 2020. South Africa can – and should – top up child support grants to avoid humanitarian crisis'. *The Conversation*, 31 March. Available at: https://theconversation.com/south-africa-can-and-should-top-up-child-support-grants-to-avoid-a-humanitarian-crisis-135222.

Beech, P. 2020. Z, V or "Nike swoosh" – what shape with the COVID-19 recession take?. *World Economic Forum*, 19 May. Available at: https://www.weforum.org/agenda/2020/05/z-u-or-nike-swoosh-what-shape-will-our-covid-19-recovery-take/.

Casale, D. and Shepherd, D. 2020. *The gendered effects of the ongoing lockdown and school closures in South Africa: Evidence from NIDS-CRAM Waves 1 and 2*. Working Paper 5. Cape Town, p. 30.

Francis, D., Ramburuth-Hurt, K. and Valodia, I. 2020a. *Estimates of employment in South Africa under the five-level lockdown framework*, 4. Johannesburg: Southern Centre for Inequality Studies, Wits University. Available at: https://www.wits.ac.za/media/wits-university/faculties-and-schools/commerce-law-and-management/research-entities/scis/documents/SCIS%20Working%20Paper%204.pdf.

Francis, D., Ramburuth-Hurt, K. and Valodia, I. 2020b. South Africa needs to focus urgently on how COVID-19 will reshape its labour market. *The Conversation*, 20 June. Available at: https://www.wiego.org/blog/informal-employment-and-global-financial-crisis-middle-income-country.

Francis, D. and Valodia, I. 2020. South Africa's budget to deal with COVID-19 fails to pave way for more equal society. *The Conversation*, 25 June. Available at: https://theconversation.com/south-africas-budget-to-deal-with-covid-19-fails-to-pave-way-for-more-equal-society-141458.

Francis, D. and Webster, E. 2019. Poverty and inequality in South Africa: critical reflections. *Development Southern Africa* 36(6), pp. 788–802. doi: 10.1080/0376835X.2019.1666703.

Madhi, S., Van den Heever, A., Francis, D., Valodia, I., Veller, M. and Sachs, M. 2020. South Africa needs to end the lockdown: here's a blueprint for its replacement. *The Conversation*, 9 April. Available at: https://theconversation.com/south-africa-needs-to-end-the-lockdown-heres-a-blueprint-for-its-replacement-136080.

National Treasury. 2020a. Budget Review 2020. Pretoria, South Africa: National Treasury of South Africa. Available at: http://www.treasury.gov.za/documents/National%20Budget/2020/review/FullBR.pdf.

National Treasury. 2020b. Supplementary Budget Review 2020. Pretoria, South Africa: National Treasury of South Africa. Available at: http://www.treasury.gov.za/documents/National%20Budget/2020S/review/FullSBR.pdf.

National Treasury. 2021. *Budget Review 2021*. Pretoria, South Africa: National Treasury of South Africa. Available at: http://www.treasury.gov.za/documents/National%20Budget/2021/review/FullBR.pdf.

Sachs, M. 2021. Fiscal Dimensions of South Africa's Crisis. Working Paper Number 15. Johannesburg: Southern Centre for Inequality Studies, Wits University. Available at: https://www.wits.ac.za/media/wits-university/faculties-and-schools/commerce-law-and-management/research-entities/scis/documents/Sachs-2021-Fiscal%20dimensions%20Working%20Paper%2015.pdf.

Sguazzin, A. 2021. As covid cases surge, South Africa eschews weekend vaccination. *Bloomberg*, 1 July. Available at: https://www.bloomberg.com/authors/ABwnnzA9x6k/antony-sguazzin.

Smialek, J. 2020. Forget swooshes and V's. The economy's future is a question mark. *The New York Times*, 29 May. Available at: https://www.nytimes.com/2020/05/29/business/economy/economy-recovery-forecast-coronavirus.html.

South Africa's Eminent Scientists. 2021. Vaccines for South Africa. Now. *The Daily Maverick*, 2 January. Available at: https://www.dailymaverick.co.za/article/2021-01-02-vaccines-for-south-africa-now/.

Statistics South Africa. 2020. Quarterly Labour Force Survey Quarter 2: 2020. Statistical Release P0211. Pretoria, South Africa: Statistics South Africa. Available at: http://www.statssa.gov.za/publications/P0211/P02112ndQuarter2020.pdf.

Statistics South Africa. 2021a. Gross domestic product: First quarter 2021. Pretoria: Statistics South Africa. Available at: http://www.statssa.gov.za/publications/P0441/P04411stQuarter2021.pdf.

Statistics South Africa. 2021b. Quarterly Labour Force Survey Quarter 1: 2021. Statistical Release P0211. Pretoria, South Africa: Statistics South Africa. Available at: http://www.statssa.gov.za/?page_id=1854&PPN=P0211&SCH=72943.

Statistics South Africa. 2021c. Quarterly Labour Force Survey Quarter 4: 2020. Statistical Release P0211. Pretoria, South Africa: Statistics South Africa. Available at: http://www.statssa.gov.za/?page_id=1854&PPN=P0211&SCH=72942.

Statistics South Africa. 2021d. Statistics of liquidation and insolvencies (preliminary): December 2020. P0043. Pretoria: Statistics South Africa. Available at: http://www. statssa.gov.za/publications/P0043/P0043 December2020.pdf.

Sulla, V. and Zikhali, P. 2018. *Overcoming poverty and inequality in South Africa: An assessment of drivers, constraints and opportunities*. Washington: International Bank for Reconstruction and Development/The World Bank. Available at: http:// documents.worldbank.org/curated/en/530481521735906534/pdf/ 124521-REV-OUO-South-Africa-Poverty-and-Inequality-Assessment-Report-2018-FINAL-WEB.pdf.

Valodia, I. 2020. Covid-19: Bold programmes are neede to mitigate the economic crisis. *The Daily Maverick*, 23 March. Available at: https://www.dailymaverick. co.za/article/2020-03-23-the-risks-of-economic-inaction-on-covid-19-are-significantly-high/.

Van den Heever, A., Valodia, I., Veller, M., Madhi, S.A. and Venter, W.D.F. 2021. South Africa's vaccine quagmire, and what needs to be done now. *The Conversation*, 2 July. Available at: https://theconversation.com/south-africas-vaccine-quagmire-and-what-needs-to-be-done-now-163784.

Webster, E., Valodia, I. and Francis, D. 2020. Towards a southern approach to inequality: inequality studies in South Africa and the global south'. In E. Webster, I. Valodia and D. Francis (Eds) *Inequality Studies from the Global South*. 1 ed. London: Routledge. Available at: https://www.routledge.com/Inequality-Studies-from-the-Global-South/Francis-Valodia-Webster/p/book/9780367235680.

CURRICULUM CHANGE AND TEACHING INNOVATIONS IN HEALTH SCIENCES: AN ESSENTIAL REQUIREMENT IN THE ERA OF PANDEMICS

Scott Smalley

Hellen Myezwa

Paula Barnard-Ashton

12.1 INTRODUCTION

South Africa instituted a country-wide lockdown on 27 March 2020 at midnight as a tactical response to the rapidly spreading COVID-19 pandemic. Overnight, all aspects of society changed, including academic teaching and learning. Students and staff were confined to their homes. The Government Gazette, law in South Africa, required all citizens to remain at home unless provided a transport permit for essential services such as healthcare, police, essential goods and services, and military activities. One could leave their home only for food, medical supplies, or medical emergencies. A curfew was instituted from 20:00 to 07:00. South Africa instituted Level 5 Lockdown, one of the strictest lockdowns of any country during the early days of the pandemic.

Two weeks prior to the nationwide lockdown, the University of the Witwatersrand Faculty of Health Sciences had experienced the first health science student testing positive for COVID-19. An uncertain future began for the academic staff involved in supporting one of the first cases in the nation with wide-reaching decisions that ultimately led to the suspension of school activities and the end to normal teaching and learning.

Soon after, the entire university closed its doors with students sent home and all staff requested to work from home. Only essential clinical and academic staff were provided travel permits to access campus on a need-only basis. To continue the academic year (January to November), remote online learning became the new normal and an emergency teaching response was developed. The pandemic had immediate and profound effects on management, teaching and learning and content delivery methods. This chapter explores the crossroads and interdependency of health science education during the COVID-19 pandemic.

12.2 OBJECTIVES

The objectives of the chapter are:

- To describe the impact of COVID-19 on the educational programme and curriculum (content and delivery).
- To describe the impact of the pandemic on pedagogy in the faculty.
- To explore and describe the innovations in response to an unexpected pandemic.
- To align the innovations to educational theory and approach.
- To describe the epistemology theoretical perspective methodology and actual methods used.
- To identify the barriers and facilitators to learning.
- To make recommendations for future preparedness.
- To document the impact of staff (socially and at work).

12.3 THEORETICAL UNDERPINNINGS FOR EDUCATIONAL CHANGE

In health professions education literature, constructivist and behaviourist theories are dominantly proposed but the application of other theories such as adult, transformative, experiential, social, information processing, collaborative, cognitive, behavioural and contextual learning theories are evident (Gewurtz et al, 2016; Kauffman and Mann, 2014; Torre et al, 2006). In most faculties of health sciences, the predominant theory is constructivist learning theory in both the undergraduate and the postgraduate space. However, there is a belief that the social cognitivist theory emerges quite strongly in clinical practice (Kauffman and Mann, 2014). The learning methods include a problem-oriented approach (Jay, 2014), reflective practice (Myezwa et al, 2017), multiple perspectives in learning and context and content dependency (Green-Thompson et al, 2012; MacFarlane and Green-Thompson, 2006). Clinical competencies in health science education are acquired through the application of behaviourist learning theory using competency-based curricula (Hassan, 2007).

In health professions curricula, the foundational knowledge has not changed. However, with the emergence of the COVID-19 pandemic, educators were required to adapt, adopt and alter the delivery of teaching and learning (Kedraka and Kaltsidis, 2020). The crisis forced students to learn from home as lockdown took effect and thus distance learning emerged as the new normal. For both students and academics, technology became instantiated at all levels in terms of availability, accessibility, utility and synthesised engagement. There are two contrasting positions in literature regarding twenty-first-century learning; one is that nothing has changed, while the other is that everything has changed especially when digital technology in education is considered (Kereluik et al, 2013). The content which educators delivered may not have changed in this pandemic emergency, but the engagement with teaching and learning with students, services, community, academics and leadership has changed dramatically. Times of crisis stimulate rapid change which results in innovation and promotes teaching and learning agility. The response to teaching and learning during a pandemic and the resultant 'Lived 21st Century Learning Framework' (Figure 12.1) that emerged from an unfolding crisis showcases one such strategy.

12.4 CURRICULUM RESPONSE: TEACHING AND LEARNING AGILITY IN TIMES OF CRISIS

Despite loud and supported calls to discard the behaviourist industrialist legacy lingering in higher education (Foley and Masingila, 2014), healthcare teaching and learning has retained the emphasis on the pre-clinical years of memorising facts lectured by older assumed knowledgeable professors with an often-tenuous transition to clinical apprenticeship with the adage 'see one, do one, teach one'. This produced students who could be observed and measured for their foundational knowledge, skills and attitudes (Ertmer and Newby, 2013; Kereluik et al, 2013). The meta-knowledge abilities such as creative thinking, real-world problem solving, skilled communication and collaboration for dynamic results were lacking. The COVID-19 pandemic finally forced the displacement of classroom teaching with remote online learning, igniting a drive towards social constructivism (Dewey, 1916). The pandemic caused upheaval in clinical training with healthcare students involved in disaster management. Learning during the pandemic led students to direct, personal experiences with real-world issues, allowing students to create meaning, not simply acquire knowledge (Ertmer and Newby, 2013).

The recipe for curricula transformation has been well described with the Lancet Commission of Education of Health Professionals for the 21st Century (Frenk et al, 2010) recommending transformative learning through competency-driven pedagogies related to local context, interprofessional education with non-hierarchical models, use of technology-enhanced learning, creation of interactive teams with social and justice accountability. Lave and Wenger's (1991) Legitimate Peripheral Participation situates learning within the community of practice for healthcare students to build on experiential learning by locating learning firmly in the real world and community.

12.4.1   The Lived Twenty-First Century Learning Framework

To survive and thrive through a crisis, students need to develop not only their foundational professional knowledge and clinical skills but also the cross-cutting twenty-first century humanistic and meta knowledge and skills as presented by Kereluik et al's (2013) twenty-first-century learning framework. The COVID-19 pandemic asks both educators and students, *what do we need to know now, how do we act on this knowledge* and *what values do we espouse with this knowledge and action?*

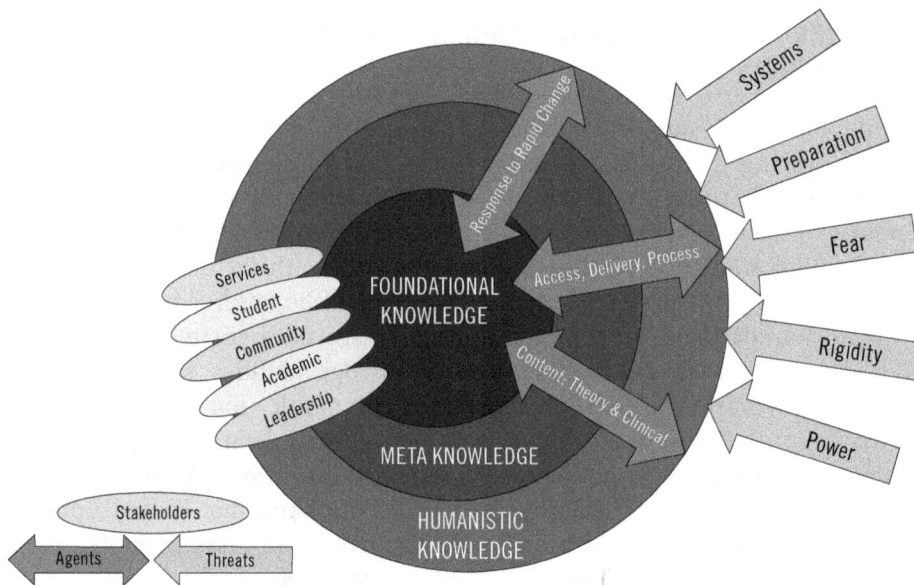

Figure 12.1 The Lived 21st Century Learning Framework: Learning through a pandemic

At the onset of the COVID-19 pandemic, it was important to find a model that would craft the principles and premises that shaped decision-making in a time when decisions were impulsive and lacking evidentiary support. This was new territory, but by drawing on current education theory for direction, and using the Kereluik et al (2013) integration of twenty-first-century learning frameworks to house the education principles of situated learning advocated by Kolb (2005) and Lave and Wenger (1991) to leverage social-constructivism, we were able to formulate the Lived 21st Century Learning Framework: Learning through a pandemic (Figure 12.1).

Foundational knowledge and skills have always been at the centre of any curriculum but do not necessarily lead to skilled practitioners who are adaptable and innovative thinking enough to cope with the demands and uncertainty of a crisis. Meta knowledge hones the twenty-first-century skills of collaboration through skilled communication, real-world problem solving, critical and reflective thinking, agility, creativity and innovation in practice. By situating activities that build meta knowledge within a community of practice, we develop the humanistic knowledge of our students. Paramount during a crisis is the humanistic knowledge of the students, academics, clinicians, administrators and managers; as the cultural competence, ethical, emotional awareness and active participation in the work of their profession contributes to alleviating the burden. The agents of change that emerged within The Lived 21st Century Learning Framework (Figure 12.1) had the potential to push the full overlap (ideal) of the three types of knowledge or pull them into discrete and delineated constructs to be developed and applied independently.

Through understanding the agents of change, identifying the threats and engaging all stakeholders as a community of practice within a situated learning context (Table 12.1), we get closer to embedding foundational knowledge in the process of innovation to adapt (meta) together with shared accountability and resultant responsive action within the community of practice (humanistic). All learners thrive rather than survive.

Table 12.1 Comparison of independent vs overlapping knowledge construction

	Independent knowledge construction	**Overlapping knowledge construction**
Foundational	A lecture on infection control and how to put on PPE.	Students participate in a situational analysis in groups at various sites. Students have to research PPE and infection control prior to the situational analysis and in their group plan how they will conduct the analysis. They have the option of videoing a journey through their clinical placement, interviewing staff and patients at various points, observe PPE procedures, checking on supply chains, etc. The students need to submit a report on the situation for their placement that will also be given to the placement supervisors/management, with recommendations.
Meta	Students produce a group video on how to don and doff, dispose, and manage the PPE resources. Or produce a pamphlet on infection control.	
Humanistic	The students engage in the clinical and non-clinical spaces and are required to adapt and use the foundational and meta knowledge associated with the concept of infection control and PPE.	

The next section considers the agents of change and the perspectives of the stakeholders in navigating the decisions and factors that charted our teaching and learning path during the COVID-19 crisis.

12.5 COLLECTIVE EXPERIENCE OF TRANSITIONING AND INNOVATION

Health science curricula in the twenty-first century are a collective experience of transitioning and innovations during a pandemic. The perspective of the student, the academic, community, leadership and management and support services must be considered, while addressing three fundamental agents of change: the response to rapid change; access, delivery and process; and finally, content: theory and clinical practice.

12.5.1 Response to Rapid Change: Management and Systems

The coronavirus pandemic was unprecedented. In the University of the Witwatersrand Faculty of Health Sciences, the response to the first case among students and staff was panic and almost palpable fear. One of the drivers was that we were dealing with an unknown: *What was this virus? How would it affect and infect us? What do we need to do?* The information about the virus was changing by the hour with unclear and changing positions about *How long it lasts on surfaces? How is the virus transmitted? Does wearing a mask mitigate or reduce the risk?* Facts were overshadowed by fake news and no clear audit of the situation. Our first response was to regroup, put facts on the table and communicate evidence-based information to the faculty, students and stakeholders, thus substantiating the need to move and act fast in the crisis (Illanes et al, 2020).

University leadership timely decisions and communication were imperative to direct the response to the COVID-19 pandemic. Five key areas became evident: dealing with staff, both for the preparedness of emergency online learning and managing staff and student anxiety; access and equity difficulties; online engagement; and the logistical implications related to safety, connectivity and keeping essential services going. The unfolding complexities of the disparities among students became starkly evident, thus revealing a more complex milieu of problems that needed nimble but adaptive problem-solving. What emerged, in retrospect, one can recognise as the formation of nerve centres (Illanes et al, 2020) which responded to the many questions asked by both students and staff. Questions such as:

- *Will my fees be reimbursed as I am no longer on campus?*
- *Can I return to campus and collect my belongings? (The assumption was that lockdown would be temporary)*
- *How will I complete my clinical exposure, assessments and my degree?*

All the elements of management surfaced and were part of the adaptive response. Tenets of systems thinking were at play, such as analysis of internal and external processes and cause and effect chains within the environment (Drack and Apfalter, 2007). Clear, consistent, constant and transparent communication was one of the key responses to the questions of uncertainty and fear experienced by the community (Edmondson, 2020). This response was undertaken at every level and to every stakeholder, while against the backdrop of an ever-changing environment: *the lockdown levels, policy and regulatory framework, shifting needs, misinformation in the general public as well as political and business responses that were both facilitatory (mobilising necessary capital) and inhibitory (as evidenced in corruption around the much needed and essential personal protective equipment).*

Important learning points in the response involved the use of the chain of command and flexibility to develop new structures as needed. The university has a clear organisational structure, but in crisis, there is need for flexibility (Heitz, 2020). Clarity and breaking down of barriers of command and control as well as harnessing the available resources was essential. What was evident and effective was devolved decision-making in response to the crisis.

The university set up teams (Figure 12.2) looking at the different needs at the central level. In the faculty, the formal structures linked the central university to the faculty. The emergence of germane and naturally occurring nerve centres (Illanes et al, 2020) followed within the faculty.

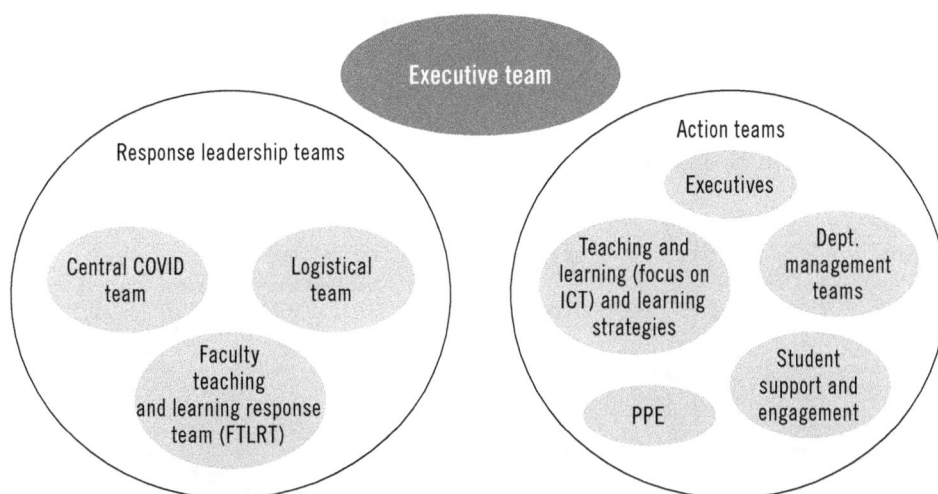

Figure 12.2 The university's working teams/nerve centres

Academic members of departments that would ordinarily work independently coalesced around needs that emerged as key responses to the pandemic; such as the need for PPE for safety – its financing, sourcing and delivery. Each node or nerve centre of operation undertook function around their purpose. These functions included *flexibility in planning* which was paramount; *leadership* at all levels was important, efficient and timely *action, communication,* clarity of aims of each portfolio and *organising* the key action resulting in clear outputs.

Often there was a need to apply a cycle of 'pause, assess and anticipate' (D'Auria and De Smet, 2020) as new information came in. The complexity of the response required non-traditional alliances. For example, a logistics team coalesced that included housing, health, academic, transport, cleaning, catering, clinical services and management to collaborate in one common space.

Following a change in systems, the next simultaneous adjustment was to the curriculum. The pandemic altered teaching and learning in profound measures, at a rapid rate not seen before in modern times.

12.5.2 Access, Delivery and Process

The move to remote online learning and digital apartheid

Czerniewicz et al (2020) highlighted that access to education has a direct relationship to longevity and positioned this as a threat to survival post pandemic if some students were 'left behind' due to the now well-illuminated inequality and equity issues that existed long before the crisis but became critical in the face of the 'pivot' to remote online learning. Barnard-Ashton (2018) defines digital apartheid *'as the degree to which students experience barriers to engaging in digital activity which places the students at a learning and achievement disadvantage when compared to peers who have digital affordances supporting their learning'*. Digital apartheid can be viewed through three dimensions (Figure 12.3) as described by Barnard-Ashton et al (2018).

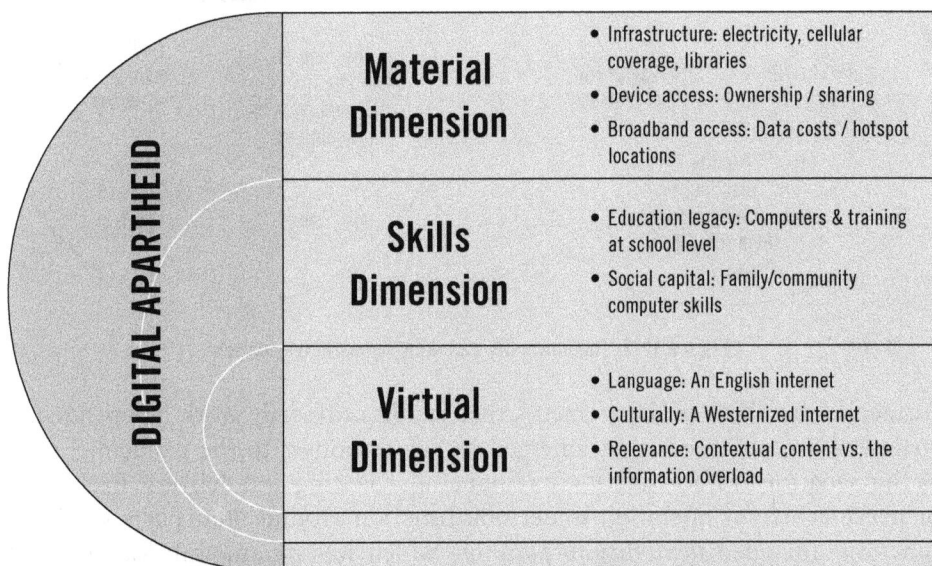

Figure 12.3 The dimensions of digital apartheid (Barnard-Ashton et al, 2018)

When thrust into a crisis, it is important to have a model that allows rapid analysis of the students' and lecturers' ability to participate in the rapid remote online learning that was proposed as the only way to save the academic year.

The **material dimension** risks to participation are typically the first to be identified and addressed. Many countries have stable access to network bandwidth with ubiquitous Local-Area Networks (LAN), fibre or cellular coverage. South Africans are severely compromised, as the four monopoly mobile network operators charge almost the highest fee/gigabyte of data in Africa and leave many rural and high-density areas with weak coverage. Without intervention, this makes remote online teaching and learning almost impossible for both the lecturers and the students. Providing students and staff with mobile data supported the access to data, but those in weak cellular signal areas were still compromised. Other infrastructure challenges included the unstable power, with regular load shedding or overload blackouts, particularly during the winter months, and the closure of all public spaces, particularly libraries which offer internet access, computers and access to knowledge resources. Learning from a mobile phone proved inadequate, raising the need for the urgent deployment of laptop computers. The University instituted an emergency device loan scheme and couriered these to students' homes as needed.

The 'missing middle' (defined as those students who were not wealthy enough to afford to pay all their financial obligations but were also outside those who could be fully subsidised by the state) and professional staff were hardest hit as low-income and bursary students were prioritised for access to loan devices and academic staff were seen as the priority for working from home. Many households now had all family members trying to work and study from home, sharing devices and bandwidth. Going forward, it is becoming evident that every student should own a laptop computer at the start of their enrolment, and staff should shift away from fixed-desk computing towards more flexible solutions.

The **skills dimension** risk is a greater threat to the first-year students and academics who have focused on face-to-face teaching prior to lockdown. There are many digital literacy open educational resources available to assist students in 'catching-up' to the level of their peers. What was evident was the peer-to-peer support that allowed some students to bridge their skills gap rapidly. For academics, however, the simple digital literacy skills did not equip them sufficiently to teach online nor understand the nature of distance and online pedagogy that supports student participation and active learning behaviours. Professional learning communities emerged in platforms such as Microsoft Teams and the Learning Management Systems which offered webinars, How-to guides, Q&A forums and provided a peer-support environment for day-to-day queries, challenges and sharing of ideas. The Faculty Remote Learning Guide was a Microsoft Team created by the Faculty Teaching and Learning Response Team as a central hub for managing the rapid transition to remote online learning.

All academics were invited to the guide which has evolved with the changing needs of the academic platform as shown in Figure 12.4.

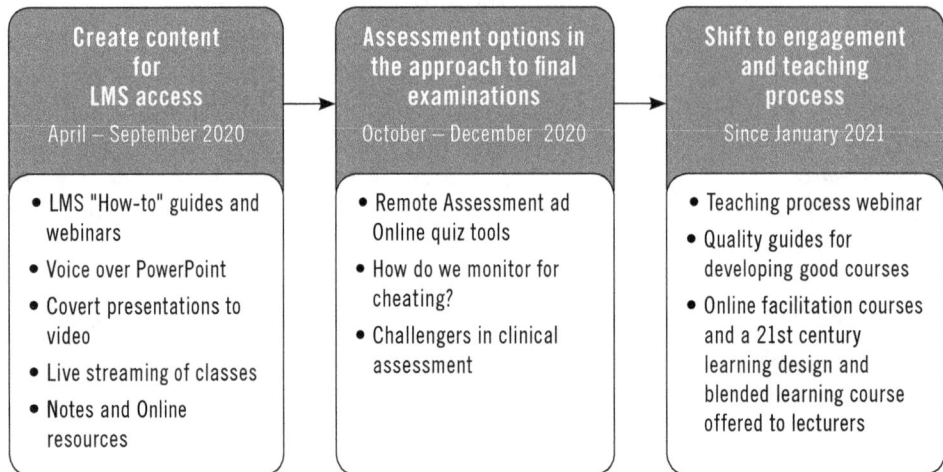

Create content for LMS access	Assessment options in the approach to final examinations	Shift to engagement and teaching process
April – September 2020	October – December 2020	Since January 2021
• LMS "How-to" guides and webinars • Voice over PowerPoint • Covert presentations to video • Live streaming of classes • Notes and Online resources	• Remote Assessment ad Online quiz tools • How do we monitor for cheating? • Challengers in clinical assessment	• Teaching process webinar • Quality guides for developing good courses • Online facilitation courses and a 21st century learning design and blended learning course offered to lecturers

Figure 12.4 FHS Remote Learning Guide focus since April 2020

The **virtual dimension** risk is complex and challenging (Barnard-Ashton, 2018). This dimension considers the impact of pushing students towards an English language internet and virtual learning environments that are not easily translated into multiple languages that would support diversity. Additionally, when using English, the internet is directed towards sites that foster a westernised style, resource design and cultural context. While this is a historic challenge, it became an exacerbated concern when students were isolated from peers and the social learning structures that traditionally assisted in breaking down these virtual dimension barriers. This requires a long-term and national approach to decolonising the virtual dimension; however, the short-term strategy was to ensure that the navigation pathways and structure of the learning environment were simple and meaningful to the student. Students were pointed directly to applicable online resources as opposed to having to do individual searches and online research around their learning topics. In a time of stress, pointing students directly to pre-selected resources negates the time-spent and confusion in learning and language complexity that results from having to search through culturally biased and unfamiliar semantics.

Curriculum delivery process

As the impact of the pandemic became apparent, the focus shifted to how we could save the academic programme. The main principle was to look at the curriculum and identify how to deliver the content. Each programme assessed how they could provide the theoretical content and later the practical or clinical components. Timetables were adjusted to align with the lockdown regulations. The timetable underwent several iterations influenced by programme needs, individual preferences and direction from different levels of the university's hierarchy. It took time for the university to coalesce in its response in one direction. The student voice was apparent and had to be taken into consideration, often affecting changes such as timing, i.e. when the online programme could start, concessions around assessment schedule and structure. As clarity on roles, responsibilities and policies became clearer, an emergency response plan and a teaching and learning plan for the COVID pandemic emerged.

12.5.3 Content: Theory and Clinical Practice

Evolving pedagogies during the pandemic

Teaching pedagogies had to shift from the context of face-to-face contact sessions to online remote learning situations along with risk mitigated clinical teaching in the hospitals and clinics during the height of the pandemic. Teaching methods had to adapt, evolve, and assimilate the content in relation to the COVID-19 context. Reliance on Experiential Learning Theory (ELT) (Kolb and Kolb, 2005) with the four-cycle model provided a basis for pedagogies to stimulate learning. Kolb and Kolb describe four stages of learning with students entering the cycle at one of four places with direct experience, active reflection on the experience, developing insight, hypotheses and conclusions through abstract conceptualisation and testing this through active experimentation (Kolb and Kolb, 2005). Learning occurs through the transformation of experience.

The ELT model portrays two dialectically related modes of grasping experience – Concrete Experience (CE) and Abstract Conceptualization (AC) – and two dialectically related modes of transforming experience – Reflective Observation (RO) and Active Experimentation (Kolb and Kolb, 2005).

Clinical cases taught through online forums or even WhatsApp chat platforms engaged the learner with simulated clinical experience, necessitating abstract conceptualisation forming hypotheses for the clinical problem. Open online chat sessions allow for reflection where the student considers their contribution, compared to fellow student answers. This is followed by direct clinical practice in the hospital setting for active testing and experimentation of their management plans.

By using ELT principles, educators could provide students with learning opportunities for abstract conceptualisation and reflective observation through online learning. This method blended with clinical practice, gives chance for concrete experience and active experimentation.

A return to clinical training

Intense negotiations occurred in South Africa for ministerial permission to allow clinical students to return to campus to re-engage in clinical training and rotation placements during the lockdown. Six weeks after Level 5 Lockdown was implemented, health science students returned to clinical training. This decision was promoted by health science academics, supported by the university leadership, with a well-developed risk mitigation plan provided to the Health and Higher Education Ministers. In contrast, clinical students in other countries were close to the end of their clinical training when the pandemic reached peak case numbers, with final year students in Europe graduating early to join the workforce. In South Africa, the academic year had just begun when the pandemic arrived, therefore national COVID-19 case numbers were initially low and, in time, exponentially increased when students re-entered the clinical teaching space. This presented several challenges, including preparing clinical training sites, student safety with the provision of personal protective equipment (PPE), adjusting learning objectives, limited availability of preceptors for teaching due to the demand of COVID-19 patients, and the need to build student resilience and overall change management.

Pandemic preparedness for the educator, student and clinical site became paramount (O'Byrne et al, 2020). Academic coordinators quickly became crisis management experts and were involved with redesigning the curriculum to include hospital site assessment preparedness and checklists for risk mitigation. This included identifying training sites able to accept students after a six-week hiatus due to lockdown and ensuring students could be placed in low-risk training situations (Wilkinson et al, 2020). Clinical coordinators had to negotiate space for students at clinical sites which resisted accepting students. In these placements, the staff were inundated with COVID-19 patients, had many ill clinicians, and a limited supply of PPE. Provision of PPE for students was an immediate problem, as shortages existed for all healthcare workers. Many health science faculties, through efforts of staff and students, were able to source PPE donations. The Faculty of Health Sciences comprises seven schools, namely the schools of Anatomy, Clinical Medicine, Dentistry, Pathology, Physiology Public Health and Therapeutic Sciences, which collectively gathered available funding to purchase back-up PPE from emergency budget sources. Many relied on provision provided from already stretched resources of hospitals and clinics. Shortages of PPE led to multiple use of 'one-time use' items such as surgical and N95 masks (O'Byrne et al, 2020).

During the pandemic, the number of patients presenting with common medical conditions dropped to very low numbers compared to patients with COVID-19 symptoms. This drastically altered the student learning experience for meeting well-established learning outcomes based on conditions that form the student's future professional scope of practice. Therefore, learning objectives became fluid with learning situated directly in the here and now for student involvement in COVID-19 cases and the sequala of the virus on comorbidities. Lave and Wegner's (1991) community of practice supports clinical competence to develop and foster in a rapidly changing clinical environment and compressed time frame. Students as legitimate peripheral participants became directly involved in disaster management and well-versed in recognising and treating a new zoonotic virus.

Pedagogies in the clinical platform also adapted with blended learning as a dynamic method for teaching and learning. Many programmes incorporated hybrid learning with three days in the clinical area, to reduce risk and exposure with two days of online learning for theory and simulated clinical cases.

Preparing and educating students on COVID-19

Student resilience and change management needed to become part of the health science curriculum for current and future students to be prepared for inevitable pandemics. Few health science faculties include disaster preparedness in the curriculum (O'Byrne et al, 2020), leaving students vulnerable and unprepared for the pandemic.

Using an online learning management system (Ulwazi/Canvas), the Health Science Faculty introduced a COVID-19 Handbook to prepare students for the return to campus and subsequent re-engagement with clinical training during the pandemic (Smalley, 2020). The online Handbook was accessible to all students and staff, easily updated with changing regulations, policy, and COVID-19 related information. The Handbook was included in the student orientation, with a section dedicated to resilience with video workshops.

Another aspect of change management was the need to develop a system for identifying positive COVID-19 cases in the student body and subsequent quarantine/isolation procedures to ensure the safety of the student and campus population. A COVID-19 screening app was used for daily screening of all students and staff entering campus and attending clinical sessions for symptoms, exposure or testing positive to COVID-19. The Handbook presented a risk table with various scenarios if a student had low-risk exposure (>1m from positive or suspected COVID-19 patient or person, <15 minutes duration in a closed environment and wearing appropriate PPE for the encounter) or high-risk exposure (<1m from positive or suspected COVID-19 patient or person, >15 minutes duration in a closed environment and not wearing appropriate PPE for the encounter) or developed symptoms of COVID-19 indicative of a Person Under Investigation to initiate a PCR COVID-19 test, or had a positive COVID-19 test (Smalley, 2020).

Assessment

When a pandemic alters the normal teaching and learning practices, it is important to review the theoretical underpinnings of assessment practice. The pandemic paved the way for programmatic assessment to become a pragmatic means to measure and assess student learning when faced with limited sessions for large group assessment activities, disruptions in clinical learning and unexpected timelines (Van der Vleuten, 2012). Multiple, low stakes, high quality, valid and reliable measurements can be implemented online and face-to-face. A challenge during a pandemic is the need to make curricular decisions without all the information. However, having a programmatic assessment allows for flexibility as many activities, weighted in small increments, combine to make the final mark. The assessment plan should be developed alongside the curriculum as an intentional educational design (Schuwirth and Van der Vleuten, 2004). This can involve designing multiple assessment methods, both formative and summative, with different assessment tools like portfolios and work-based assessments, administered to incorporate context and authentic learning even in a changing educational landscape as experienced during a pandemic (Figure 12.4).

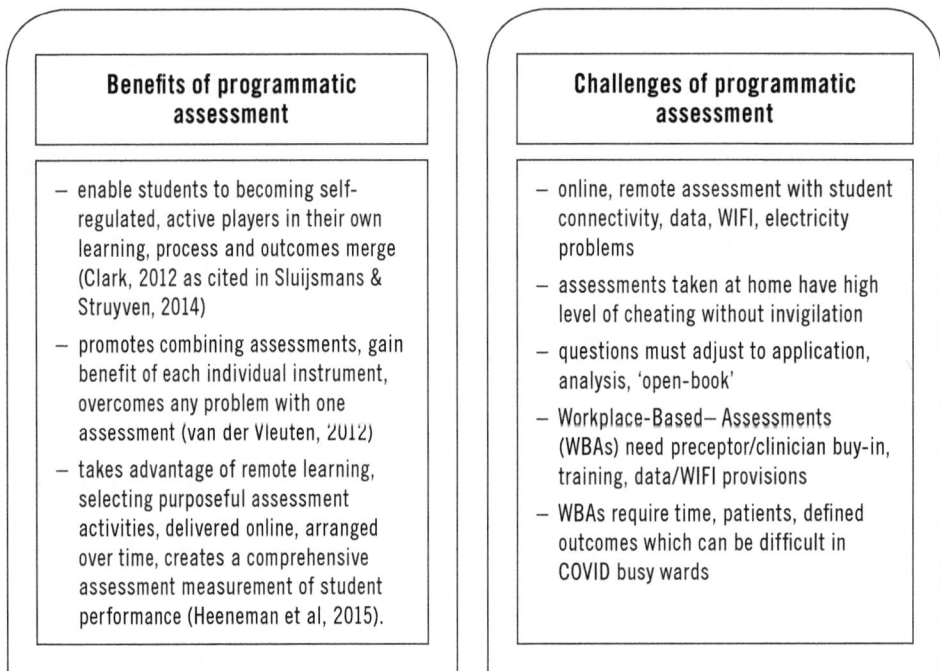

Benefits of programmatic assessment	**Challenges of programmatic assessment**
– enable students to becoming self-regulated, active players in their own learning, process and outcomes merge (Clark, 2012 as cited in Sluijsmans & Struyven, 2014) – promotes combining assessments, gain benefit of each individual instrument, overcomes any problem with one assessment (van der Vleuten, 2012) – takes advantage of remote learning, selecting purposeful assessment activities, delivered online, arranged over time, creates a comprehensive assessment measurement of student performance (Heeneman et al, 2015).	– online, remote assessment with student connectivity, data, WIFI, electricity problems – assessments taken at home have high level of cheating without invigilation – questions must adjust to application, analysis, 'open-book' – Workplace-Based– Assessments (WBAs) need preceptor/clinician buy-in, training, data/WIFI provisions – WBAs require time, patients, defined outcomes which can be difficult in COVID busy wards

Figure 12.4 Benefits and challenges of programmatic assessment

Even more so during a pandemic, with students and educators disconnected from face-to-face sessions, there is the need for continual feedback, optimising learning opportunities and reducing limitations. Assessment for learning in a programmatic assessment plan must provide students with meaningful information on their performance, allowing the learner to be an owner of their progression (Heeneman et al, 2015). Feedback must go both ways, with educators needing continual feedback from students on the assessment process and meeting objective outcomes during such a disruption.

12.6 CONCLUSION

Health professions education will not return to pre-pandemic habits as we experienced during the COVID-19 pandemic. There is complexity in responding to the effects of a pandemic within these three fundamental curricula areas requiring a responsive, dynamic, and integrated educational environment.

Reviewing approaches to health science education acknowledges different learning theories and during a pandemic forces innovation to promote learning agility in times of crisis. The curricula became a living entity with the organic creation of the Lived 21st Century Learning Framework during the upheaval. There was a constant push and pull of the three main pillars, with the three areas of knowledge threatened and supported by stakeholders. Confusion in time gave way to a common purpose to complete the academic year with learning objectives both altered for the context and maintained for the common purpose.

Surviving and thriving in health professions education is possible through a crisis.

12.7 SELF-ASSESSMENT QUESTIONS

1. What are the three types of knowledge indicated by Kereluik et al (2015) that were embedded in the Lived 21st Century Learning Framework: Learning through a pandemic?
2. What pragmatic approach to assessment emerged during the pandemic?

12.8 REFERENCES

Barnard-Ashton, P.M., Adams, F., Rothberg, A. and McInerney, P. 2018. Digital apartheid and the effect of mobile technology during rural fieldwork. *South African Journal of Occupational Therapy* 48(2), pp. 20–15. Available at: http://www.sajot.co.za/index.php/sajot/article/view/505/314.

Barnard-Ashton, P.M. 2018. The Integration of Blended Learning into the Undergraduate Occupational Therapy Curriculum. Thesis, University of the Witwatersrand. Available at: http://wiredspace.wits.ac.za/handle/10539/26984.

Czerniewicz, L., Agherdien, N., Badenhorst, J., Belluigi, D., Chambers, T., Chili, M., De Villiers, M., Felix, A., Gachago, D., Gokhale, C., Ivala, E., Kramm, N., Madiba, M., Mistri, G., Mgqwashu, E., Pallitt, N., Prinsloo, P., Solomon, K., Strydom, S., Swanepoel, M., Waghid, F. and Wissing, G. 2020. A wake-up call: Equity, inequality and COVID-19 emergency remote teaching and learning. *Postdigital Science and Education* 2, pp. 946–967. doi: https://doi.org/10.1007/s42438-020-00187-4.

D'Auria, G. and De Smet, A. 2020. Leadership in a crisis: Responding to the coronavirus outbreak and future challenges. Available at: https://www.mckinsey.com/business-functions/organization/our-insights/leadership-in-a-crisis-responding-to-the-coronavirus-outbreak-and-future-challenges?cid=eml-web.

Dewey, J. 1916. *Democracy and Education: An Introduction to the Philosophy of Education* (Unabridged Replication – 2004). New York: Dover Publications.

Drack, M. and Apfalter, W. 2007. Is Paul A. Weiss' and Ludwig von Bertalanffy's system thinking still valid today? *Systems Research and Behavioral Science: The Official Journal of the International Federation for Systems Research* 24, pp. 537–546.

Edmondson, A.C. 2020. Don't hide bad news in times of crisis. *Harvard Business Review,* 06 March. Available at: https://hbr.org/2020/03/dont-hide-bad-news-in-times-of-crisis.

Ertmer, P.A. and Newby, T.J. 2013. Behaviorism, cognitivism, constructivism: Comparing critical features from an instructional design perspective. *Performance Improvement Quarterly* 26(2), pp. 43–71.

Foley, A. and Masingila, J. 2014. Building capacity: challenges and opportunities in large class pedagogy (LCP) in Sub-Saharan Africa. *Higher Education: The International Journal of Higher Education and Educational Planning* 67(6), pp. 797–808.

Frenk, J., Chen, L., Bhutta, Z.A., Cohen, J., Crisp, N., Evans, T., Fineberg, H., Garcia, P., Ke, Y., Kelley, P., Kistnasamy, B., Meleis, A., Naylor, D., Pablos-Mendez, A., Reddy, S., Scrimshaw, S., Sepulveda, J., Serwadda, D. and Zurayk, H. 2010. Health professionals for a new century: Transforming education to strengthen health systems in an interdependent world. *The Lancet* 376(9756), pp. 1923–1958.

Gewurtz, R.E., Coman, L., Dhillon, S., Jung, B. and Solomon, P. 2016. Problem-based learning and theories of teaching and learning in health professional education. *Journal of Perspectives in Applied Academic Practice* 4(1). doi: 10.14297/jpaap.v4i1.194.

Green-Thompson L.P., McInerney P., Manning D.M., Mapukata-Sondzaba N., Chipamaunga, S. and Maswanganyi, T. 2012. Reflections of students graduating from a transforming medical curriculum in South Africa: a qualitative study. *BMC Medical Education* 12, pp. 1–9.

Hassan, S. 2007. How to develop a core curriculum in clinical skills for undergraduate medical teaching in the school of medical sciences at Universiti Sains Malaysia? *The Malaysian Journal of Medical Sciences* 14, p. 4.

Heeneman, S., Pool, A.O., Scuwirth, L.W.T., Van der Vleuten, C.P.M. and Driessen, E.W. 2015. The impact of programmatic assessment on student learning: theory versus practice. *Medical Education* 49, pp. 487–498. doi: 10.1111/medu.12645.

Heitz, C., Laboissiere, M., Sanghvi, S. and Sarakatsannis, J. 2020. Public Sector Practice: Getting the next phase of remote learning right in higher education, *McKinsey & Company*. Available at: https://www.mckinsey.com/industries/ public-and-social-sector/our-insights/getting-the-next-phase-of-remote-learning-right-in-higher-education.

Illanes, P.L., Jonathan, M.A., Sanghvi, S. and Sarakatsannis J. 2020. Coronavirus and the campus: How can US higher education organise to respond? Available at: https://www.mckinsey.com/industries/public-and-social-sector/our-insights/ coronavirus-and-the-campus-how-can-us-higher-education-organize-to-respond.

Jay, J. 2014. Problem-based learning – A review of students' perceptions in an Occupational Therapy undergraduate curriculum. *South African Journal of Occupational Therapy* 44, pp. 56–61.

Kauffman, D.M. and Mann, K.V. 2014. Teaching and learning in medical education: How theory can inform practice. In T.J. Swanwick (Ed). 2014. *Understanding medical education: Evidence, theory and practice.* 2nd Ed. Wiley & Sons, West Sussex. Chapter 2.

Kedraka, K. and Kaltsidis, C. 2020. Effects of the COVID-19 pandemic on university pedagogy: students' experiences and considerations. *European Journal of Education Studies* 7(8). doi: http://dx.doi.org/10.46827/ejes.v7i8.3176.

Kereluik, K., Punya, M., Chris, F. and Laura T. 2013. What knowledge is of most worth: Teacher knowledge for 21st century learning. *Journal of Digital Learning in Teacher Education* 29(4), pp. 127–140. doi: 10.1080/21532974.2013.10784716.

Kolb, A.Y. and Kolb, D.A. 2005. Learning styles and learning spaces: enhancing experiential learning in higher education. *Academy of Management Learning & Education* 4(2): pp. 193–212.

Lave, J. and Wenger, E. 1991. *Situated learning: Legitimate peripheral participation*: Cambridge University Press.

MacFarlane, C. and Green-Thompson, L. 2006. Medical student education in emergency medicine: new model from South Africa. *Emergency Medicine Australasia* 18, pp. 276–281.

Myezwa H., Maleka D., McInerney P., Potterton J. and Watt, B. 2017. 'He has a life, a soul, a meaning that extends far deeper than his medical assessment....': The role of reflective diaries in enhancing reflective practice during a rural community physiotherapy placement. *African Journal of Health Professions Education* 9, pp. 54–56.

O'Byrne, L. et al. 2020. Medical students and COVID-19: the need for pandemic preparedness. *J Med Ethics* 46, pp. 623–626. doi:10.1136/medethics-2020-106353.

Schuwirth, L.W.T. and Van der Vleuten, C.P.M. 2004. Changing education, changing assessment, changing research? *Medical Education* 38, pp. 805–812. Available at: http://onlinelibrary.wiley.com/doi/10.1111/j.1365-2929.2004.01851.x/epdf.

Smalley, S. 2020. Wits COVID-19 Handbook. Ulwazi Learning Management System, The University of the Witwatersrand. Available at: https://ulwazi.wits.ac.za/courses/19776.

Torre, D.M., Daley, B.J., Sebastian, J.L. and Elnicki, D.M. 2006. Overview of current learning theories for medical educators. *The American Journal of Medicine* 119, pp. 903–907. doi: 10.1016/j.amjmed.2006.06.037.

Wilkinson, L., Boyles, T., Moosa, S., Muller, M. and Cooke, R. 2020. COVID-19 Primary Care Facility Preparedness Guide. Johannesburg Metro Health District, Gauteng Department of Health, South Africa.

Van der Vleuten, C.P.M., Schuwirth, L.W., Driessen, E.W., Dkjkstra, K., Tigelaar, D., Baartman, L.K.J., Van Tartwijk, J. 2012. A model for programmatic assessment fit for purpose. *Medical Teacher* 34, pp. 205–214. doi:10.3109/0142159X.2012.652239.

eHEALTH IN THE ERA OF PANDEMICS

Maurice Mars

Richard E. Scott

13.1 INTRODUCTION

Mankind has been 'plagued' by epidemics and pandemics throughout history, a state that continues with the WHO currently listing 20 pandemic or epidemic diseases (World Health Organization, 2020b). Given the primarily geographic distinction between epidemics (an illness in excess of normal expectancy occurring within a *community* or *region*) and pandemics (an illness occurring *worldwide and crossing international boundaries*) the impacts described in this chapter, and the technology responses, will be similar for epidemics and pandemics varying primarily in scale and locale.

As a result of this most recent pandemic (COVID-19), many social, economic, and health-related impacts have been experienced throughout the globe. With the tacit ingenuity and determination of humankind, many strategies have been devised and solutions implemented. Amongst these has been the broader application of information and communication technologies (ICT) to facilitate the delivery of health and healthcare, and healthcare-related activities (surveillance, education, research).

ICT refers to technologies that provide access to information through telecommunications. These have evolved from the telegraph and telephone, through radio and television, to the Internet, wireless networks, cell phones, and other communication media. These ICTs have spawned generations of technology applications (audio-video conferencing; cellular connectivity; 'social networks'; etc.) used to communicate health-related information (audio files; image files; video files; data files) to interested parties (healthcare workers, healthcare managers, data analysts, researchers, policy- and decision-makers, and now the general populace).

'The use of information and communication technologies (ICT) for health' is the WHO definition of eHealth (World Health Organization, 2020a), with health broadly defined as 'a state of complete physical, mental and social well-being' and 'not merely the absence of disease or infirmity' (World Health

Organization, 2020c). A number of other terms have been used for aspects of eHealth: telemedicine, telehealth, mHealth, and most recently digital health (or dHealth). There is an ongoing debate and some confusion over the meaning of these words, compounded by the fact that while each has a nuanced difference, they are frequently and incorrectly, used synonymously (Scott and Mars, 2019).

The most recent of these terms, dHealth, also has varying definitions. The WHO describes it as a 'a broad umbrella term encompassing eHealth, (which includes mHealth), as well as emerging areas, such as the use of advancing computing sciences in "big data", genomics and artificial intelligence' (World Health Organization, 2019). Alternatively it is 'the fusion of technologies that blur the lines between the physical, digital, and biological spheres' (Schwab, 2017).

Most simply eHealth is comprised of four components: health informatics (data accumulation, storage, analysis, and diffusion of resulting information), telehealth (delivery of health and health-related services), e-learning (technology enabled and enhanced training), and e-commerce (business aspects of health and healthcare), Figure 13.1 (Scott and Mars, 2015). Such distinction is fading as many applications often merge two or more of these components. This chapter focuses primarily on one component of eHealth, telehealth, and adopts the broad description of the World Health Organization: Telehealth is–

> [the] delivery of health care services, where patients and providers are separated by distance. Telehealth uses ICT for the exchange of information for the diagnosis and treatment of diseases and injuries, research and evaluation, and for the continuing education of health professionals (World Health Organization, 2016).

Encompassed within the broader practice of telehealth is the more focussed practice of telemedicine, defined as '[a] medical service provided remotely via information and communication technology' (Economics Europe, 2018).

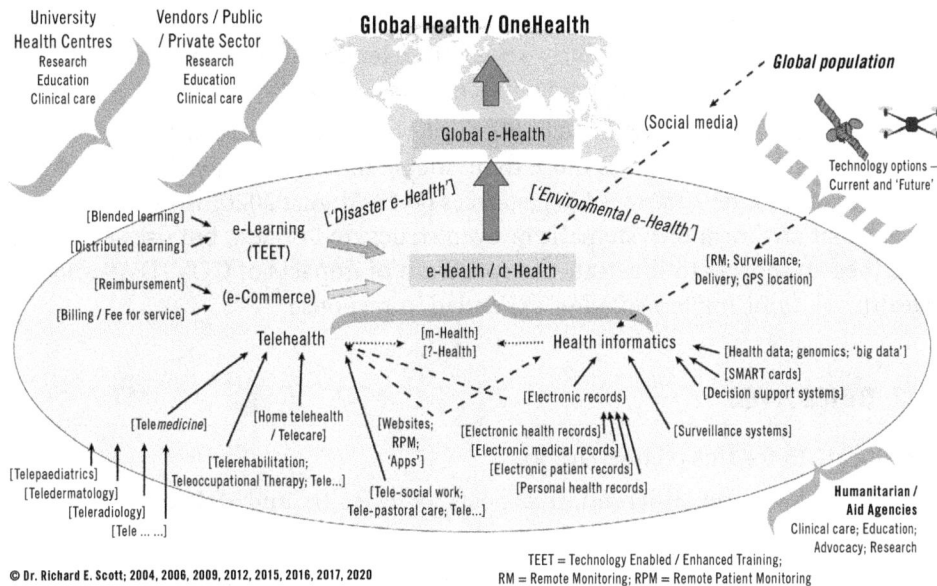

Figure 13.1 Summary illustration of the breadth of eHealth / dHealth, the global users and influencers, and the relationship with Global Health or OneHealth (recognising the zoonotic aspects of population health)

eHealth is able to use any form of ICT device (e.g., desktop PC, laptop, iPad, smart device, sensors) and covers preventative, promotive, and curative aspects of health (Scott and Mars, 2015). It can use simple or complex multimedia and is interactive: e.g., synchronous – 'real-time' person-to-person or person-to-software engagement; asynchronous – delayed messaging such as email; or hybrid – 'near real time' such as instant messaging; or sequential use of both modes – an email followed by a telephone call. eHealth can also engage and link all types of users (from highly trained clinicians to minimally trained community healthcare workers, managers, researchers, patients, and the general population), and is capable of being used as an alternate or complementary approach for almost any health issue imaginable (Scott and Mars, 2015).

Despite recent disruption to 'face-to-face' delivery of healthcare, such delivery will not disappear. Healthcare providers continue to stoically struggle, often with inadequate facilities and a lack of personal protective equipment (PPE), to deliver healthcare in this fashion (Bong et al, 2020; Ranney et al, 2020). eHealth has certainly come to the fore during this pandemic, but as often stated, such technology is not a replacement for traditional healthcare, merely another tool available to be used as and when appropriate. COVID-19 has simply highlighted just how appropriate that can be.

Pandemics create fundamental change in the way people live, work and relate to each other. This is particularly so when eHealth is used to ameliorate the negative impacts of epidemics and pandemics.

The pace of COVID-19-related publications has been unprecedented. A simple PubMed search saw resources more than double in just two months; from 4 208 resources on 15 June 2020 to 9 470 resources on 13 August 2020. This chapter does not attempt any form of systematic or even structured review, but uses examples from these resources to illustrate the spectrum of impacts of COVID-19 and the eHealth solutions implemented or expanded in response.

13.2 OBJECTIVES

The objectives for this chapter are to:

- Introduce and differentiate aspects of eHealth and dHealth, and sub-components of eHealth.
- Summarise ways in which eHealth, in particular telemedicine, has been, is being, or could be used in addressing impacts of epidemics and pandemics.
- Briefly introduce and describe some challenges to the integration of eHealth into routine health and healthcare delivery globally.

13.3 EHEALTH AND PANDEMICS – ICARES

For convenience, the acronym ICARES (Information, Clinical, Administration, Research, Education, and Surveillance) is used as a guide to describe the many ways in which eHealth has been, and can be, used in addressing epidemics and pandemics such as COVID-19. ICARES serves merely as a convenient 'rule of thumb' as there is overlap between categories.

13.3.1 Information Applications

Information is considered knowledge (obtained from investigation, study, or instruction) concerning a particular fact or circumstance that is exchanged using ICT. The information can be shared within and between many groups; health professionals, health experts (modellers and managers), decision- and policy-makers, patients, and the population.

Although not universal, many journals altered their processes to facilitate timely access to data, research, and information related to COVID-19, thereby potentially facilitating policy development and speeding clinical research. This has typically involved making COVID-19-related articles open-access and freely accessible, and/or (while maintaining appropriate peer review) publishing online and in advance of any planned print publication or through pre-print servers (Horbach, 2020; Song and Karako, 2020). Editors have reviewed and revised their roles and processes, and some journals have opened new sections specifically for COVID-19, such as BMJ's Best Practice (https://bestpractice. bmj.com/topics/en-gb/3000168). During their scanning of COVID-19-related publications, the authors noted an initial predominance of opinion pieces and editorials, which gave way to observational reports, and now more structured and informative research.

Both traditional and contemporary forms of dissemination have been used to share information to inform the public, avoid panic, or encourage appropriate behaviour (physical distancing; frequent handwashing; vaccination) and lifestyle changes (mask wearing; lockdown). Many gleaned information from the television, radio, or print media (Moosa, 2020), but many also utilised mobile and non-mobile technology to share information through social media (Facebook, YouTube, TikTok, WeChat, Instagram, Twitter, WhatsApp, LinkedIn), including medical students and healthcare providers (Olum and Bongomin, 2020).

Regrettably, this also facilitates the dissemination of misinformation and disinformation (Cuan-Baltazar et al, 2020; Li et al, 2020; Scott and Mars, 2020), creating an 'infodemic' with consequent harms (public mistrust, health dangers, crime, and death) (Ball and Maxmen, 2020; Cinelli et al, 2020, Islam et al, 2020; Lally and Christie, 2020). This has led to calls for a duty of care for social media companies to detect and remove inaccurate or false online content (Lally and Christie, 2020; Tasnim et al, 2020). While controversial, this has been pursued by several social media outlets, although diligence and effectiveness can be questioned.

The almost real-time updating, streaming, and use of algorithms related to social media presents issues of bias and information overload, leading to negative social behaviour, overconcern/anxiety, cyberchondria, and other mental health concerns (Farooq et al, 2020; O'Brien et al, 2020). It also damages the utility of social media as a convenient source of information for infodemiological and infoveillance studies.

Several papers considered the pandemic appropriate for implementing disaster protocols, and highlighted the need for the greater insertion of eHealth into existing medical school curricula and disaster plans during any review and revision, as well as ensuring the necessary info- and infrastructure is in place to permit immediate response for single or concomitant disasters (Rockwell and Gilroy, 2020; Scott and Mars, 2020; Smith and Fraser, 2020). Notably, Ashcroft et al highlighted that any form of eHealth training (from simple classroom-based interactive discussion to complex multimodal simulative experiences) resulted in improved knowledge, skill and attitudes (Ashcroft et al, 2020).

13.3.2 Clinical Applications

The COVID-19 pandemic has led to a 'new normal', the new way of doing things under lockdown, quarantine and social distancing. Medical practice, like business and education, has also adapted. Patients need to be protected from unnecessary contact with others who might be infected, and health professionals (a scarce commodity) need to be protected from avoidable contact with potentially infected patients. One aspect of telehealth, telemedicine, has always been seen as a way of overcoming the 'tyranny of distance' by improving access to, and the quality of, care particularly for those who live in rural and remote areas. The new normal is medicine practised, when possible and appropriate, at a distance. This has happened globally and rapidly, and across many specialities and allied health and support services (Bidmead and Marshall, 2020). In the United States, Amwell reported a 2 000% increase in visits on its platform before the end of April 2020. Over six weeks in March and April 2020, Langone Health in New York had a 4 345% increase in non-urgent video doctor visits, and virtual urgent care triage grew by 683% (Kaplan, 2020).

Telemedicine has involved triage, assessment and management of new cases, patient follow-up, monitoring, and screening. Triage, a well-established approach, has now been used via telephone or video call to avoid unnecessary human contact and travel for the protection of both the patient and health professional. It assists those who seek advice about COVID-19 and their need for testing or treatment, and helps determine if those with other medical conditions, both urgent and non-urgent, need to attend physically for care.

The assessment and management of new cases have followed the conventional forms of real-time interaction by synchronous video-conference or asynchronous store and forward telemedicine. Both have been extended through the use of applications not designed for clinical use (Skype, Facetime, Zoom, WhatsApp, WeChat, Facebook). There is also growing use of direct-to-consumer websites where patients can purchase a clinical service. Concerns around, for example, record-keeping, privacy and authentication for direct-to-consumer services remain.

Where appropriate, follow-up has migrated to the telephone or video-link, although problematic where health facilities are not online, or no electronic medical records exist. Allied to this is access to repeat medications. Such situations need further investigation. Monitoring takes many forms, some of which have been addressed through the use of mobile phones for ongoing contact with quarantined individuals and the use of mobile phone applications. Screening has not been confined to telephone triage. Lockdown and the fear of infection also affect mental health, and mobile phone and web-based mental health screening tools have been used for virtual assessments.

Prior to the pandemic implementation, uptake and growth of telemedicine had been slow, and subject to much speculation and research. Factors that should be taken into account when planning and implementing a successful and sustainable telemedicine service are well summarised in the Momentum list of '18 critical factors for successful telemedicine' (Momentum, 2015). They include: needs analysis; eHealth readiness assessment; financial and business plans; change management and implementation plans; and evaluation and monitoring plans; plus supportive legal, regulatory and remunerative settings.

Necessity has been the 'mother of invention'. The reality of needing to rapidly find solutions to care provision has led many clinicians who were previously ambivalent to, or even opposed to, telemedicine to become users. Some have adopted telemedicine by joining existing telemedicine services, while others have started services *de novo*. These new services are unlikely to have gone through rigorous planning and are in effect spontaneous services which fulfil the immediate needs of the health professionals, patients and health services.

What has enabled this rapid increase in telemedicine use? Health professionals have seen the benefits of telemedicine for themselves and their patients, as have funders who have expanded and improved its remuneration. Regulators have even adapted or relaxed pre-pandemic rules and regulations to facilitate its use. For example, definitions and rules related to where telemedicine can be practised, by whom, for whom, and for which conditions have been amended. This relaxation of legal and ethical regulations, guidelines, and ICT governance rules within organisations has had a profound effect. However the changes have frequently been made with the caveat that they are temporary, and have differed across the world. Some have altered requirements for the existence of a prior physician-patient relationship, others the way in which such a relationship can be established, or the need for physical examination. Rules and guidelines related to liability and responsibility for patient care, continuity of care, and unsolicited patient-initiated teleconsultation have been amended. Social media and instant messaging applications previously deemed unsuitable because of privacy and data security concerns have been approved. That ethical standards can be changed for expediency is in itself a moral and ethical conundrum and will be the subject of future debate.

A positive spinoff of the COVID-19 telemedicine surge is that, of necessity, many health professionals have been exposed to consulting 'electronically', and become aware of the related legal and ethical issues. They have, in many instances, found solutions for themselves and have independently identified the need for guidelines for using ICTs in their practice. Even those who have been sceptical, like some physiotherapists who had argued that theirs is a hands-on profession and telemedicine is inappropriate, have rapidly developed guidelines for video-consultation during the pandemic (Chartered Society of Physiotherapy, 2020).

Telemedicine is now a part of the 'new normal'. Can the clock be reset and should it be reset? Will the regulators revert to their previous positions? Will the widespread use of telemedicine remove the stigma that regulators have spuriously attached to telemedicine; that it is something new, unproven and thus potentially dangerous, and therefore requires stronger regulation than other forms of medical care to protect the patient and the professional? Irrespective of this, telemedicine has come of age and shown itself to be an essential component of health systems and providers' response to pandemics and epidemics.

13.3.3 Administrative Applications

The use of ICT for the administration of patient health services is mainly around various information systems. These include electronic medical records, scheduling, billing, radiology, picture archiving, laboratory and pharmacy information systems, surveillance reporting, data storage systems, and learning management systems for education. Each of these usually has associated legally and ethically mandated administrative functions, standard operating procedures, IT governance rules and data access and privacy rules.

For some clinicians, their adoption of telemedicine has exposed them to some of these for the first time. It has obliged them to learn and follow the relevant legal, ethical, and clinical guidelines for telemedicine. This has involved issues such as developing appropriate standard operating procedures, record keeping of synchronous and asynchronous consultations in the absence of an EMR, re-evaluating their data security measures and the security of the software used, adaptation of their routine workflow to include video-conferencing and phone triage, the consent process, implementing ePrescription, understanding new billing procedures, and in some countries licensure.

13.3.4 Research Applications

As described under 'Information', ICTs have and will continue to be used to disseminate research findings which, during epidemics and pandemics, can have immediate effects on medical practice, research, and policy. The literature also described or exemplified ways in which COVID-19 has impacted the performance and process of research itself, and how ICT has been used to facilitate or stimulate research into aspects of COVID-19 (vaccines, epidemiology) as well as responses to the pandemic (effectiveness of masks, physical distancing).

eHealth has been used to continue or facilitate research and initiate new research partnerships. Thus, virtual Communities of Practice have provided interactive fora for confidential or open sharing of data, facilitating exchange of ideas, and building new collaborations (McLoughlin et al, 2018). Simply the ability to share diverse data amongst agencies and researchers is considered crucial for activities such as contact tracing (Moorthy et al, 2020).

More esoteric research has also been stimulated, such as the use of drones for the delivery of PPE, drugs, blood, and other items (Demuyakor, 2020; Van Veelen et al, 2020). Research into drug repurposing to identify therapeutically potent molecules from pre-existing molecules has been pursued, using computer-based simulation (Muralidharan et al, 2020).

Underappreciated issues stimulated by COVID-19 that impact the performance and process of health research were identified, such as the difficulty in maintaining funding, facilities, and resources for early-career (graduate, post-doctoral) and seasoned (professional, academic) research positions and projects (Ahmed et al, 2020; Cheng and Song, 2020). The impact of lockdowns on experimental and time-sensitive studies was noted, where 'working from home' is simply not an option. Further complications associated with visas, repatriation, and travel bans for international students or researchers expecting to begin research abroad were identified. The only solution for some has been to await the re-opening of universities and research laboratories. The specific role of eHealth in addressing these concerns and issues is a rapidly evolving area.

Regarding specific research issues, the WHO identified research trends and gaps in COVID-19 related research (Zhang and Shaw, 2020). Eight knowledge gaps were highlighted: (1) human-animal interface, (2) clinical considerations, (3) vaccines, (4) behaviour and education, (5) transmission, (6) therapeutics, (7) healthcare workers, and (8) ethical considerations. Additional gaps were also noted: pandemic governance, incorporation of epidemic and pandemic issues in disaster response, risk assessment methodologies, supply chain management, and business continuity planning. The need for multidisciplinary research into many other areas (long-term care, economics of pandemics, sociology, ecology) was also recognised, amongst many more research issues, some of which will involve application of eHealth.

13.3.5 Educational Applications

While there is nothing new or novel about using ICTs for aspects of distance education, the impact of COVID-19 on the delivery of education within healthcare has been broad and deep (Hilburg et al, 2020). The pandemic has affected every setting (international, regional, national and institutional), every educational forum (conferences, workshops, seminars, classes, and clinical placements), every educational level (undergraduate, graduate, postgraduate, and professional), every health-related occupation (physicians, nurses, allied health professionals, volunteers), and every assessment mechanism (written examinations; objective structured clinical examinations; open-book examinations). Impacts have affected contemporary education (university programmes; continuing professional development), as well as COVID-19 specific education (proper PPE use and patient care; mental health of those in long-term or repeated periods of isolation; handling stress of challenging healthcare delivery and increased patient fatalities).

In an attempt to compensate, eHealth responses have been swift, grand, or basic, but always innovative, and ostensibly successful. Many activities have been transferred to 'fully online' delivery, or faced cancellation or indefinite postponement. Basic responses have often involved the use of learning management systems and video conferencing solutions (Kanneganti et al, 2020; Moszkowicz et al, 2020). Examples of swift and grand responses have included China making over 24 000 online courses accessible to university students, and Russia reporting over 70% of its universities had transferred to educational processes online (The World Bank, 2020). While superficially impressive, the true utility and effectiveness of these actions have yet to be reported, as have healthcare-specific aspects. However, past research from high and low-quality studies has shown online e-learning to be equivalent, possibly superior, to traditional learning and skills gained (George et al, 2014). The potential for permanent transition to online learning has also been raised, heightened by recent risk-laden moves to return students to campuses (Marris, 2020).

Although social media have been applied for medical education for more than a decade, such tools are gaining renewed interest. Thus innovative uses of social network platforms and smartphones have occurred (Latif et al, 2019).

Some authors did address the 'elephant in the room' – the likelihood that in many instances the principles behind sound development and delivery of distance education have been ignored in the rush (Scott et al, 2017). These principles include aspects such as 'Clarify Purpose and Conduct a Needs Assessment', although the purpose and need may be considered self-evident given COVID-19. But others, such as 'Allow Adequate Time and Technology for Development', 'Pilot Before Implementing', or 'Create Different Resources for Different Groups' have certainly not been universally performed. Traditionally delivered content cannot be simply transferred to online delivery (Ortiz, 2020; Seymour-Walsh et al, 2020). Healthcare-related teachers and trainers not only need to understand the adult-focused learning theory and teaching approaches that leverage the unique learning styles and strengths of adult learners (andragogy), but also the many technologies and tools that can enable and enhance delivery, and require training in order to utilise them effectively and efficiently.

An opportunity that remains to be debated is the potential to pool resources. In-service presentations, lectures, etc., could be delivered by national or even international expert faculty, avoiding the need to produce local material at each training site, and potentially raising the standard of education with subsequent healthcare benefits. This is often not pursued due to the emotive, almost proprietary, belief in the need for 'local' training. However, this aspect need not be sacrificed if local perspective is also provided by local educators.

Finally, beyond these educational concerns, issues of discrimination and social exclusion will have occurred despite best efforts to avoid this. Thus individuals from lower economic echelons may not have had the financial status or skill set allowing them unfettered availability of and access to technology (smartphones versus basic or feature phones; laptops; datapads; webcams) or the necessary connectivity (bandwidth; speed; duration) to avail themselves of many – any – opportunities. These issues may be of particular concern to developing countries and vulnerable populations.

The longstanding debate about 'fitting' eHealth into formal medical school curricula may also be ending. Stimulated by COVID-19, a new medical school is now formally teaching its inaugural class of medical students via Zoom on how to give remote care (Augenstein, 2020). Similarly, the longstanding didactic and face-to-face paradigm of health-related education, including professional conferences and continuing professional development (CPD), is also being challenged, with existing research showing that lectures actually result in the lowest level of behavioural change (Stancic et al, 2003).

13.3.6 Surveillance Applications

The WHO describes public health surveillance as '[a]n ongoing, systematic collection, analysis and interpretation of health-related data essential to the planning, implementation, and evaluation of public health practice'. (World Health Organization, 2020d). eHealth (or digital) technologies are already an integral part of many routine passive and active surveillance activities (reporting networks, satellite remote monitoring, syndromic surveillance) and the benefits of eHealth for data acquisition and analysis are well established.

The global growth in use of eHealth offers increasing opportunities for surveillance (Budd et al, 2020), with data exchange occurring both within and between national and international jurisdictions around the world. For example, daily international reporting of new cases, deaths and recoveries, at national and sub-national levels, has occurred during the COVID-19 pandemic. Rapid analysis of such data supports the formulation and implementation of appropriate national policies, strategies and actions. However, this requires data exchange from different sources using, currently, varied national and international data standards and reporting formats, creating significant interoperability (exchange) challenges which will require resolution as broader use of eHealth continues.

Contact tracing has also moved further into the eHealth realm. Methods include (1) mobile phone apps that may communicate with nearby phones via Bluetooth or be used to collect personal health, travel and other data,

(2) geolocation using GPS and cellphone towers to determine where the phone has been and which other phones were in that location at that time, or to confirm that those under quarantine have not left home, (3) monitoring people's movements through requiring the use of QR codes to enter businesses and public transport, with the information sent to local authorities, and (4) in combination with analysis of closed-circuit television (CCTV) and credit card receipts. Each of the digital contact tracing methods has shortcomings and concerns about privacy, confidentiality and data security, which vary from country to country. The worth of these methods is still to be assessed.

Event-based surveillance, defined as 'the organised collection, monitoring, assessment and interpretation of mainly unstructured *ad hoc* information regarding health events or risks, which may represent an acute risk to human health' is facilitated by eHealth (World Health Organization, 2014). This includes satellite image analysis, environmental and ecological surveillance, and analysis of 'digital' media – newspapers, websites, and social media (Twitter, instant messaging apps).

Pharmacovigilance, a form of surveillance, involves the detection, assessment, understanding and prevention of adverse reactions or any other medication related problems. This is relevant during pandemics caused by novel agents which require new treatment regimens, vaccine development, or drug repurposing. An example of the latter is the controversial use of chloroquine and hydroxychloroquine. Pharmacovigilance is supported through the use of eHealth and international databases of adverse events.

13.4 CHALLENGES TO eHEALTH INTEGRATION

Specific challenges vary by jurisdiction but include a plethora of issues that include: an absence of thoughtful and complete country and region eHealth strategies, and lack of necessary infrastructure and infostructure. Strategies typically lack detailed alignment of health needs with specific eHealth solutions, lack stable and long-term budgetary allocation, and lack dependable healthcare provider compensation. Infrastructure (from reliable electricity to functionally and equitably available connectivity) is typically lacking. Infostructure considerations (all other needs beyond physical hardware and software infrastructure) fail to address issues such as relevant, adequately trained, and equitably distributed health and ICT human resources, and a conducive legal, regulatory and ethical setting.

Currently, to permit response to COVID-19, many countries have modified, eased, or suspended prior legal, regulatory and ethical barriers to eHealth application, but the longevity of these approaches post-pandemic is unclear (Bashshur et al, 2020; Keesara et al, 2020). Global legal issues also arise and include abiding by accepted international laws such as the International Health Regulations, flaunted by many countries in their rush to close national borders (Habibi et al, 2020).

Without careful consideration and resolution of such challenges at the local, national, and international levels, true integration of eHealth (telehealth, telemedicine, e-learning, health informatics, and dHealth aspects) will continue to flounder, placing effective and global response to future epidemics and pandemics in jeopardy.

13.5 CONCLUSION

eHealth, in its broadest sense, will continue to be used to mitigate negative impacts of disasters, including pandemics. Some elements (discrimination, social exclusion, misinformation, disinformation, excessive exposure through social media) will remain a challenge. Greater research to mitigate these aspects is needed.

Although not truly embedded within any single healthcare system, the historical and contemporary depth and breadth of the application of eHealth is great, whether for information, clinical, administrative, research, education, or surveillance needs. Beyond its 'day-to-day' applications eHealth has a clear role to play in responding to epidemics and pandemics. This has been exemplified by the global response to COVID-19, although some countries have fared better than others, highlighting the often stated principle – *the time to learn is not during the disaster response period.*

While ways to apply eHealth for ICARES have been honed or developed, these have typically been urgently responsive rather than carefully planned. Implementation of e-records, design of virtually-delivered programmes and courses, development of eHealth systems, and thorough analysis of big data, all typically require many months. The clearest lesson from the world's response to COVID-19 has been the need for eHealth to be effectively and efficiently integrated within resilient national healthcare systems, and the systems of global health agencies, NOW – prior to the next event. In this way 'we' – the public, patients, providers, and policy-makers – will be primed and able to use these tools when and as needed, not struggling to develop, understand, and apply them on the fly.

13.6 SELF-ASSESSMENT QUESTIONS

1. Define eHealth and list the six broad areas in which it can be used to address the impacts of epidemics and pandemics.

2. The COVID-19 pandemic has led to an unparalleled increase in the practice of telemedicine – medical service provided remotely using information and communication technologies (ICT). What are some of the reasons for this?

13.7 REFERENCES

Ahmed, M.A., Behbahani, A.H., Brückner, A., Charpentier, C.J., Morais, L.H., Mallory, S. and Pool, A.H. 2020. The precarious position of postdocs during COVID-19. *Science* 368(6494), pp. 957–958.

Ashcroft, J., Byrne, M.H., Brennan, P.A. and Davies, R.J. 2020. Preparing medical students for a pandemic: a systematic review of student disaster training programmes. *Postgraduate Medical Journal* 97(1148), pp. 368–379. doi: 10.1136/postgradmedj-2020-137906.

Augenstein, S. 2020. Telehealth course is 'Part of the Future' at Hackensack Meridian School of Medicine at SHU. Available at: https://www.shu.edu/news/telehealth-is-part-of-future-at-school-of-medicine.cfm.

Ball, P. and Maxmen, A. 2020. Battling the infodemic. *Nature* 581, pp. 371–374.

Bashshur, R., Doarn, C.R., Frenk, J.M., Kvedar, J.C. and Woolliscroft, J.O. 2020. Telemedicine and the COVID-19 Pandemic, Lessons For The Future. *Telemedicine and e-Health* 26(5), pp. 571–573.

Bidmead, E. and Marshall, A. 2020. Covid-19 and the 'new normal': are remote video consultations here to stay? *British Medical Bulletin*, ldaa025.

Bong, C.L., Brasher, C., Chikumba, E., Mcdougall, R., Mellin-Olsen, J. and Enright, A. 2020. The COVID-19 pandemic: Effects on low-and middle-income countries. *Anesthesia and Analgesia*. doi: 10.1213/ANE.0000000000004846.

Budd, J., Miller, B.S., Manning, E.M., Lampos, V., Zhuang, M., Edelstein, M., Rees, G., Emery, V.C., Stevens, M.M., Keegan, N., Short, M.J., Pillay, D., Manley, E., Cox, I.J., Hetmann, D., Johnson, A.M. and McKendry, R.A. 2020. Digital technologies in the public-health response to COVID-19. *Nature Medicine* 26, pp. 1183–1192.

Chartered Society Of Physiotherapy. 2020. COVID-19: guide for rapid implementation of remote consultations. Available at: https://www.csp.org.uk/publications/covid-19-guide-rapid-implementation-remote-physiotherapy-delivery.

Cheng, C. and Song, S. 2020. How early-career researchers are navigating the COVID-19 pandemic. *Molecular Plant* 13(9), pp. 1229–1230.

Cinelli, M., Quattrociocchi, W., Galeazzi, A., Valensise, C.M., Brugnoli, E., Schmidt, A. L., Zola, P., Zollo, F. and Scala, A. 2020. The Covid-19 social media infodemic. arXiv preprint arXiv:2003.05004. Available at: https://arxiv.org/pdf/2003.05004. pdf?fbclid= IwAR08xVUpifbp5Q KhwP3FPqu7J6o AswtPoLJIiG6pIgumFfQfnVRmI5Z8Sho.

Cuan-Baltazar, J.Y., Muñoz-Perez, M.J., Robledo-Vega, C., Pérez-Zepeda, M.F. and Soto-Vega, E. 2020. Misinformation of COVID-19 on the internet: infodemiology study. *JMIR Public Health and Surveillance* 6(2), p. e18444.

Demuyakor, J. 2020. Ghana Go Digital Agenda: The impact of zipline drone technology on digital emergency health delivery in Ghana. *Humanities* 8(1), pp. 242–253.

Economics Europe. 2018. Regulatory Approaches to Telemedicine. London: General Medical Council. Available at: https://www.gmc-uk.org/-/media/documents/regulatory-approaches-to-telemedicine_docx-73978543.docx.

Farooq, A., Laato, S. and Islam, A.N. 2020. Impact of online information on self-isolation intention during the COVID-19 pandemic: Cross-sectional study. *Journal of Medical Internet Research* 22(5), p. e19128.

George, P.P., Papachristou, N., Belisario, J.M., Wang, W., Wark, P.A., Cotic, Z., Rasmussen, K., Sluiter, R., Riboli–Sasco, E., Car, L.T. and Musulanov, E.M. 2014. Online eLearning for undergraduates in health professions: a systematic review of the impact on knowledge, skills, attitudes and satisfaction. *Journal of Global Health* 4(1), p. 010406.

Habibi, R., Burci, G.L., De Campos, T.C., Chirwa, D., Cinà, M., Dagron, S., Eccleston-Turner, M., Forman, L., Gostin, L.O., Meier, B.M. and Negri, S. 2020. Do not violate the International Health Regulations during the COVID-19 outbreak. *The Lancet* 395(10225), pp. 664–666.

Hilburg, R., Patel, N., Ambruso, S., Biewald, M.A. and Farouk, S.S. 2020. Medical education during the COVID-19 pandemic: Learning from a distance. *Advances in Chronic Kidney Disease*. doi: https://doi.org/10.1053/j.ackd.2020.05.017.

Horbach, S.P. 2020. Pandemic Publishing: Medical journals strongly speed up their publication process for Covid-19. *Quantitative Science Studies* 1–12, pp. 1056–1067.

Islam, M.S., Sarkar, T., Khan, S.H., Mostofa Kamal, A.H., Hasan, S.M.M., Kabir, A., Yeasmin, D., Islam, M.A., Amin Chowdhury, K.I., Anwar, K.S. and Chughtai, A.A. 2020. COVID-19-related infodemic and its impact on public health: a global social media analysis. *The American Journal of Tropical Medicine and Hygiene* 103(4), pp. 1621–1629.

Kanneganti, A., Sia, C.H., Ashokka, B. and Ooi, S.B.S. 2020. Continuing medical education during a pandemic: An academic institution's experience. *Postgraduate Medical Journal*. doi: 10.1136/postgradmedj-2020-137840.

Kaplan, B. 2020. Revisting health information technology ethical, legal, and social issues and evaluation: telehealth/telemedicine and COVID-19. *International Journal of Medical Informatics.* doi: https://doi.org/10.1016/j.ijmedinf.2020.104239.

Keesara, S., Jonas, A. and Schulman, K. 2020. Covid-19 and health care's digital revolution. *New England Journal of Medicine* 382(23), p. e82.

Lally, C. and Christie, L. 2020. COVID-19 misinformation. UK. Parliament Post. Available at: https://post.parliament.uk/analysis/covid-19-misinformation/.

Latif, M.Z., Hussain, I., Saeed, R., Qureshi, M.A. and Maqsood, U. 2019. Use of smart phones and social media in medical education: trends, advantages, challenges and barriers. *Acta Informatica Medica* 27(2), pp. 133–138.

Li, H.O.Y., Bailey, A., Huynh, D. and Chan, J. 2020. YouTube as a source of information on COVID-19: a pandemic of misinformation? *BMJ Global Health* 5, p. e002604.

Marris, E. 2020. Millions of students are returning to US universities in a vast unplanned pandemic experiment. *Nature* 584(7822), pp. 510–512.

Mcloughlin, C., Patel, K.D., O'Callaghan, T. and Reeves, S. 2018. The use of virtual communities of practice to improve interprofessional collaboration and education: findings from an integrated review. *Journal of Interprofessional Care* 32(2), pp. 136–142.

Momentum. 2015. Eighteen critical success factors for deploying telemedicine. Available at: http://telemedicinemomentum.eu/wpcontent/uploads/2014/05/Momentum_CSFs_v01_6may2014.pdf.

Moorthy, V., Restrepo, A.M.H., Preziosi, M.P. and Swaminathan, S. 2020. Data sharing for novel coronavirus (COVID-19). *Bulletin of the World Health Organization* 98(3), p. 150.

Moosa, M. 2020. News in the COVID-19 crisis: Where do South Africans get their news, and is it trustworthy? Findings from the 2019 South African Reconciliation Barometer. IJR Policy Brief No 27. Available at: https://media.africaportal.org/documents/IJR-Policy-Brief-No-27-News-in-the-Covid-19-crisis.pdf.

Moszkowicz, D., Duboc, H., Dubertret, C., Roux, D. and Bretagnol, F. 2020. Daily medical education for confined students during COVID-19 pandemic: A simple video conference solution. *Clinical Anatomy.* doi: 10.1002/ca.23601.

Muralidharan, N., Sakthivel, R., Velmurugan, D. and Gromiha, M.M. 2020. Computational studies of drug repurposing and synergism of lopinavir, oseltamivir and ritonavir binding with SARS-CoV-2 Protease against COVID-19. *Journal of Biomolecular Structure and Dynamics*, pp. 1–6. doi: 10.1080/07391102.2020.1752802.

O'Brien, M., Moore, K. and McNicholas, F. 2020. Social media spread during Covid-19: the pros and cons of likes and shares. *Irish Medical Journal* 113(4), pp. 52–52.

Olum, R. and Bongomin, F. 2020. Social media platforms for health communication and research in the face of COVID-19 pandemic: A cross-sectional survey in Uganda. medRxiv. doi: https://doi.org/10.1101/2020.04.30.20086553.

Ortiz, P.A. 2020. Teaching in the time of COVID-19. *Biochemistry and Molecular Biology Education* 48(3), p/ 201.

Ranney, M.L., Griffeth, V. and Jha, A.K. 2020. Critical supply shortages—the need for ventilators and personal protective equipment during the Covid-19 pandemic. *New England Journal of Medicine* 382(18), p. e41.

Rockwell, K.L. and Gilroy, A.S. 2020. Incorporating telemedicine as part of COVID-19 outbreak response systems. *American Journal of Managed Care* 26(4), pp. 147–148.

Schwab, K. The Fourth Industrial Revolution: what it means, how to respond. 2016. *World Economic Forum*, 2017.

Scott, K.M., Baur, L. and Barrett, J. 2017. Evidence-based principles for using technology-enhanced learning in the continuing professional development of health professionals. *Journal of Continuing Education in the Health Professions* 37(1), pp. 61–66.

Scott, R.E. and Mars, M. 2019. Here we go again-'digital health'. *Journal of the International Society for Telemedicine and eHealth* 7, p. e1 (1–2).

Scott, R.E. and Mars, M. 2020. Behaviour change and e-health-looking broadly: A scoping narrative review. *Studies in Health Technology and Informatics* 268, pp. 123–138.

Scott, R.E. and Mars, M. 2015. Telehealth in the developing world: current status and future prospects. *Smart Homecare Technology and TeleHealth* 3, pp. 25–37.

Seymour-Walsh, A.E., Bell, A., Weber, A. and Smith, T. 2020. Adapting to a new reality: COVID-19 coronavirus and online education in the health professions. *Rural and Remote Health* 20(2), 6000. doi: https://doi.org/10.22605/RRH6000.

Smith, N. and Fraser, M. 2020. Straining the system: Novel coronavirus (COVID-19) and preparedness for concomitant disasters. *American Journal of Public Health* 110(5), pp. 648–649.

Song, P. and Karako, T. 2020. COVID-19: Real-time dissemination of scientific information to fight a public health emergency of international concern. *Bioscience Trends*. doi: 10.5582/bst.2020.01056.

Stancic, N., Mullen, P.D., Prokhorov, A.V., Frankowski, R.F. and McAlister, A.L. 2003. Continuing medical education: what delivery format do physicians prefer? *Journal of Continuing Education in the Health Professions* 23(3), pp. 162–167.

Tasnim, S., Hossain, M.M. and Mazumder, H. 2020. Impact of rumors and misinformation on COVID-19 in social media. *Journal Of Preventive Medicine And Public Health* 53(3), pp. 171–174.

The World Bank. 2020. How countries are using edtech (including online learning, radio, television, texting) to support access to remote learning during the COVID-19 pandemic. Available at: https://www.worldbank.org/en/topic/edutech/brief/how-countries-are-using-edtech-to-support-remote-learning-during-the-covid-19-pandemic.

Van Veelen, M.J., Kaufmann, M., Brugger, H. and Strapazzon, G. 2020. Drone delivery of AED's and personal protective equipment in the era of SARS-CoV-2. *Resuscitation* 152, pp. 1–2.

World Health Organization. 2014. Early detection, assessment and response to acute public health events: implementation of early warning and response with a focus on event-based surveillance: interim version. (No. WHO/HSE/GCR/LYO/2014.4).

World Health Organization. 2016. Analysis of third global survey on eHealth based on the reported data by countries, 2016. Available at: https://www.who.int/gho/goe/telehealth/en/.

World Health Organization. 2019. WHO guideline: recommendations on digital interventions for health system strengthening: web supplement 2: Summary of findings and grade tables. (No. WHO/RHR/19.7).

World Health Organization. 2020a. eHealth at WHO. Available at: https://www.who.int/ehealth/about/en/.

World Health Organization. 2020b. Emergencies – Disease Outbreaks. Available at: https://www.who.int/emergencies/diseases/en/.

World Health Organization. 2020c. Preamble to the constitution of the World Health Organization as adopted by the international health conference, New York, 19 June 1946, signed 22 July 1946. Official Records of the World Health Organization.

World Health Organization. 2020d. Public health surveillance. Available at: https://www.who.int/immunization/monitoring_surveillance/burden/vpd/en/.

Zhang, H. and Shaw, R. 2020. Identifying research trends and gaps in the context of covid-19. *International Journal of Environmental Research and Public Health* 17(10), p. 3370.

DATA SCIENCE AND ARTIFICIAL INTELLIGENCE IN THE MANAGEMENT OF COVID-19: THE GAUTENG DEPARTMENT OF HEALTH, A SHOWCASE

Bruce Mellado, PhD

14.1 INTRODUCTION

Scientific inquiry is becoming increasingly data-intensive as it endeavours to understand more and more complex problems of nature and society. These questions entail navigating through the complex multi-dimensional space of data and model parameters. The scientist is faced with the requirement to model complex systems in a setup where pre-existing knowledge of the subject is not sufficient to enact a complete model of underlying microscopic interactions which could predict the macroscopic suite of phenomena that need to be observed and measured.

The perpetual tension between scientific inquiry into the complex underlying microscopic picture and the need for solutions to practical problems in the form of tangible predictions needs to be resolved on solid scientific grounds. This represents a challenge that requires a well-defined methodological framework. The latter needs to unequivocally spell out the role of theory and data and how data is used in order to enrich the theoretical knowledge which reflects the underlying dynamics that the data itself is a manifestation of.

In this light, the question emerges as to what the role of the data itself is in building predictive models. This question ultimately boils down to epistemological interrogations that are not necessarily discussed often enough in modern science. This conversation revolves around the dynamic unity between theory and experiment which ultimately drives scientific enquiry, as to how theory and data interact with each other in order to reach higher epistemological syntheses. The researcher needs to be cognisant that the thought process that channels the scientific inquiry follows a certain interpretation of the scientific method, regardless of whether this occurs consciously or unconsciously. In the era of data-intensive science, it has become more important than ever to bring these methodological interrogations to the fore.

More often than not, semi-empirical approaches are required in order to set up modelling that has immediate applicability in use cases. *Prima facie*, semi-empirical methodologies appear to combine theoretical and empirical knowledge in a somehow ad-hoc fashion, on a case-by-case basis. The reality is that the implementation of semi-empiricism, even if unintentionally, responds to underlying dynamics between theory and practice. Its practical value needs to be unpacked in the context of epistemological considerations. In fact, one can argue that semi-empiricism is not necessarily imposed upon scientists as a temporary measure. The use of semi-empiricism transcends and does not necessarily emerge as the result of inadequate pre-existing knowledge of the subject, nor the urgent need to provide modelling solutions. There are serious methodological considerations that underpin semi-empiricism. Semi-empiricism, which will be detailed and implemented here, is radically different from pure empiricism. The latter positions itself very differently with respect to theoretical or previously accumulated knowledge.

A classic epitome in the realm of modern physics of the semi-empirical approach is the modelling of the structure of the proton in order to predict the production of particles in high energy collisions, such as the Large Hadron Collider. Matter is made of atoms. Atoms in turn are made of a nucleus and electrons revolving around it. The nucleus is composed of protons, which are positively charged and their cousins, the neutrons, which are neutral. The proton has been studied for over 100 years and it is known to be a composite particle that contains within itself a complex structure of other more elementary particles. Calculations used to compute the probability of particle production in the collisions of protons are highly complex and are derived from a well-established theory of interactions. However, the structure of the proton itself, which is an essential input to these calculations, remains a complex system that is derived from the data, as opposed to purely theoretical calculations. The structure of the proton to date is extracted from the data on the basis of a semi-empirical procedure that incorporates rigorous mathematics which emerges from the theory of fundamental interactions in conjunction with relatively simple and flexible mathematical functions designed to learn from the data.

Data science incorporates a wealth of advanced analytics techniques and methodologies and has emerged as a separate field in its own right. Data science thrives in interdisciplinary environments, as it provides a framework of scientific methods and algorithms which enables researchers to organise, analyse and extract synthetic models.

Data science alone, without domain knowledge, is not in a position to provide a self-sustainable modelling system. This is an essential consideration when implementing data science methodologies and algorithms in the context of domain-specific data flows. The interaction between data science tools and domain knowledge is also to be understood from the standpoint of the above-mentioned epistemological considerations. Therefore, the integration of data science in domain-specific inquiries requires a clearly stated methodological foundation. It is problematic to engage in advanced analytics without reflecting on questions of the scientific method.

Modelling the COVID-19 pandemic is intrinsically a multi-disciplinary exercise. The increasing amount and multidimensionality of data calls for a multi-disciplinary and holistic approach towards handling the intricacies associated with modelling a complex system. The particular case discussed here requires input from experts including epidemiologists, clinicians and practitioners, physicists, applied mathematicians, statisticians, software engineers, sociologists, and data scientists.

This chapter covers the use of techniques derived from data science and artificial intelligence (AI) for the modelling and management of the COVID-19 pandemic. Work with the Gauteng Province Department of Health and Department of Economic Development will be used as a showcase to illustrate outputs, when relevant. While most of the conclusions drawn will have illustrations drawn from the South African context, ensuing methodological considerations are applicable in a more general setup.

14.2   OBJECTIVES

The chapter will cover five sections touching upon the following aspects:

- Discuss the basic methodological tenets of the role of AI and data; basics of modelling complex systems and methodological considerations, where theory and empirical evidence complement each other.

- Discuss the interdisciplinary character of modelling the COVID-19 pandemic.

- Following this exposé of methodological considerations, three case studies of the use of AI to handle multi-dimensional data streams are succinctly described.

- Modelling of hot spots and clusters of cases using data from the Department of Health using un-supervised machine leaning.

- The use of Recurrent Neural Networks to provide algorithms for the early detection of waves and resurgences.

- Modelling the rollout of the vaccine in the South African context with the help of Deep Neural Networks and deep learning.

14.3   METHODOLOGICAL CONSIDERATIONS AND THE ROLE OF AI

Scientific enquiry entails moving from the simplest concepts to the most complex, as knowledge of the system under investigation becomes more profound and the theoretical understanding more self-consistent and predictive. The scientific method that underpins this knowledge flow has been debated considerably over the centuries, with two extreme schools of thought emerging. Pure empiricism of the Baconian type argues that experience is the only source of knowledge. Theoretical knowledge would have a secondary, if a role at all. In this light, theoretical knowledge is viewed rather as a bias that may deflect the scientist away from the essence of nature. Empiricism does not appreciate the importance of abstraction and theoretical thinking in the advancement of knowledge, and as a result, it remains one-sided. On the other side of the spectrum is the idealistic view that only theoretical expertise is the real source of knowledge and that experimentation may be inherently misleading. Whereas there are two main types of idealism, objective and subjective, experimentation plays a secondary role in generating knowledge, even if it is the material world that the researcher endeavours to explain. The idealistic worldview believes that abstractions, concepts and notions emanate from the world of ideas alone and that the material world is segregated from theory. Experimentation is viewed as a passive element in the process of knowledge generation, where experimentation is intended to prove or disprove a theory while remaining detached from the former. Idealism does not appreciate the fact that even the most obscure abstractions result from the complex and dynamic interplay between theory and experiment as science moves from less advanced to more advanced syntheses. In contrast to what idealistic belief upholds, theoretical abstractions are ultimately the result of theoretical thinking developed on the basis of experimental material and for the purpose of explaining the objective material world. Hence, a more balanced methodology is required to regulate the interplay between theory and experimentation, as the ultimate goal of the scientific endeavour is to understand the laws that govern the constant evolution of nature and society. It is necessary to view and articulate the interrelation between theory and experiment in the form of a dynamic unity, instead of over-emphasising one over the other.

The use of data science has become ubiquitous in modern science, as disciplines become more and more data-intensive. Data science through machine learning provides a formidable set of tools to extract information from the data, from experience. That said, the implementation of data science techniques in particular domains also requires a conversation pertaining to the scientific method. In this context and in light of the abovementioned methodological considerations, it is very important to establish a distinction between learning from the data and model building. Machine learning provides the scientist with the ability to create mathematical models on the basis of training adaptive algorithms on data sets. Strictly speaking, when a machine learning algorithm, such as a neural network, is trained on a data set, a number of parameters are derived with which a mathematical model is extracted. It is essential not to confuse this machine learning mathematical function with modelling as a predictive construction. The latter is a more complex synthesis of pre-existing knowledge and the additional insight provided by machine learning trained on data sets. To the extent that purely empirical approaches are not suitable to scientific enquiry, data science through machine learning is not in a position to solve the fundamental problems of a field just on the basis of training on data alone. Data science is effective in extracting hidden correlations in vast data sets but are, however, more advanced with respect to classical approaches, it does not preclude the essential role that pre-existing domain knowledge has in solving new problems. Data science through machine learning enhances the ability of the researcher to learn from the data, but does not replace theoretical knowledge of the domain. Data science enters the abovementioned dynamic unity of theory and experimentation by augmenting the capacity to extract information from the data. It is in this sense that data science comes in to accelerate the transition from less advanced to more advanced syntheses.

In the context of the discussion of scientific method, it is important to address different methodologies in machine learning. Three of these are the most discussed: supervised, semi-supervised and unsupervised training. The different methodologies correspond to different levels of modelling knowledge, where unsupervised learning assumes the least amount of prior knowledge of the system.

Supervised learning, or full supervision, has the task to learn a training set made of pairs of points. Let $X = (x_1, ..., x_n)$ be a set of n points, where $x_i \in X$ for all $i \in [n] := 1, ..., n$. The points are pulled from a common distribution on X and are random variables that are independent and identically distributed. The objective of unsupervised learning is to find interesting structure in the class of data X or an underlying density that may have generated it. In supervised learning, one needs to define $Y = (y_1, ..., y_n)$, where $y_i \in Y$ are referred to the labels of the examples x_i. It is also assumed that the pairs (x_i, y_i) are also randomly sampled over $X \times Y$. Full supervision often aims at solving a problem of classification. This is performed through generative or discriminative algorithms. Generative algorithms model how the data is generated, where the conditional probability $p(x|y)$ is inferred. By contrast, discriminative algorithms are not really concerned with how x is generated, but rather concentrate on modelling $p(y|x)$. Logistic regressions are commonly used to achieve this goal.

Semi-supervision contains elements of both supervised and unsupervised learning. Labelled data is provided but not for all the data sets. In this setup the data set $X = (x_i)_{i \in [n]}$ is split into two samples. This includes the points $X_l := (x_1, ..., x_l)$ that are assigned labels $Y_l := (x_1, ..., x_l)$ and the points $X_u := (x_{l+1}, ..., x_{l+u})$ for which labels are not provided.

Unsupervised learning uses algorithms on data that is not labelled with the intent of unveiling hidden patterns or clusters of data with certain commonalities without significant prior knowledge. The use of unsupervised learning does not necessarily imply complete absence of prior knowledge of the system. As will be seen below in this chapter, unsupervised learning can be successfully implemented when the general features of the temporal evolution of the system are known, but the scientist lacks information about the specifics of the microscopic picture.

In this chapter, showcases are presented that use the three types of machine learning described here.

14.4   THE INTERDISCIPLINARY CHARACTER OF MODELLING THE PANDEMIC

Modelling a pandemic corresponds to modelling complex systems with many degrees of freedoms and unknowns. We will comment below on generic methodological of modelling complex systems in a situation such as the COVID-19 pandemic. In this section, we will focus on the inherently interdisciplinary character of the problem at stake.

Figure 14.1 illustrates the ecosystem that is entailed in providing evidence-based modelling to this complex modelling problem. A showcase of such an ecosystem has been the work of the Gauteng Premier COVID-19 Advisory Committee. The starting point of the investigation remains the input data in combination with pre-existing domain knowledge. This includes a wide variety of data pertaining to, but not limited to, the epidemiological and clinical picture and how it evolves in time. The time evolution of the abovementioned observables carries critical information in order to unearth the underlying dynamics of the complex system under study. As the evolution of the pandemic is the result of a complex interaction of the susceptible population with the virus. Input data, such as mobility, social sentiment and many others, also play a critical role in the ecosystem of inputs required to predict the evolution of the system. These inputs need to be processed by a wide range of specialists and experts in the domain knowledge of relevance.

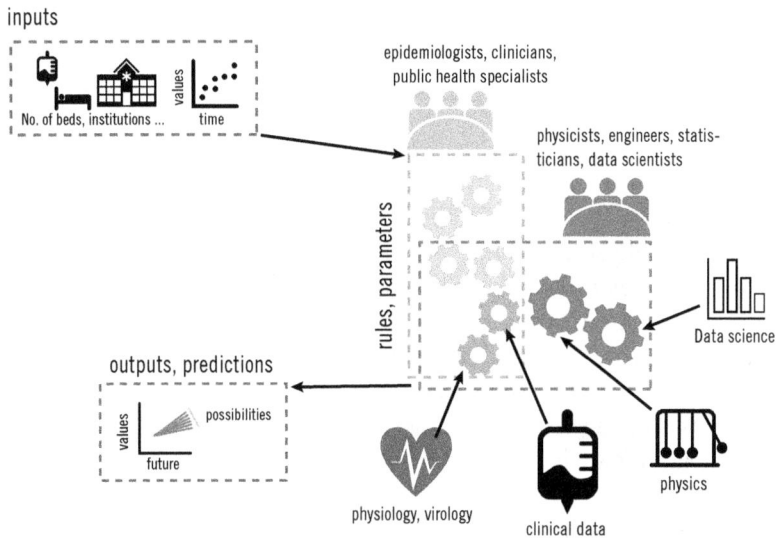

Figure 14.1 Block diagram of the thought process entailed in the processing inputs to arrive at a synthetic set of outputs and predictions

Figure 14.1 also illustrates the inherently interdisciplinary character of the ecosystem described here. To a zeroth approximation, one is allowed to assume that the flow of inputs is dominated by epidemiological and clinical data. Even in this setup, inputs need to be analysed and processed by an interdisciplinary team or teams of specialists.

The differential equations that dictate the temporal and spatial evolutions require a well-defined physical picture, as modelling the pandemic is equivalent to understanding a complex system with interactions between many subjects. This physical picture needs to be articulated through a mathematical apparatus that is functional, robust and predictive. Predictions need to be confronted with data, where data in turn corrects the model through constant validation and calibration. Data science techniques, including machine learning, are instrumental in streamlining the process of extraction of information from the data, whenever appropriate. In a dynamic complex system, regular calibration is paramount.

Domain knowledge is essential to data analysis. This requires that the team has constant input from epidemiologists, clinicians and practitioners. The perspective of managers and policy-makers is also relevant here. Modelling needs to evolve together with the data and, therefore, it necessitates domain knowledge for it not to departure from the objective reality that it is intended to describe.

14.5 UNDERSTANDING HOT SPOTS, A SHOWCASE FOR AI-DRIVEN MODELLING

One of the most complex problems that face us in determining the evolution of the pandemic is the role and characterisation of hot spots, or clusters of positive cases. The physical picture behind the generation of hot spots is particularly complex, where local factors play a central role in the creation and evolution of these hot spots. The overall physical picture used here to model the pandemic as a whole is split into two types of transmission processes. Random local transmission is a stochastic process that can be modelled with classical compartmental models. Random local transmission is driven by mobility patterns of infected subjects and how these interact with the susceptible population. We refer to this type of transmission as stochastic and its most salient characteristics can be averaged over relatively large swaths of territory. In the period between waves, a certain equilibrium is reached between the rate of infection and the local reproductive numbers so that the number of new cases per unit of time can be relatively stable over an extended period of time. The conditions of equilibrium are specific to each geo-spatial ecosystem, where parameters cannot be transported from country to country. However, the equilibrium is unstable from the standpoint of classical mechanics. External disturbances, such as super-spreader events or sudden change in societal behaviours (most prominently, family-oriented events), have proven to be those external factors that disrupt the equilibrium, leading to waves. When the equilibrium is ruptured, random local transmission accelerates leading to the creation of hot spots. The acceleration in the creation of hot spots is an unequivocal attribute of waves. The crux of the matter here is that the modelling of the random local transmission is not applicable to the formation of hot spots nor their evolution in time and space. Hot spots are the result of complex local interactions within communities. As such, every hot spot carries the idiosyncrasy of the community it develops in. As a result, modelling requires a different approach, where important parameters need to be extracted from the data across time and space. This calls for the use of machine learning through unsupervised learning.

Hot spot analysis represents an advanced statistical approach that can be effectively utilised for outbreak analytics and visualisation. It can equip public health policy- and decision-makers with updated, real-time assessment of the pandemic trends and its future projected trajectories. Furthermore, it can complement classical epidemiological surveys, leading to the identification of patterns that would be otherwise classified as low-risk ones. In conclusion, hot spot analysis has been highly helpful in promptly recognising high-risk clusters, and to adopt/adjust proper public health measures. Since the COVID-19 pandemic is a highly changeable and constantly under a flux situation, we can anticipate that hot spot analysis can aid stakeholders in making informed, evidence-based and data-driven decisions.

A Gaussian Mixture model is an algorithm that operates by generating k two-dimensional Gaussian probability distributions, where k is a hyperparameter specified. Thus, we are required to generate means, μ_i, standard deviation, σ_i, and weighting, ϕ_i, where the index specifies the i_{th} Gaussian cluster. In this setup, the probability of a new case occurring at point x_i is the sum of probabilities of all clusters:

$$p(x) = \sum_{i=1}^{k} \phi_i N(x|\mu_i, \sigma_i),$$

where N is the normal distribution.

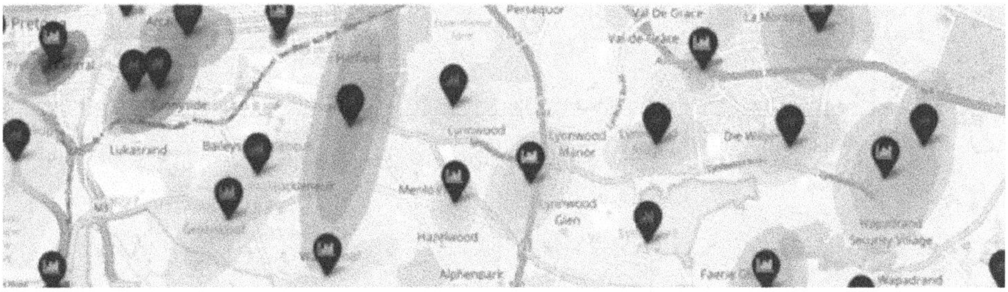

Figure 14.2 Geo-spatial distribution of hot spots in the City of Tshwane during the first wave

We generate the set of normal distributions (with associated weights, means and standard deviations) with an algorithm that optimally fits the probability distributions given the set of already known COVID-19 cases and their coordinates.

For every point x_i for each cluster, calculate the probability that that point came from a certain cluster:

$$\gamma_{ik} = \frac{\phi_k N(x_i|\mu_k, \sigma_k)}{\sum_{j=1}^{K} \phi_j N(x_i|\mu_j, \sigma_j)}.$$

Now that we have γ_{ik}, we can update the mean, standard deviation and weight of the k_i cluster as follows:

$$\phi_k = \sum_{i}^{N} \frac{\gamma_{ik}}{N},$$

$$\mu_k = \sum_{i}^{N} \frac{\gamma_{ik} x_i}{\gamma_{ik}},$$

$$\sigma_k^2 = \sum_{i}^{N} \frac{\gamma_{ik}(x_i - \mu_i)^2}{\gamma_{ik}}.$$

Figure 14.2 displays the geo-location and size of hot spots following the prescription described here, where a snapshot of the situation with the pandemic during the first wave in the City of Tshwane is given. The ellipsoids around the centre of the clusters give a measure of their size according to different confidence levels.

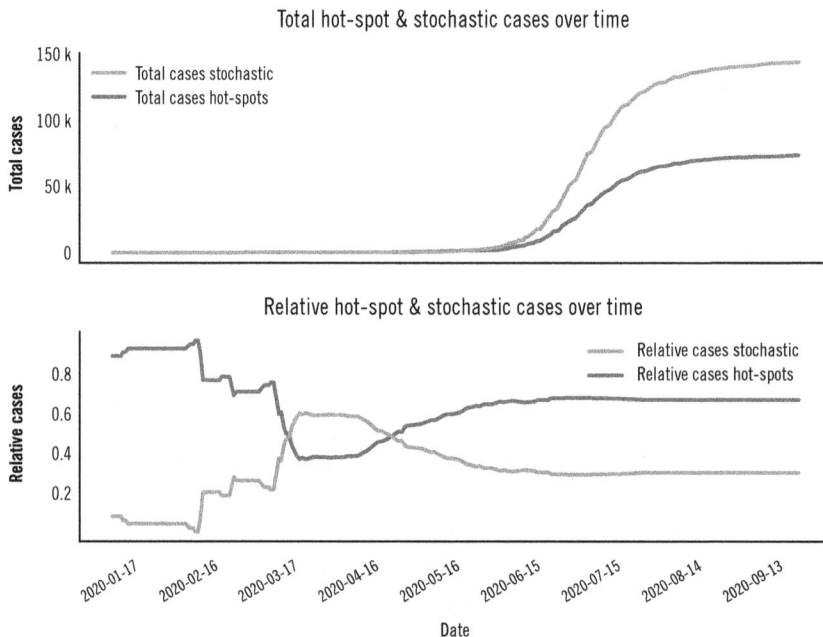

Figure 14.3 Composition of cases in the province of Gauteng during the first wave (see text)

Figure 14.3 shows the composition of the positive cases. Cases are classified into two types: cases that are associated with hot spots and cases that are not. The latter constitutes what is referred to as the stochastic contribution where these cases are more or less randomly distributed throughout geo-spatially. The first wave reached a peak in Gauteng in mid-July 2020. By then, about two-thirds of all cases were ascribed to hot spots.

Once the latent variables of the Gaussian probability distributions (weights, means, standard deviation) have been found through the processing of COVID-19 cases in locations in Gauteng, it is important to verify which are hot spots, or highly infectious areas of the province. An aspect to consider is whether the clusters found follow the Susceptible-Infection Curve, which model the number of susceptible people who get infected, over time, within a given area. The equation is as follows:

$$SI(t) = \frac{\alpha}{1 + e^{-\beta(t-\delta)}},$$

where α is the total number of susceptible cases within a cluster, β is the rate of transmission of a given disease, and δ is the duration of the disease, or the time that it takes for the function to deviate from a single exponential growth. One can fit this curve to each cluster to generate these parameters for the i_{th} cluster, giving more properties to accurately filter clusters into hot spots. The model is applicable as we expect a small increase of infection cases in the early stages of a susceptible population, and then a sharp increase as the disease spreads rapidly throughout the cluster. A plateau is expected once all susceptible people within a cluster are infected.

A problem encountered in modelling the COVID-19 pandemic is that SIRD models generally function stochastically. However, pockets of cases usually developing in high-density areas undergo independent, rapid infection which does not fit into the overarching model. This micro-system cluster is referred to as a hot spot and undergoes independent non-stochastic hot spot dynamics. In order to classify a specific group of cases in an area as a hot spot the cases must first be grouped and their characteristics modelled, using each groupings characteristics to define a hot spot cluster.

It therefore follows that in order to produce informative predictions for governmental policy- and decision-makers, such as estimate numbers of hospital beds, use of intensive care units wards and when the peak will occur, the hot spot cluster cases must be extracted from the data the stochastic SIRD model is calibrated on. The model then is able to interpret the progression of COVID-19 without the inconsistencies incurred by the non-conforming hot spot cases.

This is done by extracting the daily ratio of stochastic cumulative cases from the total cases in all clusters and applying this ratio to the recorded data before it is used to inform the model.

14.6   THE USE OF AI FOR THE DEVELOPMENT OF EARLY DETECTION ALGORITHMS

The nature of the way the virus spreads causes cases to come in waves. It is crucial to be able to have an early alert system to identify when another wave of cases is about to occur. The availability of a variety of newly developed indicators allows for the exploration of multi-feature prediction models for case data.

Two early detection algorithms were developed in partnership with the Gauteng Department of Health. First, an algorithm based on classical analytics and epidemiological models with short-term predictivity was released before the advent of the second wave.[1] A second, multi-dimensional early detection algorithm was released in March 2021, before the advent of the third wave in SA.[2] We will describe the latter below.

Ten indicators were selected as possible features for our prediction model. The model chosen is a Recurrent Neural Network (RNN) with Long Short-Term Memory (LSTM). RNNs with LSTM are known to be good time-series predictive models, especially for multi-feature model architectures that require a memory component without the gradient descent pitfalls of a normal RNN. Here we describe the development of an early detection system that functions by predicting future daily confirmed cases-based features that include mobility indices, stringency indices and epidemiological parameters. The model was trained on the intermittent period in between waves one and two in all of the South African provinces. The COVID-19 case prediction parameter chosen was the daily change in cases dTCt. The chosen model was trained on data in the interim period between two COVID-19 case peaks. This caused the system to be able to predict daily cases accurately during the interim period, however, when there is a COVID-19 case peak, the system is unable to recognise the behaviour of the features in relation to the prediction parameter dTCt. The inability of the model to predict the daily cases as soon new waves emerge has been taken advantage of to develop the early detection system. Here supervised learning is used.

Using data from in between the first and second waves to calibrate the model and using the second peaks data as verification of the correct functioning of the model, the system was able to accurately identify and confirm the beginning of the second wave. All provinces in South Africa were used to verify that the earlier detection system functions to identify the beginning of the second wave. The approach was used to detect subsequent waves as well.

Since the beginning of the COVID-19 pandemic, Google and Facebook have produced mobility reports that include different types of mobility indicators as a measure to understand the consequence of implemented regulation and Non-pharmaceutical Interventions (NPI) on the movement and interaction of the public. These indicators can be used as valuable inputs to the model. Each of the mobility reports includes different types of mobility indicators that are developed in using different methodologies.

The Google Mobility Report data is useful to understand the geo-spatial movement of people during the pandemic. Movement trends of people over time and over different categories of places are tracked. The report contains three location categories namely: retail, recreation, groceries, pharmacies,

---

[1]   https://www.covid19sa.org/riskindex.
[2]   https://www.covid19sa.org/riskindex-ai.

parks, transit stations, workplaces, and residential. These indicators provide a valuable resource for understanding how people interact with different types of locations. All of the Google Mobility indicators have the same overall trend with minor differences except for the residential, which has an almost opposite behaviour due to the increased numbers of people staying in their homes as a result of the pandemic.

The Facebook movement data sets were developed to assist researchers and public health experts in monitoring and tracking how populations are responding to physical distancing measures. The Facebook mobility report two complementary indicators to describe change in movement over time: 'Change in Movement' and 'Stay Put'. Each of the indicators provides different perspectives on movement trends. The Facebook mobility report methodology divides up geographical areas into equal area tiles. The 'Change in Movement' indicator measures the number of tiles people are visiting in a day in a specific region as a comparison to a baseline defined as the average number of tiles visited daily in the month of February 2021. The 'Stay Put' indicator conversely measures how many people are staying within a single tile area for the whole day as a comparison to the February baseline. People who use Facebook on a mobile device have the choice of providing their precise location. Movement Range Trends are produced by aggregating this data.

Another valuable type of indicator to be considered as a feature for the model are stringency indicators. There are a number of stringency indicators that have been developed as indications of the level or strictness of implemented regulation in a specific country or region. Arguably the most comprehensive stringency indicator that has been developed is the OxCGRT[3] stringency index. This is used as an input characterising the stringency of NPIs in South Africa and serves as input to the RNN.

The figure below displays the result risk index derived from the RNN-based early detection algorithm trained on data from the Gauteng province. The red curve corresponds to the generated risk index for the month of March 2021. The risk index remained significantly below threshold for that period of time.[4]

---

[3]   https://covidtracker.bsg.ox.ac.uk.
[4]   https://www.covid19sa.org/riskindex-ai.

Gauteng

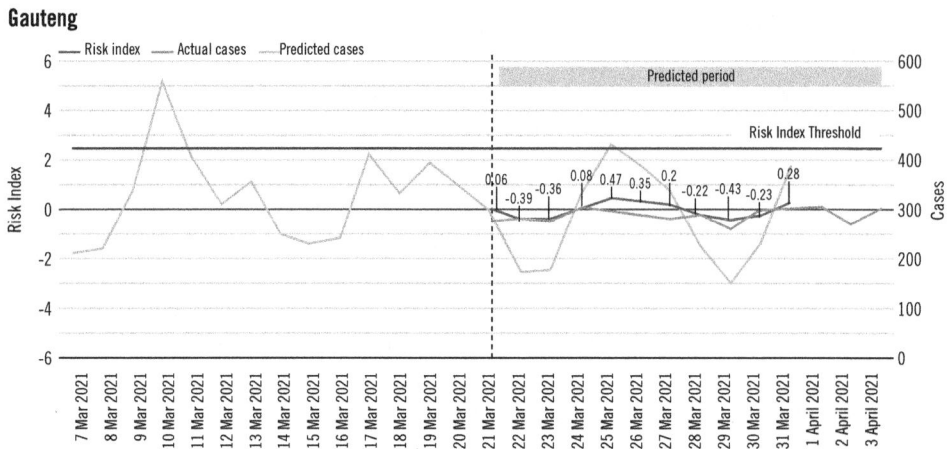

Figure 14.4 Distribution of daily cases in Gauteng compared with the prediction made by the early detection algorithm weeks before the third wave

Figure 14.4 illustrates the performance of the early detection algorithm for the Gauteng province. Here, data from the period in between the second and third waves was used to validate the performance of the algorithm. The prediction from the early detection algorithm is confronted with data that is not used in training. The relative deviation of the data from the prediction is well below the risk index threshold. This indicates that the data is consistent with the absence of a wave.

14.7   THE USE OF AI IN MODELLING THE ROLLOUT OF VACCINATION

In order to identify and prioritise target groups who can benefit most from vaccination, in the Gauteng Province pilot study, multi-dimensional data have been provided by the Gauteng Department of Health (GDoH) and are being used to characterise variables associated with severe illness. Fourteen dimensions of individual-specific characteristics have been modelled and include: age; eleven relevant comorbidities; gender and ethnicity; information pertaining to the type of hospitalisation (General Ward, ICU, High Care and Isolation) and whether the subject was discharged alive or died in care is also provided. This allows for the implementation of a supervised machine-learning classification procedure. Multi-dimensional survey data are also available and provide representative data samples with a large number of inputs pertaining to social vulnerabilities. A subset of these inputs accords with the data inputs from the GDoH and matching between the two data sets has been performed. The data sets from the GDoH contain comorbidities as an index of vulnerability that covers comorbidities relevant to COVID-19. These include diabetes, hypertension, emphysema, bronchitis, asthma, pneumonia, heart disease, stroke, HIV/AIDS and tuberculosis. The data sets provided by the GDoH contain about 5 000 points of complete patient records for the period of the first wave of COVID-19 and the beginning of the second, where the remainder of the data is becoming available. This limited data set is sufficient to train smart algorithms with relatively high efficiency.

A Deep Neural Network (DNN) has been trained to separate two classes of data sets: severe illness (ICU, High Care and Mortality) and less severe illness (subject discharged from the General Ward). A training sample with 70% of the data has been used, where a testing sample with 30% of the data has been used to validate results and to estimate potential over-training. The corresponding DNN weights have been applied to the population data provided by the Gauteng City-Region Observatory.[5] Here semi-supervision has been used to establish the populations with different risks. Figure 14.5 displays the receiver operating characteristic curve of the DNN model. The horizontal axis shows the fraction of the adult population in Gauteng, where the vertical axis displays the reduction in severe illness. The DNN model indicates that by vaccinating about 20% of the adult population, the probability of severe COVID-19 illness can be reduced by over 80%. Further refinements through multi-class labelling and enhanced data sets can improve the efficiency of the smart algorithm.

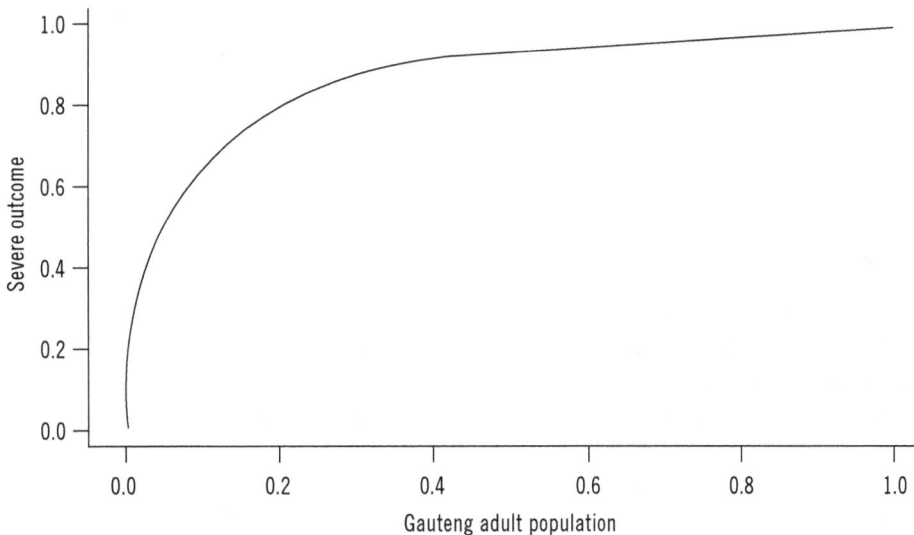

Figure 14.5 The receiver operating characteristic curve of the DNN model (see text)

5   https://www.gcro.ac.za.

The DNN output provides a dimensionless number between 0 (highest risk of severe illness) and 1 (lowest risk of severe illness). Ideally, the population is classified according to the DNN output, which can be easily achieved through an electronic system. Further, AI-derived recommendations can be elaborated, as in Table 1, for classifying the risk of severe illness (1 greatest, 5 lowest risk) by demographic interval and by co-morbidity.

Table 14.1 Vaccine target population classification based on risk, as derived from the smart algorithm. Source: Gauteng Premier's COVID-19 Advisory Committee (Mbada, 2021)

Risk group	Age (years)	Co-morbidities	Population over 18 (%)
1	>60	Hypertension, Diabetes, Cardiac Disease	3.8
2	50-60	Hypertension, Diabetes, Cardiac Disease	3.7
3	40-50	Hypertension, Diabetes, Cardiac Disease	3.7
4	>18	Any co-morbidity	18
5	>18	–	71

14.8   CONCLUSIONS

This chapter succinctly touches upon questions of methodology and the scientific method in the context of the rise of data science in data-intensive disciplines. Data science provides invaluable tools for scientists to extract insights from the data. However, purely empirical approaches are inadequate for scientific inquiry. As such, Data science requires pre-existing theoretical knowledge that emanates from the domain that machine learning algorithms are applied on. These methodological considerations are essential to correctly conceptualise the role of AI in the context of scientific inquiry. As a particular domain in knowledge moves from less sophisticated to more sophisticated syntheses, it profits from data science in extracting information from the data. That said, it is pivotal to recognise that the beginning and the end of the scientific inquiry remains the realm of domain knowledge. These methodological considerations have been applied in a number of projects related to the modelling of the pandemic in the Gauteng province. These include the modelling of hot spots, the development of early detection algorithms and the modelling of the rollout of vaccination. These have practical implications that have been used to advise policy-makers in the Gauteng province.

14.9 SELF-ASSESSMENT QUESTIONS

1. What are some of the comorbidities included in the Gauteng Department's datasets?
2. Why is the Google Mobility Report useful?

14.10 REFERENCES

Hill, A. 2020. The math behind epidemics. *Physics Today* 73, pp. 11, 28.

Kermack, W.O. and McKendrick, A.G. 1927. A contribution to the mathematical theory of epidemics. *Proc. R. Soc. A* 115, p. 700.

Mbada, M. 2021. Urbanisation and Health, Presentation given to Public Health Association of South Africa, 16 February 2021.

Mellado, B., et al. 2021. Leveraging Artificial Intelligence and Big Data to optimize COVID-19 clinical public health and vaccination roll-out strategies in Africa. *International Journal of Environmental Research and Public Health* 18(15), 7890.

Nowzari, C., Preciado, V.M. and Pappas, G.J. 2016. Analysis and control of epidemics: a survey of spreading processes on complex networks. *IEEE Control Systems Magazine* 36, pp. 26–46.

Stevenson, F., et al. 2021. Development of an early alert system for an additional wave of COVID-19 cases using a recurrent neural network with long short-term memory. *International Journal of Environmental Research and Public Health* 18(14), 7376.

Tang, L., Zhou, Y., Wang, L., Purkayastha, S., Zhang, L., He, J., Wang, F. and Song, P.X.K. 2020. A review of multi-compartment infectious disease models. *International Statistical Review* 88(2), pp. 462–513.

Wiemken, T.L. and Kelley, R.R. 2020. Machine learning in epidemiology and health outcomes research. *Annual Review of Public Health* 41, pp. 21–36.

CHAPTER 15

THE DEVELOPMENT OF VACCINES AND IMMUNOLOGICAL THERAPIES IN PANDEMICS

Charles S. Wiysonge

Glenda E. Gray

Ames Dhai

15.1 INTRODUCTION

Hundreds of millions of deaths and disability have occurred during infectious disease pandemics and other public health emergencies (Nabel, 2013). Vaccines, when available, have played a critical role in controlling disease outbreaks during times of health crises. It is easy to forget that dreadful infectious diseases such as smallpox, polio, and yellow fever used to cause millions of deaths and disability in parts of the world that are now free of these diseases, largely thanks to vaccines (Nabel, 2013; Plotkin and Plotkin, 2011). Unfortunately, even where vaccines exist, there may be substantial challenges with access, acceptance, and uptake of vaccination services (Cooper et al, 2018; Machingaidze et al, 2013; Wilson and Wiysonge, 2020). The mere existence of a vaccine may not be enough to control a pandemic: public acceptance and uptake of vaccines in large numbers for disease transmission to be interrupted is required for control, elimination, and global eradication.

Table 15.1 Processes for Infectious Disease Control and Elimination

Control	The reduction of disease incidence, prevalence, morbidity, or mortality because of deliberate efforts
Elimination of Disease	Reduction to zero, of the incidence of a disease in a defined geographical area because of deliberate interventions
Elimination of Infections	Reduction to zero of the incidence of infection caused by a specific agent in a defined geographical area as a result of deliberate efforts, e.g. measles, poliomyelitis
Eradication	Permanent reduction to zero of the worldwide incidence of infection caused by a specific agent as a result of deliberate interventions and where interventions are no longer needed, e.g. smallpox
Extinction	The specific infectious agent no longer exists in nature or in the laboratory. There are no such examples

(Adapted from 'The Principles of Disease Elimination and Eradication'
(Walter R Dowdle MMWR Supplements 1999/48(SU01); 23–7.)

Vaccines are a good strategy and an important tool in the quest for disease control. They utilise the body's natural defences to develop immunity by training the immune system to recognise the infectious agent; after the induction of an immune response by vaccination. Vaccines utilise antigens from the infectious agents to induce an immune response that will either prevent infection or alter the course of the infection or disease. After the induction of the immune responses, the body is left with a supply of memory antibodies and cells that can be activated should the individual be exposed in the future. Once enough people are immunised, outbreaks can be controlled and become less frequent, enabling even people who have not been vaccinated to be protected – what is referred to as herd immunity.

Monoclonal antibodies and other immunological therapies may play a similar, though limited, role as vaccines and may also be useful during a pandemic. Monoclonal antibodies are laboratory-produced substitutes for antibodies. COVID-19 monoclonal antibodies are created by identifying COVID-19-specific B cells of patients who have recently recovered from COVID-19 infection or by utilising mice genetically modified to have an immune system.

15.2 CHAPTER OBJECTIVES

- The primary objective of this chapter is to provide a summary of vaccine development, access, and acceptance; with a focus on COVID-19.

- The secondary objective will be to summarise existing information on monoclonal antibodies for COVID-19.

15.3 DEVELOPMENT, ACCESS, AND ACCEPTANCE OF VACCINES

15.3.1 Development of Vaccines

Development of vaccines started with the smallpox vaccine in 1796, after which it took almost a century for the next vaccine to be made (Nabel, 2013; Plotkin and Plotkin, 2011). However, since the mid-twentieth century, there has been a dramatic acceleration in the development of new vaccines. Currently, there are more than 60 licensed vaccines against about 30 infectious diseases (Ollmann Saphire, 2020; Plotkin and Plotkin, 2011; Tomori and Kolawole, 2021; Ndwandwe and Wiysonge, 2021).

The traditional approaches to vaccine development include the use of whole organisms (live attenuated or inactivated), toxoids, subunits, or conjugation (Plotkin and Plotkin, 2011). Live attenuated vaccines are made of live organisms, which through culture, under certain conditions, have lost their virulent properties. Whole cell inactivated vaccines consist of organisms that have undergone treatment with chemicals or heat, which has rendered them unable to cause disease (Plotkin, 2005). Toxoids are illness-causing components produced by pathogens that have been inactivated. For subunit vaccines, a part of the organism rather than the whole organism is used to create an immune response. Finally, conjugate vaccines are made by linking the outer polysaccharide coats of certain organisms to proteins; leading to a better immune response than the polysaccharide (Plotkin and Plotkin, 2011).

Newer approaches to vaccine development include the use of viral vectors (for recombinant vaccines) and genetic instructions (for nucleic acid vaccines). For recombinant vaccines, a gene thought to code for a protective protein is isolated and then recombined with the deoxyribonucleic acid (DNA) of a viral vector. Nucleic acid vaccines use genetic instructions, in the form of DNA or ribonucleic acid (RNA), for an infectious agent's protein that prompts an immune response. Delivering this to human cells leads to the expression of the infectious agent's proteins, triggering an immune system recognition (Plotkin and Plotkin, 2011; Callaway, 2020b).

Vaccine development usually takes years and unfolds step by step (Laher et al, 2020). It is a lengthy and expensive process, and typically takes multiple vaccine candidates and many decades to produce one licensed vaccine (Kanesa-thasan et al, 2011; Plotkin, 2005; Bekker and Gray, 2017). Because of the cost and high failure rates, vaccine developers typically follow a linear sequence of steps, with multiple pauses for data analysis or manufacturing-process checks (Plotkin, 2005). Experimental vaccine candidates are created in the laboratory and tested in animals before moving into progressively larger human clinical trials from phase 1 to 3 (WHO, 2010; Kanesa-thasan et al, 2011).

A phase 1 trial is a first-in-human study, which recruits a few hundred (or less) healthy volunteers, to assess whether a candidate vaccine is safe. Phase 2 trials are typically conducted among several hundred participants, to assess whether the candidate vaccine elicits an immune response. A phase 2 trial also gathers information on the most frequent short-term side effects of the vaccine. Thousands of volunteers are recruited in a phase 3 vaccine trial to assess whether the vaccine is effective and safe. Phase 3 vaccine trials also document the most common side effects of the vaccine being tested. Less than 10% of vaccines that go into human trials are eventually found to be safe and effective in phase 3 trials. For example, the pursuit of an HIV vaccine has been going on now for close to 40 years without success (Bekker and Gray, 2017; Laher et al, 2020). It takes on average 8–17 years and can cost up to US$1 billion to make a vaccine (Kanesa-thasan et al, 2011).

15.3.2 Licensure and Recommendations of Vaccines for Public Health Programmes

When a vaccine has been found to be safe and effective in phase 3 trials, the vaccine manufacturer would apply to national regulatory authorities (NRAs) for approval or licensure. Examples of NRAs include the South African Health Products Regulatory Authority (SAHPRA) and the United States Food and Drug Administration (FDA). The NRA reviews trial results and decides whether to license the vaccine for use in the country or not. An NRA should only license a vaccine if it is satisfied that the vaccine is safe and effective, and the vaccine's beneficial effects outweigh potential risks. Once a vaccine is licensed, and rolled out in human populations, there is a need to monitor people who receive it to collect additional data on safety and effectiveness (Ndwandwe and Wiysonge, 2021).

During a pandemic, an NRA may grant an emergency use authorisation for a vaccine prior to full approval (Kesselheim et al, 2020; Avorn and Kesselheim, 2020). In such a situation, the NRA allows an unapproved vaccine to be used for prevention of the pandemic disease when there are no approved and available alternatives (Krause and Gruber, 2020). For example, by July 2021, NRAs across the world had issued emergency use authorisations for at least 18 COVID-19 vaccines; allowing widespread use of these vaccines prior to them meeting the substantial evidence criteria for approval (Ndwandwe and Wiysonge, 2021).

When an NRA has approved a vaccine, the manufacturer can apply to the World Health Organization (WHO) for pre-qualification of the vaccine (WHO, 2010). The prequalification process is an additional check to ensure that vaccines used in vaccination programmes are safe and effective. Prequalification supports the needs of national vaccination programmes with regards to vaccine potency, thermostability, presentation, labelling, and shipping conditions. However, NRAs are responsible for regulatory oversight, testing, and release of WHO-prequalified vaccines (WHO, 2010).

The Strategic Advisory Group of Experts on Immunisation (SAGE) issues evidence-informed global recommendations for use of vaccines in vaccination programmes (Duclos et al, 2012). Other technical and narrowly focused global vaccine advisory committees (such as the Global Advisory Committee on Vaccine Safety) support SAGE. In turn, continental immunisation technical advisory groups help identify continental challenges and define priorities. Taking into consideration the local context, national immunisation technical advisory groups (NITAGs) contextualise SAGE recommendations and provide guidance to their national government (Wiyeh et al, 2018b). The NITAG in South Africa is referred to as the National Advisory Group on Immunisation (NAGI), and the one in the United States is referred to as the Advisory Committee on Immunization Practices (Ngcobo and Cameron, 2012; Schoub et al, 2010; Lee and Carr, 2018).

15.3.3 Development, Access, and Acceptance of COVID-19 Vaccines

During COVID-19 infection, the virus uses its surface spike protein to lock onto the angiotensin-converting enzyme 2 receptors on the surface of human cells. Once inside, these cells translate the virus RNA to produce more viruses. This process prompts an immune response, whereby specialised antigen-presenting cells engulf the virus and display portions of it to activate T-helper cells. The latter trigger other immune responses, including the production of antibodies and the activation of cytotoxic T cells which destroy virus-infected cells (Callaway, 2020b). Researchers have utilised traditional and new vaccine development approaches to mimic this process.

The search for effective and safe vaccines against COVID-19 has progressed at an unprecedented speed since January 2020 (Lurie et al, 2020; Steckelberg et al, 2020; Callaway, 2020a). This involved executing many steps in parallel, before confirming a successful outcome of another step, thus necessitating elevated financial risks and multiple regulatory challenges. Various governments and organisations galvanised enormous resources to address these financial risks (Lurie et al, 2020; Steckelberg et al, 2020). By July 2021, there were nearly 200 COVID-19 vaccine candidates in pre-clinical development, more than 100 vaccine candidates in clinical development, and 18 vaccines authorised for emergency use (Ndwandwe and Wiysonge, 2021). Most of the vaccines use a two-dose schedule, 21–28 weeks apart, except for one vaccine which requires only one dose for full vaccination (Sadoff et al, 2021a; WHO, 2021a; WHO, 2021b). These include two messenger RNA (mRNA) vaccines from Pfizer and BioNTech (Sahin et al, 2020) and Moderna (Anderson et al, 2020). mRNA vaccines use genetic instructions (in the form an RNA) for a coronavirus protein that prompts an immune response (Callaway, 2020b). The second group of vaccines authorised for emergency use are adenoviral vector-based vaccines developed by Johnson & Johnson (Sadoff et al, 2021a), the Gamaleya Research Institute in Russia (Logunov et al, 2020), and AstraZeneca (Ramasamy et al, 2020). Viral vector COVID-19 vaccines use a chemically weakened virus (such as the adenovirus) which is genetically engineered to produce coronavirus proteins in the body. These viruses are weakened, so they cannot cause disease. There are two types of viral vectors, those that can still replicate within cells (i.e. replicating viral vectors) (Logunov et al, 2020; Sadoff et al, 2021a) and those that cannot replicate (i.e. non-replicating viral vectors) (Ramasamy et al, 2020). The third major group of COVID-19 vaccines authorised for emergency use are whole-virus-inactivated vaccines (Ndwandwe and Wiysonge, 2021). The COVID-19 vaccines took less than 12 months from scientific concept to emergency use authorisation (Anderson et al, 2020; Sahin et al, 2020). This is an unparalleled record in vaccine development (Ndwandwe and Wiysonge, 2021). With four years from scientific concept to approval in 1967, the mumps vaccine previously held the fastest record in vaccine development (Steckelberg et al, 2020).

During the H1N1 influenza pandemic in 2009, high-income countries bought nearly all available vaccines and low and middle-income countries did not have access until the high-income countries had received enough supplies (Usdin, 2020). By the time the vaccines arrived in most low and middle-income countries, the pandemic was over. Rather than an emphasis on global access, the H1N1 influenza pandemic in 2009 portrayed high levels of vaccine nationalism (Usdin, 2020). For COVID-19 vaccines, a coalition led by WHO, the Global Alliance for Vaccines and Immunisation (Gavi), and the Coalition for Epidemic Preparedness Innovations (CEPI) was formed to head off vaccine nationalism. The COVID-19 Vaccine Global Access (COVAX) Facility is a global risk-sharing mechanism for pooled procurement and equitable distribution of eventual COVID-19 vaccines (Gavi, 2020). Opaque financing and pricing mechanisms and volumes of vaccine available to countries have inevitably led to challenges to the fair allocation of vaccines by COVAX at country level. Direct negotiations with pharmaceuticals and bilateral country agreements have augmented access and increased the timeliness of receipt of vaccines in most low and middle-income countries. Vaccine distribution to contain COVID-19 is proving to be the biggest obstacle for all health systems, both well-resourced and less resilient health systems, especially those vaccines that require extreme cold storage conditions. The Pfizer-BioNTech vaccine requires storage at -70 degrees Celsius. Most vaccination sites in low and middle-income countries do not have a system to store vaccines at this extremely low temperature. Issues of vaccine storage and maintenance of the cold chain could impact access to rural communities or areas where continuous power supply is not secure. Even vaccines with less stringent storage requirements will require a logistically complex vaccination campaign in an era of pandemic fatigue and growing vaccine hesitancy.

Access may not be the only challenge for optimal uptake of COVID-19 vaccines. Recent surveys show that a substantial proportion of people may refuse or delay taking vaccination (Cooper et al, 2021; Wiysonge et al, 2021). The delay in acceptance or the refusal of vaccines, despite the availability of vaccination services, is referred to as vaccine hesitancy (Cooper et al, 2018; Wiyeh et al, 2019). It poses significant risks not only for the hesitant people, but also the wider community. Delays and refusals of COVID-19 vaccination would make communities unable to reach thresholds of coverage necessary for containment of spread of the virus (Wiyeh et al, 2018a; Wiysonge et al, 2021). This would perpetuate community transmission of COVID-19 and keep the pandemic alive. Vaccine hesitancy is not a new phenomenon, but the proliferation of anti-vaccination misinformation through social media has given it new urgency (Wiysonge, 2019). A recent study used a cross-country regression framework to evaluate the effect of social media on vaccine hesitancy globally (Wilson and Wiysonge, 2020). The study found that misinformation online is associated with an increase in negative discussion of vaccines on social media as well as a decline in vaccination coverage over time (Wilson and Wiysonge, 2020). Thus, misinformation on social media in the context of COVID-19 may increase the number of individuals who are hesitant about getting a vaccine, even if their fears have no scientific basis. Thus, the key to countering vaccine misinformation on social media should be the removal of such misinformation (Wilson and Wiysonge, 2020).

By 15 October 2021, more than 6.7 billion doses of COVID-19 vaccines had been administered worldwide; with marked regional variation from 2.2 billion doses in China, 968.4 million in India, 820.4 million in Europe, and 645.6 million in North America, to only 170.7 million doses administered on the African continent (Ritchie et al, 2021). Overall, 47.5% of the world population has received at least one dose of a COVID-19 vaccine; with unequal uptake across continents from 59.1% in North America and 57.6% in Europe to as low as 7.6% in Africa. While national coverage is as high as 88-95% and increasing in high-income countries such as the United Arab Emirates and Portugal, most countries in Africa are still struggling to reach 5% coverage (Ritchie et al, 2021).

Through an open-label phase 3B implementation research study known as Sisonke, South Africa made the single-dose Johnson & Johnson vaccine immediately available to nearly 500 000 healthcare workers between 17 February and 17 May 2021 before the national rollout of COVID-19 vaccines in the country, which started on 17 May 2021 (Sisonke, 2021). 'Sisonke' is a Zulu word meaning 'together'. The Sisonke study was necessary to maintain a healthy work force to deal with a third wave of COVID-19 infections, which was predicted to start in May–June 2021. Halfway through the Sisonke study, SAHPRA paused vaccination to investigate extremely rare and severe blood clots detected in six out of about 6.8 million people vaccinated with the Johnson & Johnson vaccine in the USA (MacNeil et al, 2021; Mahase, 2021). However, the study resumed after approval was granted to proceed with an amended protocol to augment safety and oversight. This time, more rigorous pre-vaccination screening and post-vaccination monitoring of participants at risk of blood clotting disorders were introduced after the resumption (SAMRC, 2021). Although the decision to pause the Sisonke Study initially precipitated a rise in vaccine hesitancy, healthcare workers were later queuing in large numbers at vaccination sites across the country in the last week of the study (Sisonke, 2021). Primarily, this was achieved through widespread public and participant (both past and future) communication, education of vaccination staff and other healthcare workers, and an increase in the number of vaccination sites from the initial 46 to 93 across the country, including in rural areas (SAMRC, 2021). Following the Sisonke study, the national COVID-19 vaccination rollout started in South Africa on Monday 17 May 2021 (NDoH, 2021). Two vaccines are offered in the national rollout, the single-dose Johnson & Johnson viral-vector vaccine as well as the two-dose Pfizer-BioNTech mRNA vaccine (NDoH, 2021)). By 15 October 2021, more than 20 million doses of COVID-19 vaccines had been administered in South Africa; corresponding to a national vaccination coverage of 23% (Ritchie et al, 2021).

15.3.4 Adolescent and Childhood Vaccination

Adults were the initial target for COVID-19 vaccination in South Africa and elsewhere (NDoH, 2021; CDC, 2021; Chemaitelly et al, 2021; Levin et al, 2021). However, evidence has been accumulating on the favourable efficacy and safety of mRNA vaccines in adolescents and children (Polack et al, 2020; Frenck et al, 2021; Pfizer, 2021). The first study that provided convincing efficacy data on people younger than 18 years of age was the pivotal phase 2/3 trial of the two-dose Pfizer-BioNTech mRNA vaccine; conducted from July 2020 to October 2020 in South Africa, the United States, Argentina, Brazil, Germany, and Turkey. The mRNA vaccine was 95% effective in preventing COVID-19, with similar vaccine efficacy across all age groups (Polack et al, 2020). The second study was a phase 3 trial of the mRNA vaccine among 2260 adolescents

12–15 years old in the United States from October 2020 to March 2021 (Frenck et al, 2021). The trial reported vaccine efficacy of 100% with a favourable safety profile. Following these results, multiple Western countries have authorised the two-dose Pfizer-BioNTech mRNA vaccine for emergency use among children 12–17 years old. On 15 October 2021, the South African National Department of Health announced that children 12–17 years of age would be eligible for the Pfizer-BioNTech mRNA vaccine as from 20 October 2021. This followed approval of the vaccine for this age group by the national regulatory authority, SAHPRA (Phaahla, 2021).

In September 2021, Pfizer and BioNTech announced that a pivotal phase 2/3 trial had shown that their two-dose mRNA vaccine is safe and effective in children 5 to 11 years of age (Pfizer, 2021). This phase 2/3 trial is recruiting children aged 6 months to 11 years in the United States, Finland, Poland, and Spain. The companies plan to submit these data to national regulatory authorities across the world soon (Pfizer, 2021).

15.3.5 Booster Doses of COVID-19 Vaccines

It is currently unknown how long immunity following two doses of the Pfizer-BioNTech or a single dose of the Johnson & Johnson vaccines would last. Emerging evidence shows that the effectiveness of both vaccines against COVID-19 infections among healthcare workers is decreasing over time, probably due to a combination of both waning immunity and greater infectiousness of new variants of concern (Oliver, 2021; Sisonke, 2021).

Data available by September 2021 show that a single dose of the Johnson & Johnson viral-vector vaccine elicits durable humoral and cellular immune responses in adults for at least eight months after vaccination (Barouch et al, 2021). A booster dose of the vaccine, six months after the first dose, elicited rapid and robust increases in levels of spike-binding antibodies (Sadoff et al, 2021b). By October 2021, in South Africa, there is an increasing call from healthcare workers for a booster dose of the Johnson & Johnson vaccine, with the hope of reducing breakthrough infections and increasing protection against hospitalisation and death in this high-risk group. On 15 October 2021, the National Department of Health announced that this request is receiving attention. The department is working with the South African Medical Research Council and SAHPRA to find an evidence-informed approach for offering a booster dose for healthcare workers (Phaahla, 2021). In a related development, on 15 October 2021, an independent expert panel convened by the United States Food and Drug Administration advised the agency to authorise a booster dose of the Johnson & Johnson vaccine for people 18 years or older; with a recommendation that it should be given at least two months after the first dose (Johnson-and-Johnson, 2021).

There is also emerging evidence on the waning of humoral immunity as from six months after the second dose of the Pfizer-BioNTech mRNA vaccine (Oliver, 2021; Levin et al, 2021; Goldberg et al, 2021; Chemaitelly et al, 2021). This decrease in antibody levels seems to be more pronounced among persons 65 years of age or older and persons with compromised immunity (Levin et al, 2021; Oliver, 2021). Based on these data, the South African Ministerial Advisory Committee on COVID-19 vaccines has advised that a booster dose of the mRNA vaccine be given to individuals with immunosuppression (Phaahla, 2021). The United States also offers a booster dose of the mRNA vaccine to individuals 65 years of age or older and other high-risk groups (CDC, 2021).

15.3.6 Vaccine Uptake and Mandatory Vaccinations

Having adequate supplies of vaccines and the processes in place to administer them are just part of the battle towards achieving containment of pandemics. We have seen during the COVID-19 pandemic how anti-vaccine sentiment impacts negatively against developing vaccine confidence. The goal of decreasing onward transmission of the virus, thereby gaining wider protection of communities, will not be achieved if reluctance to vaccinate results in inadequate numbers of people presenting themselves at the vaccine sites for inoculation. A severe increase in new coronavirus infections caused by the delta variant and a decrease in vaccine uptake forced governments in many countries to make COVID-19 vaccines mandatory for healthcare workers and other high-risk groups. In addition, proof of vaccination by producing a vaccine certificate or pass or the presentation of a negative test result has been instituted in several jurisdictions globally (Reuters, 2021; Gostin et al, 2021; Gurie et al, 2021).

Courts may have regard to foreign law interpretations of provisions in their Constitutions similar to those in the South African Constitution. Although, many of these recent legislative interventions have yet to be legally tested, the context, proportionality and legitimate public health objectives would be key factors to consider when instituting mandatory vaccination measures. In almost all instances, an individual's rights to personal autonomy and various freedoms would need to be balanced against the protection of the broader community's health and safety (Stuart, 2009). In South Africa, the right to bodily and psychological integrity, which includes the right to security in and control over their body is affirmed in the Constitution (section 12(2)(*b*)) (Constitution, 1996). The Constitution also affirms the right to an environment that is not harmful to health or well-being (section 24(*a*)) and the right to freedom of conscience, religion, thought, belief and opinion (section 15(1)). Notwithstanding the entitlements inherent in these rights, most rights in the Constitution may be limited, provided the limitation is of general application, and is 'reasonable and justifiable', which means that it is rational, proportional and the least restrictive means of achieving its objective (section 36(1)).

A compulsory requirement that people who may be exposed to COVID-19 infection must be vaccinated by a scientifically proven, safe and effective vaccine which has been approved by the regulator (South African Health Products Regulatory Authority) is 'reasonable and justifiable' because of public health reasons which include that of securing protection against death and severe disease; decreasing onward transmission; reducing risk of ongoing mutations into variants of concern; relieving pressure on ICUs; and protecting healthcare workers so that they are enabled to respond to the needs of other patients who otherwise may have been turned away. Vaccinations are the least restrictive means to achieve the purpose because the current precautions requiring the wearing of masks, sanitising or washing of hands, keeping a social distance and ensuring adequate ventilation are not sufficient. Hence the limitation would be proportional to the infringement of the relevant rights. Furthermore, if adequate vaccination rates are not achieved, there would be a continuing contraction of the economy, unacceptably high unemployment rates, and restrictions on other Constitutional rights and freedoms, such as freedom of association (section 18) and freedom of movement (section 21).

The law as regards workplace protection is very clear in South Africa. The Occupational Health and Safety Act (Act 85 of 1993) makes it necessary for every employer to take reasonable measures to ensure the health and safety of its employees in the workplace (section 8(1)) and for every employer whose workers interface with the public to take reasonable measures to ensure that interface does not endanger the health and safety of the members of the public (section 9(1)). Section 12(1) requires employers to ensure a work environment that is not harmful to employees by protecting them from 'hazards emanating from listed work' and section 12(1)*(b)* requires employers to 'as far as reasonably practicable, prevent the exposure of such employees to the hazards concerned, or where prevention is not reasonably practicable, minimise such exposure'. Section 14 is specific to employee responsibilities, mandating that employees need to 'take reasonable care for the health and safety of [themselves] and of other persons who may be affected by [their] acts or omissions' (section 14*(a)*). Section 14*(c)* requires employees to 'carry out any lawful order given to [them], and obey health and safety rules and procedures, laid down by [their] employer', or a person authorised by the employer, 'in the interest of health and safety'. In terms of section 38(1)*(a)*, it is a criminal offence for an employee not to comply with the rules as set out by the employer. In June 2021, a Direction was gazetted by the Minister of Labour, allowing for employers to make COVID-19 vaccinations in certain workplaces a mandatory requirement.

15.4 DEVELOPMENT OF MONOCLONAL ANTIBODIES AGAINST COVID-19

COVID-19 monoclonal antibodies refer to laboratory-produced molecules which serve as substitutes for antibodies. COVID-19 monoclonal antibodies are created by identifying COVID-19-specific B cells of patients who have recently recovered from COVID-19 infection or by utilising mice genetically modified to have an immune system (Marovich et al, 2020). Once the B cells are identified, the immune globulin genes are recovered. These genes are then expressed to produce monoclonal antibodies. Most COVID-19 monoclonal antibodies target the viral spike protein (Marovich et al, 2020).

15.5 CONCLUSION

Vaccines have led to the eradication of smallpox, have nearly eradicated polio, and have led to major reductions in deaths and disability from many serious infectious diseases (Machingaidze et al, 2013; Wiysonge et al, 2007). A challenge in responding to pandemic diseases is that vaccines may not always exist for them or that existing vaccines may not be effective against them. The influenza pandemic of 1918–1919 is estimated to have killed more than 50 million people, and less severe influenza pandemics occurred in 1957, 1968, and 2009 (Sambala et al, 2018). In the last three influenza pandemics, vaccines were available (Guan et al, 2010; Smith et al, 2009; Lee et al, 2013; Sambala et al, 2018). COVID-19 vaccines have accelerated at a record-breaking pace. By July 2021, there were about 300 candidate COVID-19 vaccines in various stages of preclinical and clinical development, with 18 of them authorised for emergency use during the pandemic (Ndwandwe and Wiysonge, 2021). There are four main classes of COVID-19 vaccines in development: whole virus vaccines, protein-based vaccines, viral vector vaccines, and nucleic acid vaccines. The last two categories use technologies that were unproven before 2020, as no vaccine licensed at that stage used any of the two technologies.

15.6 SELF-ASSESSMENT QUESTIONS

1. Which technologies for COVID-19 vaccines were unproven before 2020?
2. What is vaccine hesitancy and how might it affect containment of spread of the virus?

15.7 REFERENCES

Anderson, E.J., Rouphael, N.G., Widge, A.T., Jackson, L.A., Roberts, P.C., Makhene, M., Chappell, J.D., Denison, M.R., Stevens, L.J., Pruijssers, A.J., Mcdermott, A.B., Flach, B., Lin, B.C., Doria-Rose, N.A., O'dell, S., Schmidt, S.D., Corbett, K.S., Swanson, P.A., 2nd, Padilla, M., Neuzil, K.M., Bennett, H., Leav, B., Makowski, M., Albert, J., Cross, K., Edara, V.V., Floyd, K., Suthar, M.S., Martinez, D.R., Baric, R., Buchanan, W., Luke, C.J., Phadke, V.K., Rostad, C.A., Ledgerwood, J.E., Graham, B.S. and Beigel, J.H. 2020. Safety and Immunogenicity of SARS-CoV-2 mRNA-1273 Vaccine in Older Adults. *N Engl J Med*.

Avorn, J. and Kesselheim, A. 2020. Regulatory Decision-making on COVID-19 Vaccines During a Public Health Emergency. *Jama* 324, 1284–1285.

Barouch, D.H., Stephenson, K.E., Sadoff, J., Yu, J., Chang, A., Gebre, M., Mcmahan, K., Liu, J., Chandrashekar, A., Patel, S., Le Gars, M., De Groot, A.M., Heerwegh, D., Struyf, F., Douoguih, M., Van Hoof, J. and Schuitemaker, H. 2021. Durable Humoral and Cellular Immune Responses Following Ad26.COV2.S Vaccination for COVID-19. *medRxiv*.

Bekker, L.G. and Gray, G.E. 2017. Hope for HIV control in southern Africa: The continued quest for a vaccine. *PLoS Med* 14, e1002241.

Callaway, E. 2020a. COVID vaccine excitement builds as Moderna reports third positive result. *Nature* 587, pp. 337–338.

Callaway, E. 2020b. The race for coronavirus vaccines: a graphical guide. *Nature* 580, pp. 576–577.

CDC. 2021. Vaccines for COVID-19. Available at: https://www.cdc.gov/coronavirus/2019-ncov/vaccines/index.html.

Chemaitelly, H., Tang, P., Hasan, M.R., Almukdad, S., Yassine, H.M., Benslimane, F.M., Al Khatib, H.A., Coyle, P., Ayoub, H.H., Al Kanaani, Z., Al Kuwari, E., Jeremijenko, A., Kaleeckal, A.H., Latif, A.N., Shaik, R.M., Abdul Rahim, H.F., Nasrallah, G.K., Al Kuwari, M.G., Al Romaihi, H.E., Butt, A.A., Al-Thani, M.H., Al Khal, A., Bertollini, R. and Abu-Raddad, L.J. 2021. Waning of BNT162b2 Vaccine Protection against SARS-CoV-2 Infection in Qatar. *N Engl J Med*.

Cooper, S., Betsch, C., Sambala, E.Z., Mchiza, N. and Wiysonge, C.S. 2018. Vaccine hesitancy – a potential threat to the achievements of vaccination programmes in Africa. *Hum Vaccin Immunother* 14, pp. 2355–2357.

Cooper, S., Van Rooyen, H. and Wiysonge, C.S. 2021. COVID-19 vaccine hesitancy in South Africa: how can we maximize uptake of COVID-19 vaccines? *Expert Rev Vaccines* 20, pp. 921–933.

Duclos, P., Durrheim, D.N., Reingold, A.L., Bhutta, Z.A., Vannice, K. and Rees, H. 2012. Developing evidence-based immunization recommendations and GRADE. *Vaccine* 31, pp. 12–9.

Frenck, R.W., Jr., Klein, N.P., Kitchin, N., Gurtman, A., Absalon, J., Lockhart, S., Perez, J. L., Walter, E.B., Senders, S., Bailey, R., Swanson, K.A., Ma, H., Xu, X., Koury, K., Kalina, W.V., Cooper, D., Jennings, T., Brandon, D.M., Thomas, S. J., Türeci, Ö., Tresnan, D.B., Mather, S., Dormitzer, P.R., Şahin, U., Jansen, K.U. and Gruber, W.C. 2021. Safety, Immunogenicity, and Efficacy of the BNT162b2 Covid-19 Vaccine in Adolescents. *N Engl J Med,* **385**, 239-250.

Gavi. 2020. COVAX. https://www.gavi.org/covax-facility, 23 November, p. 1.

Goldberg, Y., Mandel, M., Bar-On, Y. M., Bodenheimer, O., Freedman, L., Haas, E.J., Milo, R., Alroy-Preis, S., Ash, N. and Huppert, A. 2021. Waning immunity of the BNT162b2 vaccine: A nationwide study from Israel. *medRxiv* 21262423.

Guan, Y., Vijaykrishna, D., Bahl, J., Zhu, H., Wang, J. and Smith, G.J. 2010. The emergence of pandemic influenza viruses. *Protein Cell* 1, pp. 9–13.

Johnson-and-Johnson. 2021. Johnson and Johnson COVID-19 vaccine booster shot unanimously recommended for emergency use authorization by U.S. FDA Advisory Committee. Available at: https://www.janssen.com/johnson-johnson-covid-19-vaccine-booster-shot-unanimously-recommended-emergency-use-authorization-us.

Kanesa-Thasan, N., Shaw, A., Stoddard, J.J. and Vernon, T.M. 2011. Ensuring the optimal safety of licensed vaccines: a perspective of the vaccine research, development, and manufacturing companies. *Pediatrics,* 127 Suppl 1, S16–22.

Kesselheim, A.S., Darrow, J.J., Kulldorff, M., Brown, B.L., Mitra-Majumdar, M., Lee, C.C., Moneer, O. and Avorn, J. 2020. An Overview Of Vaccine Development, Approval, And Regulation, With Implications For COVID-19. *Health Aff (Millwood)* 101377hlthaff202001620.

Krause, P.R. and Gruber, M.F. 2020. Emergency Use Authorization of Covid Vaccines – Safety and Efficacy Follow-up Considerations. *N Engl J Med* 383, p. e107.

Laher, F., Bekker, L.G., Garrett, N., Lazarus, E.M. and Gray, G.E. 2020. Review of preventative HIV vaccine clinical trials in South Africa. *Arch Virol* 165, pp. 2439–2452.

Lee, B.Y., Haidari, L.A. and Lee, M.S. 2013. Modelling during an emergency: the 2009 H1N1 influenza pandemic. *Clin Microbiol Infect* 19, pp. 1014–22.

Lee, G. and Carr, W. 2018. Updated Framework for Development of Evidence-Based Recommendations by the Advisory Committee on Immunization Practices. *MMWR Morb Mortal Wkly Rep* 67, pp. 1271–1272.

Levin, E.G., Lustig, Y., Cohen, C., Fluss, R., Indenbaum, V., Amit, S., Doolman, R., Asraf, K., Mendelson, E., Ziv, A., Rubin, C., Freedman, L., Kreiss, Y. and Regev-Yochay, G. 2021. Waning Immune Humoral Response to BNT162b2 Covid-19 Vaccine over 6 Months. *N Engl J Med.*

Logunov, D.Y., Dolzhikova, I.V., Zubkova, O.V., Tukhvatullin, A.I., Shcheblyakov, D.V., Dzharullaeva, A.S., Grousova, D.M., Erokhova, A.S., Kovyrshina, A.V., Botikov, A.G., Izhaeva, F.M., Popova, O., Ozharovskaya, T.A., Esmagambetov, I.B., Favorskaya, I.A., Zrelkin, D.I., Voronina, D.V., Shcherbinin, D.N., Semikhin, A.S., Simakova, Y.V., Tokarskaya, E.A., Lubenets, N.L., Egorova, D.A., Shmarov, M.M., Nikitenko, N.A., Morozova, L.F., Smolyarchuk, E.A., Kryukov, E.V., Babira, V.F., Borisevich, S.V., Naroditsky, B.S. and Gintsburg, A.L. 2020. Safety and immunogenicity of an rAd26 and rAd5 vector-based heterologous prime-boost COVID-19 vaccine in two formulations: two open, non-randomised phase 1/2 studies from Russia. *Lancet* 396, pp. 887–897.

Lurie, N., Saville, M., Hatchett, R. and Halton, J. 2020. Developing Covid-19 Vaccines at Pandemic Speed. *N Engl J Med* 382, pp. 1969–1973.

Machingaidze, S., Wiysonge, C.S. and Hussey, G.D. 2013. Strengthening the expanded programme on immunization in Africa: looking beyond 2015. *PLoS Med* 10, p. e1001405.

Macneil, J.R., Su, J.R., Broder, K.R., Guh, A.Y., Gargano, J.W., Wallace, M., Hadler, S.C., Scobie, H.M., Blain, A.E., Moulia, D., Daley, M.F., Mcnally, V.V., Romero, J.R., Talbot, H.K., Lee, G.M., Bell, B.P. and Oliver, S.E. 2021. Updated Recommendations from the Advisory Committee on Immunization Practices for Use of the Janssen (Johnson and Johnson) COVID-19 Vaccine After Reports of Thrombosis with Thrombocytopenia Syndrome Among Vaccine Recipients – United States, April 2021. *MMWR Morb Mortal Wkly Rep* 70, pp. 651–656.

Mahase, E. 2021. Covid-19: US suspends Johnson and Johnson vaccine rollout over blood clots. *Bmj* 373, p. n970.

Marovich, M., Mascola, J.R. and Cohen, M.S. 2020. Monoclonal Antibodies for Prevention and Treatment of COVID-19. *JAMA* 324, pp. 131–132.

Nabel, G.J. 2013. Designing tomorrow's vaccines. *N Engl J Med* 368, pp. 551–60.

NDOH. 2021. Vaccine information portal. Available at: https://sacoronavirus.co.za/vaccine-updates/.

Ndwandwe, D. and Wiysonge, C.S. 2021. COVID-19 vaccines. *Curr Opin Immunol* 71, pp. 111–116.

Ngcobo, N.J. and Cameron, N.A. 2012. The decision making process on new vaccines introduction in South Africa. *Vaccine* 30 Suppl 3, pp. C9–13.

Oliver, S. 2021. Evidence to recommendation framework: Pfizer-BioNTech COVID-19 booster dose. ACIP Meeting, 23 September 2021. Available at: https://www.cdc.gov/vaccines/acip/meetings/downloads/slides-2021-9-23/03-COVID-Oliver.pdf.

Ollmann Saphire, E. 2020. A Vaccine against Ebola Virus. *Cell*, 181, 6.

Pfizer. 2021. Pfizer and BioNTech announce positive topline results from pivotal trial of COVID-19 vaccine in children 5 yo 11 years. Available at: https://www.pfizer.com/news/press-release/press-release-detail/pfizer-and-biontech-announce-positive-topline-results.

Phaahla, M.J. 2021. Remarks by Dr M J Phaahla, Minister of Health during COVID-19 Vaccination roll-out programme Media Briefing, on 15 Oct 2021. Available at: https://sacoronavirus.co.za/category/press-releases-and-notices/.

Plotkin, S.A. 2005. Vaccines: past, present and future. *Nat Med* 11, pp. S5–11.

Plotkin, S.A. and Plotkin, S.L. 2011. The development of vaccines: how the past led to the future. *Nat Rev Microbiol* 9, pp. 889–93.

Polack, F.P., Thomas, S.J., Kitchin, N., Absalon, J., Gurtman, A., Lockhart, S., Perez, J.L., Pérez Marc, G., Moreira, E.D., Zerbini, C., Bailey, R., Swanson, K.A., Roychoudhury, S., Koury, K., Li, P., Kalina, W. ., Cooper, D., Frenck, R.W., Jr., Hammitt, L.L., Türeci, Ö., Nell, H., Schaefer, A., Ünal, S., Tresnan, D.B., Mather, S., Dormitzer, P.R., Şahin, U., Jansen, K.U. and Gruber, W.C. 2020. Safety and Efficacy of the BNT162b2 mRNA Covid-19 Vaccine. *N Engl J Med* 383, pp. 2603–2615.

Ritchie, H., Mathieu, E., Rodés-Guirao, L., Appel, C., Giattino, C., Ortiz-Ospina, E., Hasell, J., Roser, M., Macdonald, B., Beltekian, D. and Roser, M. 2021. Coronavirus (COVID-19) vaccinations. Available at: https://ourworldindata.org/covid-vaccinations.

Sadoff, J., Gray, G., Vandebosch, A., Cárdenas, V., Shukarev, G., Grinsztejn, B., Goepfert, P. A., Truyers, C., Fennema, H., Spiessens, B., Offergeld, K., Scheper, G., Taylor, K.L., Robb, M.L., Treanor, J., Barouch, D.H., Stoddard, J., Ryser, M.F., Marovich, M.A., Neuzil, K.M., Corey, L., Cauwenberghs, N., Tanner, T., Hardt, K., Ruiz-Guiñazú, J., Le Gars, M., Schuitemaker, H., Van Hoof, J., Struyf, F. and Douoguih, M. 2021a. Safety and Efficacy of Single-Dose Ad26.COV2.S Vaccine against Covid-19. *N Engl J Med*.

Sadoff, J., Le Gars, M., Cardenas, V., Shukarev, G., Vaissiere, N., Heerwegh, D., Truyers, C., De Groot, A.M., Scheper, G., Hendriks, J., Ruiz-Guiñazú, J., Struyf, F., Van Hoof, J., Douoguih, M. and Schuitemaker, H. 2021b. Durability of antibody responses elicited by a single dose of Ad26.COV2.S and substantial increase following late boosting. *medRxiv*, 21262569.

Sahin, U., Muik, A., Derhovanessian, E., Vogler, I., Kranz, L. M., Vormehr, M., Baum, A., Pascal, K., Quandt, J., Maurus, D., Brachtendorf, S., Lörks, V., Sikorski, J., Hilker, R., Becker, D., Eller, A. K., Grützner, J., Boesler, C., Rosenbaum, C., Kühnle, M.C., Luxemburger, U., Kemmer-Brück, A., Langer, D., Bexon, M., Bolte, S., Karikó, K., Palanche, T., Fischer, B., Schultz, A., Shi, P.Y., Fontes-Garfias, C., Perez, J.L., Swanson, K.A., Loschko, J., Scully, I.L., Cutler, M., Kalina, W., Kyratsous, C.A., Cooper, D., Dormitzer, P.R., Jansen, K.U. and Türeci, Ö. 2020.

COVID-19 vaccine BNT162b1 elicits human antibody and T(H)1 T cell responses. *Nature* 586, pp. 594–599.

Sambala, E.Z., Kanyenda, T., Iwu, C.J., Iwu, C.D., Jaca, A. and Wiysonge, C.S. 2018. Pandemic influenza preparedness in the WHO African region: are we ready yet? *BMC Infect Dis* 18, p. 567.

SAMRC. 2021. Calling all health personnel to come forward for enrolment in the last week of the Sisonke Phase 3 b study. Available at: https://www.samrc.ac.za/media-release/calling-all-health-personnel-come-forward-enrolment-last-week-sisonke-phase-3-b-study.

Schoub, B.D., Ngcobo, N.J. and Madhi, S. 2010. The National Advisory Group on Immunization (NAGI) of the Republic of South Africa. *Vaccine* 28 Suppl 1, pp. A31–4.

Sisonke. 2021. Sisonke study: a pragmatic real world phase 3b clinical trial of the single-dose COVID-19 vaccine candidate among frontline healthcare workers in South Africa. Available at: http://sisonkestudy.samrc.ac.za/.

Smith, G.J., Bahl, J., Vijaykrishna, D., Zhang, J., Poon, L.L., Chen, H., Webster, R.G., Peiris, J.S. and Guan, Y. 2009. Dating the emergence of pandemic influenza viruses. *Proc Natl Acad Sci U S A* 106, pp. 11709–12.

Steckelberg, A., Johnson, C.Y., Florit, G. and Alcantara, C. 2020. These are the top coronavirus vaccines to watch. *Washington Post*. Available at: https://www.washingtonpost.com/graphics/2020/health/covid-vaccine-update-coronavirus/.

Tomori, O. and Kolawole, M.O. 2021. Ebola virus disease: current vaccine solutions. *Curr Opin Immunol* 71, pp. 27–33.

Usdin, S. 2020. COVAX created to try to avoid global bidding frenzy for COVID-19 vaccines. *Biocentury* 17 June, pp. 1–3.

WHO. 2010. WHO Expert Committee on Biological Standardization, sixty-first report. Procedure for assessing the acceptability, in principle, of vaccines for purchase by United Nations agencies. *WHO Technical Report Series,* 978.

WHO. 2021a. Draft landscape and tracker of COVID-19 candidate vaccines – 12 October 2021. Available at: https://www.who.int/publications/m/item/draft-landscape-of-covid-19-candidate-vaccines.

WHO. 2021b. Status of COVID-19 Vaccines within WHO EUL/PQ evaluation process. Guidance Document 18 May 2021. Available at: https://extranet.who.int/pqweb/sites/default/files/documents/Status_COVID_VAX_18May2021.pdf.

Wilson, S.L. and Wiysonge, C. 2020. Social media and vaccine hesitancy. *BMJ Glob Health,* 5.

Wiyeh, A.B., Cooper, S., Jaca, A., Mavundza, E., Ndwandwe, D. and Wiysonge, C.S. 2019. Social media and HPV vaccination: Unsolicited public comments on a Facebook post by the Western Cape Department of Health provide insights into determinants of vaccine hesitancy in South Africa. *Vaccine* 37, pp. 6317–6323.

Wiyeh, A.B., Cooper, S., Nnaji, C.A. and Wiysonge, C.S. 2018a. Vaccine hesitancy 'outbreaks': using epidemiological modeling of the spread of ideas to understand the effects of vaccine related events on vaccine hesitancy. *Expert Rev Vaccines* 17, pp. 1063–1070.

Wiyeh, A.B., Sambala, E.Z., Ngcobo, N. and Wiysonge, C.S. 2018b. Existence and functionality of national immunisation technical advisory groups in Africa from 2010 to 2016. *Hum Vaccin Immunother* 14, pp. 2447–2451.

Wiysonge, C.S. 2019. Vaccine Hesitancy, an Escalating Danger in Africa. Think Global Health; 17 December 2019. Available at: https://www.thinkglobalhealth.org/article/vaccine-hesitancy-escalating-danger-africa.

Wiysonge, C.S., Ndwandwe, D., Ryan, J., Jaca, A., Batouré, O., Anya, B.M. and Cooper, S. 2021. Vaccine hesitancy in the era of COVID-19: could lessons from the past help in divining the future? *Hum Vaccin Immunother*, pp. 1–3.

Wiysonge, C.S., Nomo, E., Ticha, J.M., Shang, J.D., Njamnshi, A.K. and Shey, M.S. 2007. Effectiveness of the oral polio vaccine and prospects for global eradication of polio. *Trop Doct* 37, pp. 125–6.

CHAPTER 16

EPIDEMIOLOGY, DIAGNOSTICS AND SURVEILLANCE: APPLICATIONS DURING PANDEMICS

Oluseyi Ajayi

Galenda J. Nagudi

Lazarus Kuonza

Peter Nyasulu

Tobias Chirwa

16.1   INTRODUCTION

An outbreak of a pneumonia-like disease among patients in Wuhan City, Hubei province of China, was reported to the World Health Organization on 31 December 2019 (Clinical Management of COVID-19 disease, Version 3, 2020; Zhu et al, 2020). By 7 January 2020, the causative agent was identified to be a novel virus which belonged to the Coronaviridae family, the order Nidovirales, and the genus Coronavirus (Paintsil and Paintsil, 2020), termed severe acute respiratory syndrome coronavirus 2 (SARS-CoV-2) (Clinical Management of COVID-19 disease, Version 3, 2020). Coronaviruses belong to a subfamily called Coronavirinae which also has four genera namely; *Alphacoronavirus*, *Betacoronavirus*, *Gammacoronavirus*, and *Deltacoronavirus* (Paintsil and Paintsil, 2020). Similar to other coronaviruses, the SARS CoV-2 is an enveloped, single-stranded, positive-sense RNA virus (Paintsil and Paintsil, 2020). Its ability to easily adapt to its host makes its transmission from human to human highly efficient (Paintsil and Paintsil, 2020). Reports from a five-year surveillance in Yunnan Province, China indicated that the SARS CoV-2 originated from bats that dwelled in caves (Paintsil and Paintsil, 2020). The SARS- CoV-2 is notably associated with high fatality and has become a pandemic evidenced by the spread from China to other countries, including Africa, due to the increased rate of air travel between China and Africa for the purpose of international trade (Paintsil and Paintsil, 2020; Zhu et al, 2020). The novel coronavirus disease 2019 epidemic (COVID-19) caused by SARS CoV-2 was declared a Public Health Emergency of International Concern (PHEIC) by the WHO on 30 January 2020 (Gilbert et al, 2020).

In Africa, the first case of COVID-19, which was asymptomatic, was reported on 14 February 2020 by the Egyptian Ministry of Health and Population in Cairo (Paintsil and Paintsil, 2020). In sub-Saharan Africa, the first case of COVID-19 was reported in Nigeria on 27 February 2020 in an Italian passenger, who had travelled to Nigeria from Italy on 25 February 2020 (Lone and Ahmad, 2020; Paintsil and Paintsil, 2020). The patient was immediately admitted on arrival to an isolation centre and contact screening was conducted (Paintsil and Paintsil, 2020).

16.2 OBJECTIVES

The objectives of this paper are:

- To reinforce the role of diseases measurement as a public health tool in strategising public health interventions to contain COVID-19 pandemic.
- To enhance the value of surveillance data, a critical element for effective control of COVID-19.
- To highlight surveillance as a cornerstone for controlling the COVID-19 pandemic globally.
- To emphasise the role of effective diagnostic as key for implementing COVID-19 interventions.
- To illustrate the interface between disease intelligence model and an effective surveillance rapid COVID-19 detection and how this can mitigate the spread of the pandemic.

16.3 STRATEGIES FOR PANDEMIC PREPAREDNESS AND RESPONSE

The effective management of the COVID-19 pandemic depends on the level of preparedness and how equipped a nation is (Paintsil and Paintsil, 2020). A component of the World Health Organization (WHO) frameworks called the 2018 State Party Self-Assessment Annual Reporting (SPAR) has been adopted for all African countries (Paintsil and Paintsil, 2020). SPAR assesses the core capacities of all African countries which are requisite to detect, assess, notify and report events as well as responding promptly to public health risks and emergencies of national and international concern (WHO, nd). The International Health Regulations (IHR) core capacities however include national legislation, policy and financing; coordination and not-for-profit (NFP) communications; surveillance; response; preparedness, risk communication; human resources and laboratory (Bertrand et al, 2015). Indicators under each core capacity are scored based on the levels of increasing capacity and decreasing vulnerability, which ranges between 0 to 100 (Paintsil and Paintsil, 2020). By 2018, eight countries attained a SPAR score of 60 and above out of 100. They include Algeria which scored 80, Egypt scored 82, Morocco scored 75, Rwanda scored 67, Mauritius scored 62, South Africa scored 66, Tunisia scored 66, and Sudan scored 65. The Central African Republic and the Comoros were the countries with the least capability and were the most vulnerable to IHR hazards, with a SPAR score of 13 and 19, respectively (Paintsil and Paintsil, 2020).

On 3 February 2020, the Africa Centers for Disease Control and Prevention (Africa CDC) created the Africa Task Force for Novel Coronavirus (AFCOR) to coordinate the preparedness and response to the inevitable entry and spread of SARS-COV-2 across African Union member states (Lone and Ahmad, 2020). AFCOR, in collaboration with the WHO, identified six strategic areas of preparedness to enable countriesto efficiently tackle the pandemic: '(a) laboratory diagnosis; (b) surveillance, screening at points of entry and cross-border activities inclusive; (c) prevention and control of infections in health facilities; (d) clinical management of people with severe COVID-19; (e) risk communication and community engagement; and (f) supply chain management and stockpiles.' (Lone and Ahmad, 2020).

Despite efforts made by African states to put in place measures to manage the pandemic, numerous challenges still exist in most of the countries. One of the major challenges has been the limited laboratory equipment and supplies for SARS-CoV-2 testing. This has resulted in the underestimation of the true magnitude of the epidemic in most of the countries. Similar to the Ebola epidemic that occurred in 2014 in West Africa, there is variability in the application of screening measures to detect SARS-CoV-2 infection among travellers, with more stringent precautions being taken at the airports as compared to land or sea points of entry (Lone and Ahmad, 2020). Overall, due to the variability of virus entry in different countries at different time points, countries in Africa are experiencing varied stages of the pandemic, hence the conceptualisation of the actual epidemiology will only be possible at the end of the pandemic (Lone and Ahmad, 2020). Continued health education targeting the general population is necessitated to assist in COVID-19 prompt detection, reporting and responding (Lone and Ahmad, 2020).

The WHO dashboard provides global COVID-19 statistics on a daily basis, including the distribution of the cases by geographical regions and by country. On 28 February 2021, the dashboard showed a total of 384 956 new COVID-19 cases, and a cumulative total of 113 315 218 confirmed cases and 2 520 550 deaths. The figure below shows the number of confirmed COVID-19 cases by WHO region.

Americas	50,426,060
	confirmed
Europe	38,674,452
	confirmed
South-East Asia	13,517,009
	confirmed
Eastern Mediterranean	6,388,249
	confirmed
Africa	2,840,208
	confirmed
Americas	1,620,580
	confirmed

Source: World Health Organization

▨ Data may be incomplete for the current day or week.

Mar 31   Jun 30   Sep 30   Dec 31

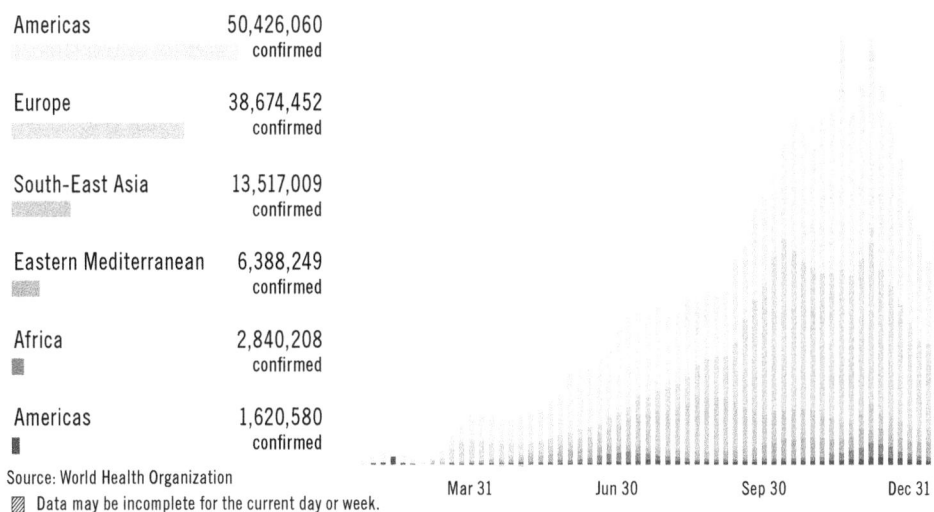

Figure 16.1 Number of COVID-19 confirmed cases by WHO region as of 28/02/2021

South Africa

On 5 March 2020, South Africa's first confirmed COVID-19 case was diagnosed. This was a South African citizen who had returned from a trip to Italy a few days earlier(Pressure and Wilfond, 2020). By 26 March 2020, a total of 1 170 people across South Africa had tested positive for COVID-19, prompting the government to implement a national lockdown in order to reduce the spread of the infection. At the time when the first lockdown was declared, the doubling time, defined as the period required for the number of cases in the epidemic to double, had gone down to two days (Pressure and Wilfond, 2020). Measures that were implemented during the national lockdown included the closure of learning institutions, restriction of international and intercity travel, limiting gatherings and encouraging the general population to socially distance and practise hand hygiene (Pressure and Wilfond, 2020).

At the beginning of the epidemic, a consortium of 10 government and university laboratories was formed and named the South African Network for Genomics Surveillance of COVID (SANGS_COVID) (Giandhari et al, 2020). The purpose for the formation was to monitor genomic changes to the coronavirus as the epidemic spread across the South African population.

The spread of the COVID-19 epidemic has been quite diverse across the provinces in South Africa. The Western Cape and Eastern Cape provinces experienced rapid increases in numbers of cases during the early phases of the epidemic, followed by the KwaZulu-Natal and Gauteng provinces (Giandhari et al, 2020). The early rapid growth of the epidemic in the Western Cape province was largely attributed to super spreader events among essential workers in the retail and the manufacturing industries (Pressure and Wilfond, 2020). In KwaZulu-Natal, a rapid increase in COVID-19 cases and deaths were linked to localised transmission of the virus in a large private hospital in Durban, the third-largest city in the country (Giandhari et al, 2020). The execution of early lockdown measures and widespread use of non-pharmacological interventions (NPIs), significantly slowed down the spread of the virus in South Africa (Pressure and Wilfond, 2020).

16.4   EPIDEMIOLOGY

The estimated median incubation period for COVID-19 is 4–5 days, with a range of 2–14 days (Clinical Management of COVID-19 disease, Version 3, 2020). The SARS-CoV-2 virus can be transmitted from people who do not manifest any clinical symptoms, but the extent of transmission has not been well-documented (Jassat et al, 2020; Clinical Management of COVID-19 disease, Version 3, 2020). A study reported that an infected person potentially has the ability to spread the virus to two other people (Kochhar and Salmon, 2020; Clinical Management of COVID-19 disease, Version 3, 2020). On the other hand, a systematic review reported a global reproductive number ranging from 1–5 as of June 2020; this is referred to as the reproduction number, Ro (Thiede et al, 2020). A reproductive number is the value that estimates the risk of an infected individual transmitting an infection to other uninfected susceptible individuals they come into contact with (Girdler-Brown and Murray, 2020). Given that SARS-CoV-2 was a novel virus, everyone in the population was deemed to be susceptible, especially during the early phases of the epidemic (National Institute For Communicable Diseases, 2020). The older population and those with comorbidities are said to be at a higher risk of getting infected with SAR-CoV-2 (Clinical Management of COVID-19 disease, Version 3, 2020). The first wave of SARS-COV-2 was highest at the beginning of July 2020. The second wave followed in November 2020 and was at its peak in January 2021(NICD, 2021).

The basic reproduction number for COVID-19 has been reported to vary significantly, depending on multiple factors such as country, population characteristics and stage of the epidemic. This means an individual infected with the SARS-CoV-2 has the ability to infect one to five other people. A study done in South Africa reported an average reproductive number of 1.39 in the month of May 2020 (Giandhari et al, 2020). The National Institute for Communicable Disease (NICD), whose core function is to conduct public health surveillance in the South African population, estimated the reproduction numbers for COVID-19 for the different national lockdown levels/stages (Table 16.1).

Table 16.1 A summary of the reproductive number as per the national lockdown stage in South Africa

National lockdown stage	Reproductive number	95% CI
5	1.13	1.07–1.60
4	1.26	1.06–1.50
3	1.02	1.00–1.04
2	0.84	0.74–0.95
1	0.99	0.93–1.04

The results presented in Table 16.1 have limitations as they could be affected by a number of factors that affect mortality which include: time taken to identify COVID-19 deaths, time lag between the onset of symptoms and death reporting, usage of dexamethasone treatment and nasal oxygen (National Institute For Communicable Diseases, 2020).

16.5   SURVEILLANCE

WHO defines surveillance as the process of systematic collection, collation and analysis of data with prompt dissemination to those who need to know to allow for relevant action to be taken (WHO, 2006). Surveillance can be either active or passive. Passive surveillance involves regular submission of disease records collected from patients by responsible institutions (World Health Organization, 2004). Active surveillance, on the other hand, involves the active solicitation of reports or cases of disease in the health facilities or in the community (World Health Organization, 2004). The sole objective of a disease surveillance system is to ensure information is effectively and efficiently collected for a timely response so as to prevent or stop further disease spread (Surveillance and Systems, 2001). There is no doubt that COVID-19 has challenged most if not all country disease surveillance systems in their readiness to handle an epidemic. In South Africa, the National Institute for Communicable Diseases (NICD), a division of the National Health Laboratory Services (NHLS), is mandated to manage and carry out surveillance on public health communicable diseases at both national and regional levels (Randall, 2020).

On 1 April 2020, in response to the emergence of COVID-19 the NICD introduced a new surveillance system named DATCOV (National Institute For Communicable Diseases (NICD) week 6, 2021). DATCOV is a hospital-based sentinel surveillance system whose purpose is to monitor trends in COVID-19 hospitalisations and to describe clinical characteristics and outcomes of patients hospitalised for COVID-19 (Jassat et al, 2020). A total of 638 health facilities comprising of 387 from the public sector and 251 from the private sector were reporting to DATCOV as of 13 February 2021 (National Institute For Communicable Diseases (NICD) week 6, 2021). A total of 209 870 admissions were reported from the 638 hospitals across all nine provinces of South Africa (National Institute For Communicable Diseases (NICD) week 6, 2021). It was also observed that the number of admissions in the second wave surpassed those in the first wave in both the public and private health facilities (National Institute For Communicable Diseases (NICD) week 6, 2021). The figure below shows the graph of the variation in hospital admissions per epidemiological week populated by the NICD from DATCOV reports. The four provinces that accounted for the largest number of admissions were Gauteng, KwaZulu-Natal, Eastern Cape and Western Cape (National Institute For Communicable Diseases (NICD) week 6, 2021).

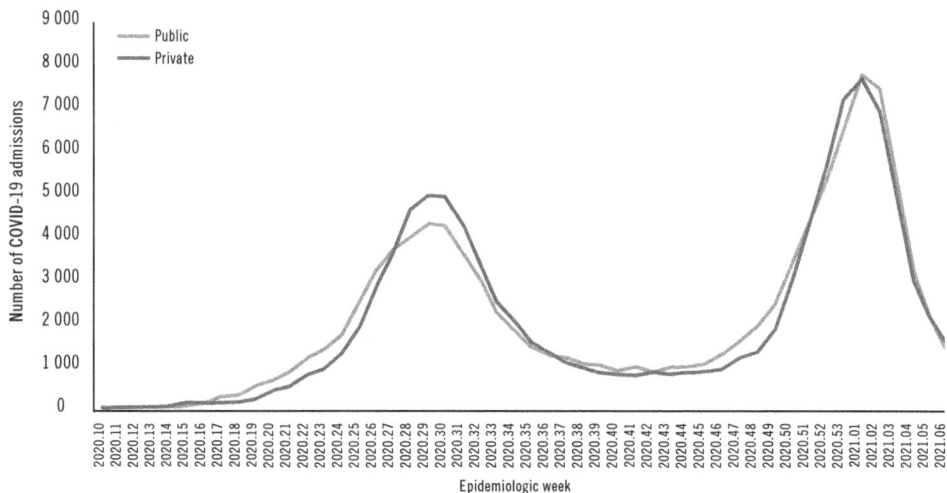

Figure 16.2 Number of COVID-19 hospital admissions in South Africa, 5 March 2020–13 February 2021

One of the essential tools that has been widely utilised to control the spread of COVID-19 is contact tracing. Contact tracing is the process where individuals exposed to an infectious person are identified, assessed and monitored to prevent further disease transmission (South Africa National Department of Health, 2020). In June 2020, the National Health Department published guidelines on contact tracing for COVID-19. The document highlighted that the areas of emphasis were community engagement, focus on the phases of the epidemic, case targeting and contact tracing and monitoring (South Africa National Department of Health, 2020). The guidelines' purpose was to give guidance on how contact tracing is to be implemented, managed, monitored and evaluated in South Africa (South Africa National Department of Health, 2020). A range of 7–14 days prior to the index case's onset of symptoms or from when they tested positive forms all possible places and sources of exposure. The table below shows the recommended contact tracing techniques according to the epidemic phase.

Table 16.2 Recommendations of contact tracing techniques according to epidemic phase by the National Health Department in South Africa

Phase	Characteristics of the phase	Contact tracing level
Phase 0 (preparedness): No Covid-19 case	• No reported cases in province/district/sub-district.	Aim: Preparedness Sensitise the population to the idea of outbreak control measures including contact tracing, quarantine, individual and community social distancing.
Phase 1 (containment): Early stage outbreak	• One or more imported cases. • Limited local transmission cases related to imported cases.	Aim: Prevent sustained transmission Conduct contact tracing (contact identification for all confirmed cases, contact listing and classification, choose contact follow-up approach and do daily contact follow-up). All contacts of confirmed and probable eases should be identified, quarantined and traced through phone calls and/or home visits.
Phase 2 (containment): Expanding outbreak	• Increasing number of imported cases. • Increased focal spread but all cases linked to known transmission chains. • Outbreak clusters with a known common exposure.	Aim: Contain and slow transmission Intensify contact tracing and adherence to quarantine as much as possible. If resources reach limit, prioritise contacts follow-up with the highest risk exposures, particularly health workers and vulnerable populations. All contacts of confirmed and probable cases should be identified, quarantined and monitored through self-reporting, phone calls and/or home visits in case of failure to self-report.

➡

Phase	Characteristics of the phase	Contact tracing level
Phase 3 (containment and mitigation): Advancing outbreak	• Localised outbreaks start to merge. • One or more cases or deaths occur outside known transmission chains. • Sustained person to person transmission - multiple generations in transmission chains. • Cases are detected among severe acute respiratory illness (SARI) case with no known exposure.	Aim: Slow transmission to delay and reduce outbreak peak and burden on health services Halt contact tracing in all outbreak areas and implement targeted screening and testing. Trace contacts only in districts/sub-districts reporting first cases where containment might still be possible or among high-risk vulnerable contacts. All contacts of confirmed and probable cases should be identified, quarantined and monitored through self-reporting, phone calls and/or home visits in case of failure to self-report.
Phase 4 (mitigation): Large outbreak with nationwide transmission	• Widespread sustained community transmission • Multiple generation transmission chains can be identified but most cases occurring outside of chains • Community-wide transmission throughout all or nearly all of the districts.	Aim: Reduce mortality among severe cases All contacts of confirmed and probable cases should be identified, quarantined and monitored through self-reporting, phone calls and/or home visits In case of failure to self-report. Halt contact tracing activities with few exceptions, determined by the need and value for doing so, such as outbreaks in hospitals. The national authorities could decide to continue tracing contacts only in newly infected areas and intensify active case finding in health facilities and communities.

Advantages and disadvantages of active and passive forms of surveillance being carried out in South Africa are outlined in Table 16.3.

Table 16.3 Advantages and disadvantages of the active and passive forms of surveillance

Type of surveillance	Advantages	Disadvantages
Hospital sentinel surveillance	– Requires limited resources – Easy management – Provides a basic understanding of disease burden – Provides accurate disease burden as records are based on reliable laboratory results – Information collected can be used to monitor disease trends and plan public health programmes	– Facilities reporting need reliable laboratory results – Demands a great deal of data management – Unable to identify incident rates of disease – The information collected is not representative of the whole country – Data quality issues may arise if staff collecting that data is not well trained or overwhelmed by the workload – Usually has poor timeliness
Contact tracing	– Gives the opportunity to monitor disease after community exposure – Timely data collection – Gives a clear picture of what is happening in the community as it unfolds – Provides more complete data	– Resource intensive – Requires skilled and committed staff – Expensive and logistically difficult to maintain – Demands a great deal data management

In addition, there are other surveillance indicators that have been implemented to monitor different elements of the COVID-19 pandemic in South Africa. Examples include the following:

- **New cases per day** – reported nationally every day, including geographic distribution. This provides daily insight on the number of infected people daily.
- **Testing rate** – number of COVID-19 tests per 100 000 population, also monitored daily. This provides a picture of both the willingness of individuals to report at health facilities to get tested and also the testing capacity at the health facilities.
- **Positivity rate** – Percentage of positive tests of all tests conducted. This indicator provides a reflection of the level of disease transmission. However, care should be taken to investigate a rapid increase in positivity rate as it may be as a result of increased testing capacity.
- **COVID-19 mortality** – COVID-19 deaths per 100 000 population (includes community deaths). This indicator provides insight into what deaths are attributed to COVID-19.

From the data collected from sentinel hospital surveillance below are some statistics obtained from the reports provided from 5 March 2020 to 13 February 2021.

Table 16.4 Number of reported in-hospital admissions and deaths by age and gender
(NICD COVID-19 Hospital surveillance week 6 2021 report)

Age (years)	ADMISSIONS				DEATHS			
	Female	Male	Unknown	Total	Female	Male	Unknown	Total
0-4	1389	1651	7	3047	50	46	1	97
5-9	350	484	3	837	8	12	0	20
10-14	616	561	0	1177	13	14	0	27
15-19	1860	1003	3	2866	55	48	0	103
20-24	3353	1652	3	5008	123	90	0	213
25-29	5917	2709	4	8630	273	168	0	441
30-34	8192	4725	3	12920	513	386	0	899
35-39	9204	6561	5	15770	727	643	0	1370
40-44	8949	7794	5	16748	950	962	1	1913
45-49	10292	9448	7	19747	1441	1498	2	2941
50-54	11967	10628	2	22597	1957	2006	0	3963
55-59	12902	11217	8	24127	2815	2739	1	5555
60-64	11464	10297	8	21769	3163	3316	1	6480
65-69	9326	8164	6	17496	3155	3003	0	6158
70-74	7436	6577	12	14025	2673	2648	4	5325
75-79	5353	4332	3	9688	2030	1896	0	3926
80-84	3866	2715	4	6585	1553	1214	1	2768
85-89	2063	1274	1	3338	867	641	0	1508
90-94	903	440	1	1344	436	227	0	663
>=95	334	211	0	545	137	73	0	210
Unknown	840	658	108	1606	121	125	5	251
TOTAL	**116576**	**93101**	**193**	**209870**	**23060**	**21755**	**16**	**44831**

Table 16.5 Number of COVID-19 hospital cumulative admissions and death by province
(NICD COVID-19 Hospital surveillance week 6 2021 report)

Province	Provincial Population mid-2020*	Cumulative admissions	Cumulative Admissions/ 100,000	Cumulative deaths	Cumulative deaths/ 100,000
Eastern Cape	6734001	29384	436,4	9156	136,0
Free State	2928903	11529	393,6	2354	80,4
Gauteng	15488137	56788	366,7	10174	65,7
KwaZulu-Natal	11531628	39428	341,9	8218	71,3
Limpopo	5852553	6990	119,4	1953	33,4
Mpumalanga	4679786	7388	157,9	1775	37,9
North West	4108816	10656	259,3	1293	31,5
Northern Cape	1292786	3562	275,5	622	48,1
Western Cape	7005741	44145	630,1	9286	132,5
South Africa	**59622350**	**209870**	**352,0**	**44831**	**75,2**

16.5.1 Clinical Characteristics

Based on reviews and current guidelines, the clinical presentation of COVID-19 can be classified into mild, moderate, and severe (Amawi et al, 2020). Patients with mild (uncomplicated) COVID-19 are likely to have symptoms that include mild fever, dry cough, sore throat, respiratory irritation, tiredness, abdominal pains, body aches and malaise (feeling unwell) (Clinical Management of COVID-19 disease, Version 3, 2020; Amawi et al, 2020). Those with moderate illness usually include symptoms such as cough, shortness of breath, loss of sense of taste and smell (Clinical Management of COVID-19 disease, Version 3, 2020; Amawi et al, 2020). An unidentified proportion of infected individuals tend to have an unexpected worsened condition after about a week with clinical manifestations such as high fever, respiratory failure, septic shock, and/or multi-organ dysfunction (Clinical Management of COVID-19 disease, Version 3, 2020; Amawi et al, 2020). Some rare symptoms include nausea and diarrhoea (Clinical Management of COVID-19 disease, Version 3, 2020; Amawi et al, 2020).

16.5.2 Outcomes and Prognosis

As of July 2020 in South Africa, out of 215 855 positive cases, there were a total of 3 502 deaths (Blumberg et al, 2020). There was an unexpected surge in the number of COVID-19 cases in December, which was attributed to the emergence of a new strain called 501Y.V2 (B.1.351) (Fontanet et al, 2021).

Mostly, the COVID-19 disease progresses to a state of complete recovery. The recovery process could take a couple of weeks, especially in severe cases which is dependent on some factors such as patients' sex, age, underlying disease, and various approaches used to treat patients in different regions (Hatami et al, 2020) (Clinical Management of COVID-19 disease, Version 3, 27 March 2020). COVID-19 sometimes could progress to acute respiratory distress syndrome (ARDS), multiple organ failure and sometimes death, even though little is still known about the clinical sequelae of COVID-19 (Sigfrid et al, 2020). There is continued new evidence suggesting post-COVID fibrosis, which may lead to associated breathlessness and cough (Garg et al, 2021).

16.5.3 Reinfection

The criteria used to define reinfection appear to differ widely. Evidence from previous studies shows that people who are infected with any of the four seasonal human coronaviruses develop some protective immunity for short durations. SARS-CoV-2 appears to follow a similar pattern, suggesting that individuals who get infected with the virus can be re-infected within an average of 12 months after the first illness (Edridge et al, 2020). A recent study carried out in a single medical centre in Leicester, England reported six cases of reinfection (Richardson, 2020). The Centers for Disease Control and Prevention (CDC) uses the following criteria to define reinfection with SARS-CoV-2: 'detection of SARS-CoV2 RNA with Ct values 90 days after the first detection of viral RNA whether or not symptoms were present and paired respiratory specimens from each episode that belong to different clades of virus or have genomes with >2 nucleotide differences per month' (Richardson, 2020).

16.6   MATHEMATICAL MODELLING

Modelling can be used to make projections on how a disease is spread, understand the different factors that affect disease transmission, evaluate possible intervention strategies, and plan ahead for likely future occurrences (Serhani and Labbardi, 2020; Reddy et al, 2021). During the course of the pandemic, numerous models were developed to make short-term and long-term predictions on different aspects of the epidemic at the National and Provincial levels (Reddy et al, 2021). The models have been used to predict trends in numbers of COVID-19 cases and deaths, to estimate hospital and Intensive Care Unit (ICU) beds during peak periods, and other areas (Sheetal et al, 2020; Reddy et al, 2021).

Most of the models have been built using compartmental modelling techniques that classify the population into compartments based on the dynamic aspects of the evolution of the disease in the population, e.g. susceptible, exposed, infectious and recovered (Reddy et al, 2021). A couple of differential equations that determine how people transit from one compartment to another are defined and solved based on the assumptions about how the disease progresses, existing public health policies, demography and varied patterns among individuals in the population (Reddy et al, 2021).

The South African COVID-19 Mathematical Modelling Consortium was commissioned to support the South African government in developing, evaluating and validating models to project the spread of COVID-19 in the population, in order to support government policy and planning (Sheetal et al, 2020). The consortium considered numerous parameters and assumptions to come up with reasonable projections of the epidemic. Some of these parameters include: the frequency of undetected/undiagnosed COVID-19 infections in the population; possible local clustering of cases, estimated mortality due to COVID-19; possible behavioural changes within the population in response to the high levels of mortality; and possible changes in the epidemiology of the virus as the epidemic evolved locally and globally (Sheetal et al, 2020).

16.6.1 Short-term prediction of the total number of reported COVID-19 cases at national level

The three-parameter logistic, four-parameter logistic and Richards models (Reddy et al, 2021) were used to project the total number of COVD-19 cases at the national level.

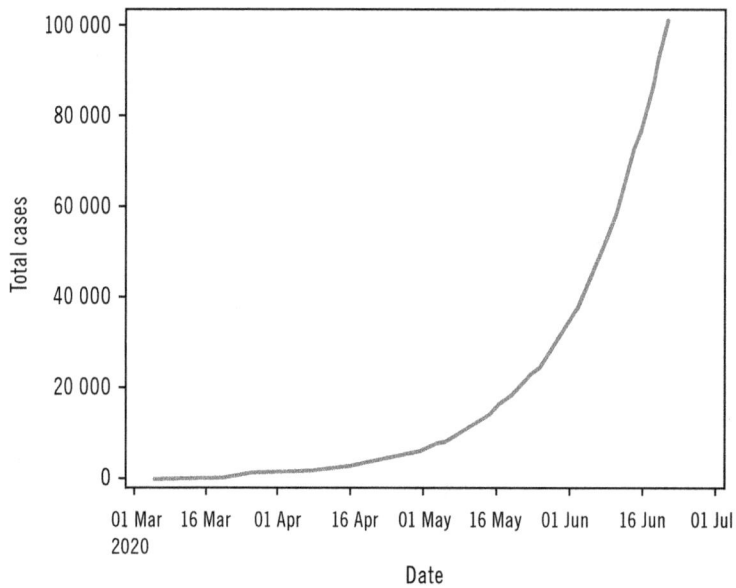

Figure 16.3 The cumulative COVID-19 cases for the period 5 March 2020 to 22 June 2020 (Reddy et al, 2021)

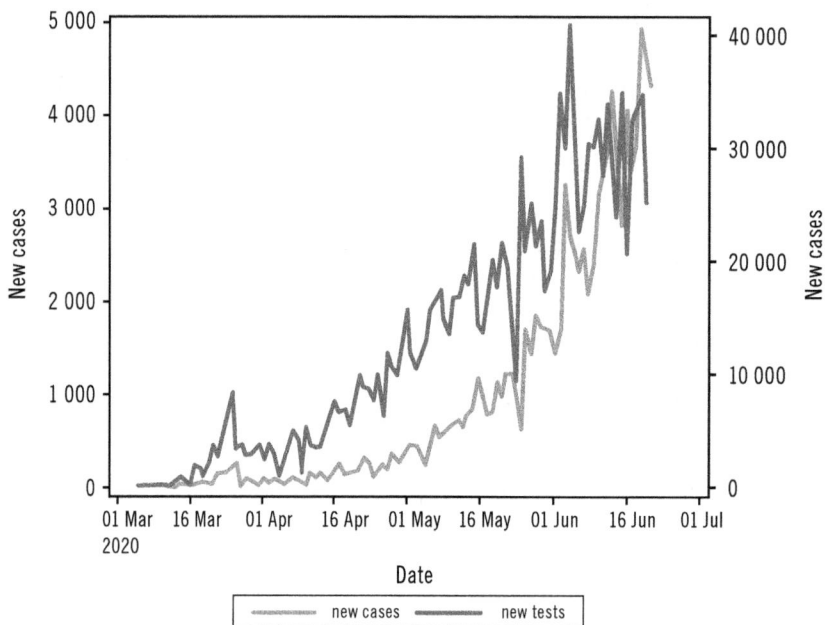

Figure 16.4 The relationship between daily COVID-19 tests and cases diagnosed for the period 5 March 2020 to 22 June 2020 (Reddy et al, 2021)

16.6.2 Short-term forecasts of the total number of reported COVID-19 cases – A province-level analysis

At sub-national levels, the pattern of the spread of COVID-19 appeared to differ for each province (see Figure 16.4). When the initial projections were done on 22 June 2020, three provinces (Western Cape, Eastern Cape and Gauteng) were responsible for 90.3% of the 101 590 cases of COVID-19 that had been reported in South Africa.

Five data-driven nonlinear growth models were considered for the Western Cape Province, namely the three-parameter logistic model, four-parameter logistic model, Weibull and Richards models, and the three-parameter logistic regression model provided the best fit to the data. Due to the significantly slower growth rate of the outbreaks in the Eastern Cape and Gauteng from 5 March 2020 until 22 June 2020, piecewise growth models were fitted to capture this change point. The three-parameter logistic model provided the best fit to the Eastern Cape data, with a change point in the growth rate at day 80 (8 June 2020). Similarly, a piecewise three-parameter logistic model was fitted to the Gauteng data with a change point at day 87 (1 June 2020). The actual observed number of cases on 26 June 2020 was 57 941, 21 938 and 31 344 in the Western Cape, Eastern Cape, and Gauteng, respectively, indicative of an underestimation of cases in Eastern Cape and Gauteng. This underestimation was more pronounced for a 10-day (1 July 2020) forecast onward, where the observed cases in the Eastern Cape and Gauteng were 29 340 and 45 944, respectively (Reddy et al, 2021).

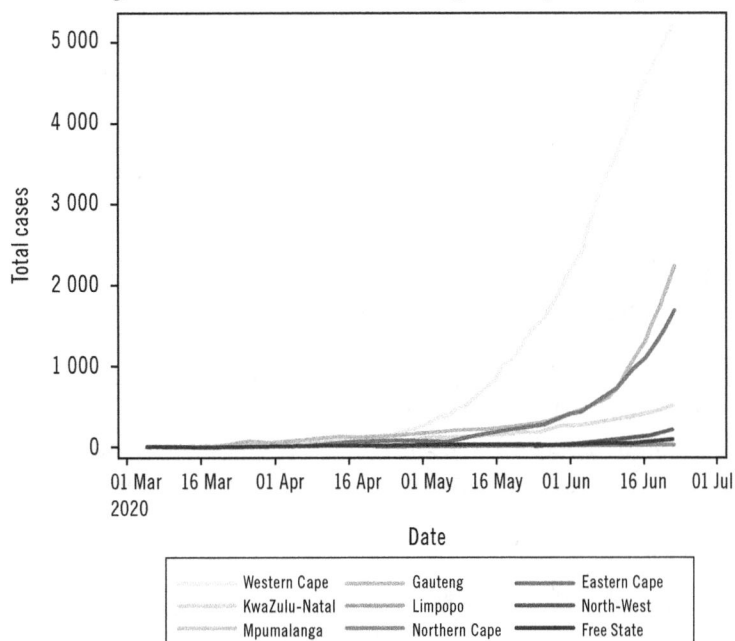

Figure 16.5 The cumulative COVID-19 cases in each of the nine provinces in South Africa for the period 5 March 2020 to 22 June 2020 (Reddy et al, 2021)

The data presented in Figure 16.5 show that models for cases and deaths provided robust and accurate short-term forecasts for a period of 10 days ahead at the national level. However, due to the fast-changing growth rate as the country approached the peak of the first wave of the COVID-19 epidemic, coupled with government-driven changes in COVID-19 control regulations and the reopening of the economy, it is important to fit models daily as new data becomes available, and that predictions are constantly updated accordingly (Reddy et al, 2021). However, it is important to note some limitations of fitting these models, which include problems of convergence between the five models and that some provinces had a late outbreak compared to other provinces that had an early outbreak (Reddy et al, 2021).

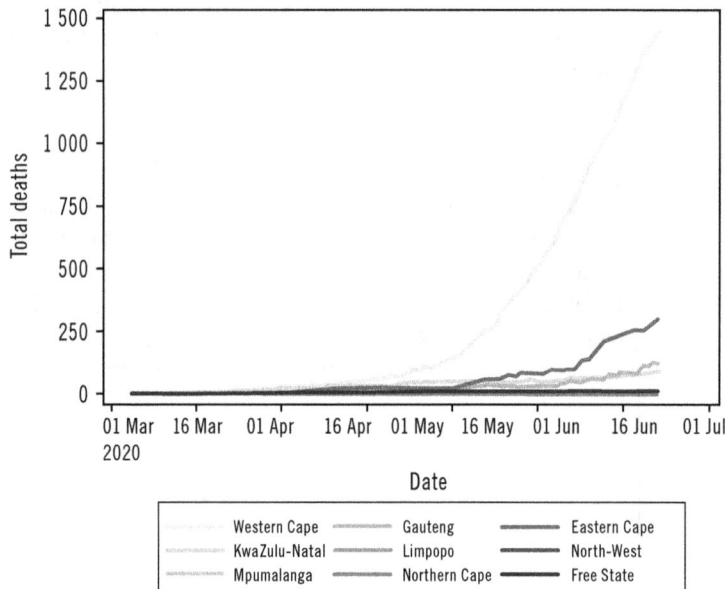

Figure 16.6 The cumulative COVID-19 deaths in each of the nine provinces in South Africa for the period 5 March 2020 to 22 June 2020 (Reddy et al, 2021)

As depicted from the short-term forecasts for the three models fitted to the cases (see Figure 16.6, Table 16.2), all three models appear to fit the observed data (within the estimation period) well with the three-parameter and four-parameter logistic models providing very similar predictions over the 30-day period ahead.

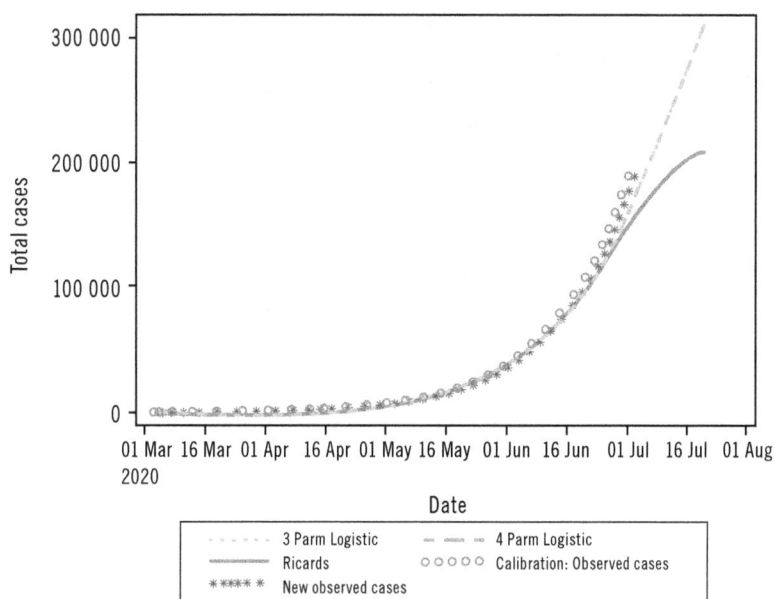

Figure 16.7 The predicted cumulative COVID-19 cases from the three-parameter logistic, four-parameters logistic and the Richards model and observed cases (Reddy et al, 2021)

A study among African countries that had availability of data, showed a significant correlation between State Party Self-Assessment Annual Reporting (SPAR) and Joint External Evaluation Indicators; as well as between Infectious Disease Vulnerability Index (IDVI) and the INFORM Epidemic Risk Index (Gilbert et al, 2020), when subjected to multivariate analysis. The study projected that Egypt, Algeria and South Africa had the highest importation risk from China, with moderate to high SPAR capacity scores (87, 76, and 62, respectively) (Gilbert et al, 2020). Additionally, different countries exhibited different functional capacity, for example 'South Africa had the maximum score for laboratory capacity (100), but a low score in risk communication (20). Conversely, Nigeria had a low score in the laboratory capacity (27) and the maximum score in the IHR Coordination capacity (100)' (Gilbert et al, 2020).

16.6.3 Diagnostics

National and International organisations such as WHO and the CDC have recommended the use of reverse transcriptase inhibitor Polymerase chain reaction (RT-PCR) as the gold standard for diagnosing COVID-19 (Lippi and Plebani, 2020; Amawi, H. et al. (2020)).

Table 16.6 The various diagnostic methods and the type of samples that is collected and tested (Lippi and Plebani, 2020; Amawi, H. et al. (2020))

SARS-CoV-2, SARS-CoV and MERS-CoV diagnose systematic assessment result.			
Viral strain	Test	Samples	References
SARS-CoV-2	rRT-PCR; E gene assay; confirmatory testing: RdRp gene assay	Respiratory samples from hospitalised patients	
SARS-CoV-2	COVID-19 IgG/IgM rapid test kit	Saliva swab samples	Commercial kit from myLAB Box
SARS-CoV-2	A colorimetric assay based on gold nanoparticles	Saliva swab	Oxford Suzhou Centre for Advanced Research (OSCAR)
SARS-CoV-2	A colorimetric assay based on gold nanoparticles coated with glycans	Saliva swab	Iceni Diagnostics
MERS-CoV	A collection of six separate, industrial, MERS CoV RNA detection kits focused on the PCR-RRT: (i) PowerChek (Kogene Biotech, Korea); (ii) DiaPlexQ (SolGent, Korea); (iii) Anyplex (Seegene), Korea) Screening: envelope gene (upE) Confirmation: ORF1a (iv) AccuPower (Bions, Korean) (v)	28 swabs alert for the other air viruses nasopharyngea	
MERS-CoV	Loopamp RNA Amplification Kit (RT-LAMP)	Laboratory isolates MERS-CoV swabs from healthy adults	
MERS-CoV	A one-step rRT-PCR assay, based on specific TaqMan	Synthesis of UpE and ORF1b	
SARS-CoV	Real-time qRT-PCR; ELISA technique	Samples obtained from 40-SARS hospitalised patients in Hong Kong	

➡

SARS-CoV-2, SARS-CoV and MERS-CoV diagnose systematic assessment result.			
Viral strain	**Test**	**Samples**	**References**
SARS-CoV	Enhanced RT-fluorescent PCR	Samples obtained from 80-SARS hospitalised patients in Hong Kong	
SARS-CoV	Quantitative, RT and, nested PCR	Samples obtained from 46-SARS hospitalised patients from Taiwan	
SARS-CoV	Western blot assay with N195 protein	274 clinical sera collected from patients with probable or suspected SARS, dengue fever, autoimmune diseases	
SARS-CoV	RT-PCR	274 clinical sera collected from Hong Kong	

16.6.4 Radiological findings

Sixty per cent of COVID-19 patients exhibited chest x-ray abnormalities, while 85% of patients had chest CT scan abnormalities (Clinical Management of COVID-19 disease Version 3, 2020). The observed pattern of these abnormalities that is classical for COVID-19 is the appearance of patchy ground-glass opacities (Clinical Management of COVID-19 disease, Version 3, 2020).

16.7 VACCINE INITIATIVES

Vaccines undoubtedly provide the most effective way to curb infectious diseases epidemics. In the current situation, we believe vaccines coupled with other public health interventions will ultimately lead to the resolution of the COVID-19 pandemic. In previous pandemics, it took years of research to develop, test and produce safe and effective vaccines for use at population level (Times, 2021). During this COVID-19 pandemic, scientists have adopted new approaches and technologies to develop effective vaccines in record time, and obtained authorisation for emergency use from relevant regulatory bodies (including WHO Emergency Use Listing) (Kochhar and Salmon, 2020; Times, 2021). By 27 February 2021, a total of 71 vaccines were undergoing clinical trials and at least 78 more were in the preclinical trials phase (Times, 2021). The number of vaccines at various stages included: 40 undergoing vaccine safety and dosage testing (Phase 1), 27 in expanded safety trials (Phase 2), 20 in large scale efficacy tests (Phase 3), six in early or limited use (Authorised), six approved for full use (Approved) and four abandoned after trials (Times, 2021).

As of June 2021, three vaccine trials have been carried out in South Africa. The first trial by the name Ox1Cov-19 Vaccine VIDA trial begun in June 2020 and was a collaboration between Oxford University, the University of the Witwatersrand and the Jenner Institute (Makoni, 2020). The second trial of a COVID-19 vaccine was by Novavax which was also a collaboration with the University of the Witwatersrand (Makoni, 2020). The enrolment began in August and included both HIV-positive and negative adults. The third vaccine trial for Ad26.COV2-S was a Johnson & Johnson product that had been conducted in two phases. Phase 3A, which was the ensemble trial was designed to evaluate safety and efficacy of a single vaccine dose versus a placebo (Makoni, 2020). The second phase (3B) was a collaboration with the South African National Department of Health and the South African Medical Research Council (SAMRC). It was conducted among health workers (Sisonke (Together) study, 2021). The aim of the study was to monitor the efficacy of the vaccine in preventing severe COVID-19 hospital admissions and deaths among healthcare workers as compared to the general unvaccinated population (Sisonke (Together) study, 2021).

16.8 CHALLENGES

Lack of information on the COVID-19 healthcare delivery, particularly for fatally-ill patients admitted to the ICUs in Africa, has been a major problem (Paintsil and Paintsil, 2020). Shortages of the SAR-CoV-2 testing kit, bed space, and intensive care units have also been reported across Africa (Paintsil and Paintsil, 2020). In the United States, there are about 336 ICU beds per million populations compared to 75 and 1 ICU bed per million populations in South Africa and Uganda, respectively. Unfortunately, most nations in sub-Saharan Africa have less than 20 ICU beds for their whole population (Paintsil and Paintsil, 2020). The ability of the coronavirus to mutate into different strains poses a challenge to the development of vaccines. Furthermore, the availability of testing kits, the infrastructure to carry out clinical trials and to manufacture therapeutic drugs which can combat COVID-19 are limited (Margolin et al, 2020).

16.9 CONCLUSION

There is a need for the African continent to learn from the COVID-19 pandemic experience in order to establish sustainable preventive measures, especially with respect to infrastructure. Some other measures include the need to organise campaigns which promote infection prevention and control practices within healthcare facilities; and the need for active surveillance activities. There is a need for more rigorous research and development, especially with substantial funding support from the government and collaborations with global institutions for defining a research plan. For instance, in settings where PCR-based testing is not available for mild illnesses, viral antigens for serological testing can be cheaply produced (Margolin et al, 2020). This ought to be done without undermining the effectiveness of partnering with inter- and intra-continental universities to build capacity in readiness for future pandemics (Paintsil and Paintsil, 2020).

16.10 SELF-ASSESSMENT QUESTIONS

1. How has the COVID-19 pandemic been handled in sub-Saharan Africa?
2. What is the way forward for COVID-19 management in sub-Saharan Africa?

16.11 REFERENCES

Amawi, H., I Abu Deiab, G., Aljabali, A.A.A., Dua, K. and Tambuwala, M.M.2020. COVID-19 pandemic: An overview of epidemiology, pathogenesis, diagnostics and potential vaccines and therapeutics. *Therapeutic Delivery* 11(4), pp. 245–268. doi: 10.4155/tde-2020-0035.

Bertrand, S., Carr, Z., Chungong, S., Cox, P., Curtin, T., Fuchs, F., Gudtschmidt, K., Hollmeyer, H., Xing, J., Kandel, N., Kawano, M., Lee, V., Mills, R., Sreedharan, R., Tshioko, F., Jabbour, J. and Hoffman, T. 2015. WHO International Health Regulations (2005) Core Capacity Workbook, A series of exercises to assist the validation of core capacity implementation levels.

Blumberg, L., Jassat, W., Mendelson, M. and Cohen, C. 2020. The COVID-19 crisis in South Africa: Protecting the vulnerable. *South African Medical Journal* 110(9), pp. 825–826. doi: 10.7196/SAMJ.2020.v110i9.15116.

Anders, D., Bamford, L., Boyles, T., Blumberg, L., Cohen, C., Gray, A., Mazanderani, A.H., Kufa-Chakeza, T., Dawood, H., Mabena, F., Mehtar, S., Mayet, N., Mendelson, M., Nel, J., Preiser, W. and Taljaard, J. 2020. Clinical Management of COVID-19 disease, Version 3. Available at:https://sahivsoc.org/Files/Clinical%20Management%20of%20COVID-19%20disease_Version%203_27March2020.pdf.

Edridge, A.W.D., Kaczorowska, J., Hoste, A.C.R., Bakker, M., Klein, M., Jebbink, M.F., Master, A., Kinsella, C.M., Rueda, P., Prins, M., Sastre, P., Deijs, M. and Van der Hoek, L. 2020. Human coronavirus reinfection dynamics: lessons for SARS-CoV-2. *Medrxiv*, pp. 1–10.

Fontanet, A., Autran, B., Lina, B., Kieny, M.P., Karin, S.S.A. and Sridhar, D. 2021. SARS-CoV-2 variants and ending the COVID-19 pandemic. *The Lance*, 397(10278), pp. 952–954. doi: 10.1016/S0140-6736(21)00370-6.

Garg, P., Arora, U., Kumar, A. and Wig, N. 2021. The "post-COVID" syndrome: How deep is the damage? *Journal of Medical Virology* 93(2), pp. 673–674. doi: 10.1002/jmv.26465.

Giandhari, J., Pillay, S., Wilkinson, E., Tegally, H., Sinayskiy, I., Schuld, M., Lourenco, J., Chimukangara, B., Lesselss, R., Moosa, Y., Gazy, I., Fish, M., Singh, L., Khanyile, K.S., Fonseca, V., Giovanetti, M., Alcantara, L.C., Petruccione, F. and De Oliveira, T. 2020. Early transmission of SARS-CoV-2 in South Africa: An epidemiological and phylogenetic report. *medRxiv*. doi: 10.1101/2020.05.29.20116376.

Gilbert, M., Pullano, G., Pinotti, F., Valdano, E., Poletto, C., Boëlle, P.Y., D'Ortenzio, E., Yazdanpanah, Y., Eholie, S.P., Altmann, M., Gutierrex, B., Kraemer, M.U.G. and Colizza, V. 2020. Preparedness and vulnerability of African countries against importations of COVID-19 : a modelling study. *Lancet* 395(10227), pp. 871–877. doi: 10.1016/S0140-6736(20)30411-6.

Girdler-Brown, B.V. and Murray, J. 2020. Epidemic reproduction numbers and herd immunity. *Southern African Journal of Public Health (incorporating Strengthening Health Systems)* 4(2), p. 59. doi: 10.7196/shs.2020.v4i2.121.

Hatami, N., Ahi, S., Sadeghinikoo, A., Foroughian, M., Javdani, F., Kalani, N., Fereydoni, M., Keshavarz, P. and Hosseini, A. 2020. Worldwide ACE (I/D) polymorphism may affect COVID-19 recovery rate: an ecological meta-regression. *Endocrine* 68(3), pp. 479–484. doi: 10.1007/s12020-020-02381-7.

Jassat, W., Cohen, C., Kufa, T., Goldstein, S., Masha, M. and Cowper, B., Slade, D., Greyling, C., Soorju, S., Kai, R., Walaza, S., Blumberg, L. 2020. Datacov: a sentinel surveillance programme for hospitalised individuals with Covid-19 in South Africa. *Covid-19 Special Public Health Surveillance* 18(1), pp. 1–15.

Kochhar, S. and Salmon, D.A. 2020. Planning for COVID-19 vaccines safety surveillance. *Vaccine* 38(40), pp. 6194–6198. doi: 10.1016/j.vaccine.2020.07.013.

Lippi, G. and Plebani, M. 2020. The critical role of laboratory medicine during coronavirus disease 2019 (COVID-19) and other viral outbreaks. *Clin Chem Lab Med* 58(7), pp. 1063–1069.

Lone, S.A. and Ahmad, A. 2020. COVID-19 pandemic–an African perspective. *Emerging Microbes and Infections* 9(1), pp. 1300–1308. doi: 10.1080/22221751.2020.1775132.

Makoni, M. 2020. COVID-19 vaccine trials in Africa. *The Lancet. Respiratory medicine* 8(11), pp. e79–e80. doi: 10.1016/S2213-2600(20)30401-X.

Margolin, E., Burgers, W.A., Sturrock, E.D., Mendelson, M., Chapman, R., Douglass, N., Williamson, A.L. and Rybicki, E.P. 2020. Prospects for SARS-CoV-2 diagnostics, therapeutics and vaccines in Africa, *Nature Reviews Microbiology* 18, pp. 690–704. doi: 10.1038/s41579-020-00441-3.

National Institute For Communicable Diseases. 2020. The initial and daily covid-19 effective reproduction number (R) in South Africa, 10 June, pp. 1–9.

National Institute For Communicable Diseases (NICD) week 6 (2021). Covid-19 Sentinel Hospital Surveillance Update. Available at: www.nicd.ac.za.

NICD. 2021. COVID-19 special public health surveillance bulletin pandemic in three districts of South Africa – preliminary 18(9), pp. 1–11.

Paintsil, E. and Paintsil, E. 2020. COVID-19 threatens health systems in sub-Saharan Africa: the eye of the crocodile. *J Clin Invest* 130(6), pp. 2741–2744.

Pressure, P. and Wilfond, B.S. 2020. The South African response to the pandemic. *The New England Journal of Medicine* 36(1), pp. 1–3.

Randall, L.M. 2020. NICD objectives. *Am J Obstet Gynecol* 73(3), pp. 465–472. doi: 10.1016/s0002-9378(16)37422-1.

Reddy, T., Shkedy, Z., Janse van Rensburg, C., Mwambi, H., Debba, P., Zuma, K. and Manda, S. 2021. Short-term real-time prediction of total number of reported COVID-19 cases and deaths in South Africa: a data-driven approach. *BMC Medical Research Methodology* 21(1), pp. 1–11. doi: 10.1186/s12874-020-01165-x.

Richardson, A. 2020. Reinfection with SARS-CoV-2: implications for vaccines. Available at: https://www.ncbi.nlm.nih.gov/pmc/articles/PMC7799323/pdf/ciaa1 866.pdf. doi: 10.1093/cid/ciaa1866.

Serhani, M. and Labbardi, H. 2020. Mathematical modeling of COVID-19 spreading with asymptomatic infected and interacting peoples. *Journal of Applied Mathematics and Computing* 66, pp. 1–20. doi: 10.1007/s12190-020-01421-9.

Silal, S., Hounsell, R., Norman, J., Pulliam, J., Beauclair, R., Bingham, J., Dushoff, J., Kassanjee, R., Li, M., Van Schalkwyk, C., Welte, A., Jamieson, L., Nichols, B. and Meyer-Rath, G. 2020. Estimating cases for COVID-19 in South Africa – Long-term national projections Report Update: 6 May 2020. Health Economics and Epidemiology Research Office. University of Witwatersrand.

Sigfrid, L., Cevik, M., Jesudason, E., Lim, W.S, Rello, J., Amuasi, J. H., Bozza, F., Palmieri, C., Munblit, D., Holter, J.C., Kildal, A.B., Russell, C.D., Ho, A., Turtle, L., Drake, T.M., Beltrame, A., Hann, K., Bangura, I.R., Fowler, R., Lakoh, S., Berry, C., Lowe, D.J., McPeake, J., Hashmi, M., Dyrhol-Riise, A.M., Donohue, C., Plotkin, D.R., Hardwick, H., Elkheir, N., Lone, N., Docherty, A.B., Harrison, E.M., Baille, K.J., Carson, G., Semple, M.G. and Scott, J.T. 2020. What is the recovery rate and risk of long-term consequences following a diagnosis of COVID-19? A harmonised, global longitudinal observational study. *medRxiv*. doi: 10.1101/2020.08.26.20180950.

Sisonke (Together) study. 2021. Available at: https://www.samrc.ac.za/news/sisonke-together-study-open-label-pragmatic-real-world-phase-3b-clinical-trial-investigational.

South Africa National Department of Health. 2020. National Guidelines on Contact Tracing for Covid-19.

Surveillance, D. and Systems, R. 2001. WHO protocol for the assessment of National Communicable Disease Surveillance and response systems. *International Organization* 16(1), pp. 237–241. doi: 10.1017/S0020818300010912.

Thiede, R., Abdelatif, N., Fabris-Rotelli, I., Manjoo-Docrat, R., Holloway, J., Janse van Rensburg, C., Debba, P., Dudeni, N., Kimmie, Z. and Le Roux, A. 2020. Spatial variation in the basic reproduction number of COVID-19: A systematic review, (November), pp. 1–12.

Times, T.N.Y. 2021. Coronavirus Vaccine Tracker. doi: 10.11164/jjsps.37.2_338_2.

WHO. 2006. Module 8: making disease surveillance work. Available at: https://www.who.int/publications/i/item/module-8-making-disease-surveillance-work.

WHO. No date. International Health Regulations, pp. 1–2. Available at: http://www.emro.who.int/international-health-regulations/about/ihr-core-capacities.html.

World Health Organization. 2004. Making disease surveillance work. Available at: https://www.who.int/publications/i/item/module-7-making-disease-surveillance-work.

Zhu, J., Zhang, Q., Jia, C., Wang, W., Chen, J., Xia, Y., Wang, W., Wang, X., Wen, M., Wang, H., Zhang, Z., Xu, S., Zhao, J. and Jiang, T. 2020. Epidemiological characteristics and clinical outcomes of coronavirus disease patients in northwest china: high-volume research from low population density regions. *Frontiers in Medicine* 7, pp. 1–9. doi: 10.3389/fmed.2020.564250.

COVID-19 IN SOUTH AFRICA: LESSONS FROM IMPLEMENTING A NEW NATIONAL HOSPITAL SURVEILLANCE PLATFORM

Waasila Jassat

Cheryl Cohen

Maureen Masha

Warren Parker

Lucille Blumberg

17.1 INTRODUCTION

At the start of the COVID-19 pandemic, South Africa, like many low- and middle-income countries, lacked a real-time national health information system to monitor COVID-19 hospitalisations. Assessing morbidity, mortality and risk factors for severe illness of emerging pathogens is essential and monitoring trends in hospitalisation provides a robust indicator of pandemic progression (Garcia-Basteiro et al, 2020). In March 2020, South Africa reported its first COVID-19 case and intensified its national response (NICD, 2020a; South Africa Government, 2020). This prompted the vision for the DATCOV hospital surveillance system at an early stage of the pandemic.

17.2 OBJECTIVES

The objectives of the chapter are:

- To describe the DATCOV hospital surveillance system for COVID-19 with regard to assessing morbidity, mortality and risk factors for severe illness for COVID-19.
- To discuss the robustness of the DATCOV hospital surveillance system as an indicator of pandemic progression.
- To explore the value of data derived from the DATCOV hospital surveillance system.
- To set out some of the lessons learnt to inform the development of pandemic tracking systems in low- and middle-income settings.

17.3 THE CONTEXT

South Africa has a publicly funded district health system which serves around 84% of the population, with a complementary private health system largely funded by health insurance schemes (Naidoo, 2012). Monitoring of national hospital-based morbidity and mortality requires data from both systems.

Like a number of low- and middle-income countries (LMIC), South Africa has not adopted a unique patient identifier approach and currently has no national health information system or electronic health record system that provides national-level data. The public health system, in particular, has limitations regarding information technology resources and human resources for data collection (Katurura et al, 2018; Akanbi et al, 2014). Following the advent of the COVID-19 pandemic, it was noted that the District Health Information System (DHIS) used by the National Department of Health (NDoH), provided only aggregate reporting of caseloads from public sector clinics and hospitals and did not allow for the collection of patient-level data on COVID-19 hospital admissions.

COVID-19 data was available through laboratory-based surveillance conducted by the National Institute for Communicable Diseases (NICD), with reports on testing and laboratory-confirmed cases at a national level. South Africa's Notifiable Medical Conditions (NMC) system requires the submission of data on all notifiable conditions, including emerging pathogens like COVID-19. Yet, it only caters for static submission of data on the day of notification without any longitudinal information on the course and outcome of the hospitalisation.

With the advent of COVID-19 cases in South Africa in March 2020, it was clear that existing surveillance systems could not be rapidly up-scaled to monitor hospitalised COVID-19 cases. Therefore, the NICD leveraged its mandate for public health surveillance and the legal requirement for all healthcare workers to report NMCs (NICD, 2020b), to engage hospitals across all provinces to report COVID-19 hospitalisations through a common system.

17.4 THE DATCOV HOSPITAL SURVEILLANCE SYSTEM

The NICD adapted and digitised the World Health Organization (WHO) COVID-19 case report forms (WHO, 2020) onto an online web-based platform accessible via mobile phone, tablet or computer. The tool included reporting on demographic data, comorbid disease, complications, treatment and outcomes of the hospital admission.

Named DATCOV, the NICD's surveillance system allowed public- and private-sector hospitals to submit data on hospitalisations for all patients diagnosed with COVID-19 (Jassat et al, 2020). The emerging data were available in real-time and informed overall caseloads and epidemiological trends to inform tracking of the disease and guide strategies including prevention, treatment and resource allocation.

DATCOV caters for longitudinal data entry at multiple time points, including at admission, daily during the hospital stay, and at outcome (discharge, transfer or death). DATCOV comprehensively tracks a patient journey by allowing for multiple admissions to be recorded for one patient, as well as mortality and outcomes occurring after discharge from hospital.

The initial DATCOV design used direct data entry on the online platform. When it was discovered that private hospital groups and the Western Cape provincial government had data already available in electronic format in existing information systems, the platform was modified to accommodate data transfer into the DATCOV database to circumvent the need to duplicate data entry processes.

The DATCOV platform was set up to allow all hospitals and provincial and national Departments of Health, access to their patients' line-lists and summary reports. Daily patient line-lists and summary reports were shared by email with the provinces and the NDoH. The data was then imported into the national data lake to feed into national COVID-19 monitoring dashboards. NICD also created various Application Programming Interfaces (APIs) to allow direct access to the database.

17.4.1 Implementation

The translation of the DATCOV system from concept to implementation was achieved in a single week and went online in late March 2020 (Jassat et al, 2020). It was piloted in eight designated COVID-19 public hospitals in early April 2020. Within the next month, private sector hospital groups and three of the country's nine provinces were implementing the system. By 15 July 2020, the National Health Council decided that DATCOV would be implemented in all public hospitals. A project team from the NDoH and NICD engaged provinces, and by early October 2020, all public and private hospitals in the country reported on DATCOV (Figure 17.1). As new hospitals enrolled, historic admissions were also captured, thus ensuring comprehensive data on hospitalisation trends. Although information technology and human resources in hospitals are uneven nationally, and internet connectivity is intermittent in some settings, even rural hospitals were able to submit data regularly. Internet data transfer rates were reduced through a revision of the system design.

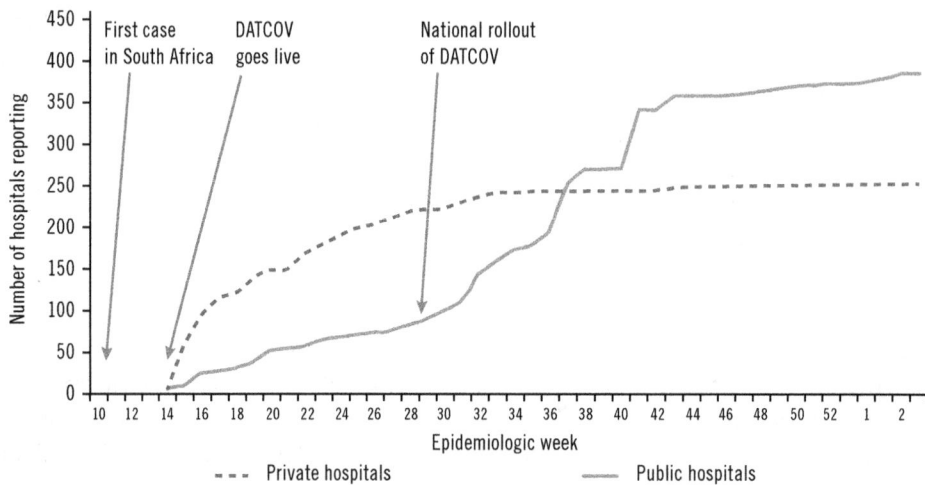

Figure 17.1 Timeline of public and private hospitals reporting to DATCOV,
5 March 2020–30 January 2021, South Africa

While there was strong commitment and uptake of the DATCOV system, it remained necessary to implement quality control measures. For DATCOV, a 15-person team was established with skills including epidemiology, public health, surveillance, data analysis and data management. Data imports contained validation checks to identify data errors and the team ran routine checks for completeness and outlying data to address missing and incorrect data.

As the COVID-19 pandemic progressed, the DATCOV system was expanded to include modules for (a) deaths occurring out of hospital, (b) surveillance in long-term residential facilities, (c) a paediatric clinical registry, and (d) follow-up for long-term symptoms and complications of COVID-19 ('Long COVID').

17.4.2 The Value of DATCOV Data

The DATCOV data has been widely used by provincial and national Departments of Health, COVID-19 Ministerial Advisory Committees and COVID-19 'war-rooms', research organisations and the media, among others, for monitoring of trends and to inform strategies and policies.

By early February 2021, 230 000 admissions had been recorded on DATCOV and the following benefits were noted:

1. DATCOV provides real-time data on COVID-19 hospitalisation nationally. It informs understanding of epidemiological trends, allows for reproductive rate modelling, informs patient-level risk factors for mortality, and improves understanding of most and least affected areas.

2. Through the DATCOV system, it is possible to monitor the progression of the pandemic in the different provinces of South Africa. This capacity served as a rapid alert for the second wave COVID-19 resurgence in November 2020, and also described health service utilisation, including general and critical care bed capacity and the need for essential supplies, including oxygen and ventilators.

3. DATCOV provided insight into hospitals with high case fatality rates, allowing for further investigation into the reasons for poor outcomes, and prioritisation of remedial actions, including additional resources, training and support.

4. The new variant, Beta (501Y.V2), predominated (Tegally et al, 2020) during the second wave of COVID-19, which peaked in January 2021. It was possible to demonstrate that there was an increase in in-hospital mortality during the second wave (Jassat et al, 2021a). Reports were available for 502 patients with readmissions more than three months after the first infection, allowing for an investigation into whether these individuals had repeat infections and thereby informing understanding of long-term immunity.

5. DATCOV data yielded valuable information for understanding the risk factors associated with COVID-19 mortality and provided relevant data on the role of comorbidities, including non-communicable diseases and co-infections with HIV and tuberculosis (Jassat et al, 2021b). This information informed COVID-19 prevention strategies for vulnerable groups, including vaccine prioritisation, and prioritised clinical guidance for hospital cases.

6. DATCOV allowed for the analysis of admissions in specific sub-populations, including healthcare workers (NIOH, 2021), paediatric (Kufa et al, 2021) and obstetric (Masha et al, 2021) populations. The data also informed guidelines for population-wide measures, including risk stratification for workplaces and considerations for reopening schools.

7. DATCOV surveillance of vulnerable populations in 43 long-term care facilities yielded important insights into the dynamics of transmission and the burden of COVID-19 mortality within these settings (Arendse et al, 2021).

8. Through DATCOV, it has been possible to follow up a cohort of COVID-19 patients post-discharge and describe 'Long COVID' sequelae (Dryden et al, 2021).

17.4.3 Lessons Learned

DATCOV was conceptualised at the start of the pandemic and, within six months, had obtained government endorsement and achieved complete coverage throughout South Africa's public and private hospital system. The lessons from implementing this surveillance system inform the development of pandemic tracking systems in low- and middle-income settings.

1. Rapid response during the early part of an evolving pandemic

The South African response to COVID-19 required rapid and decisive action towards an innovative, creative, flexible, secure and user-friendly hospital surveillance system with real-time data availability to monitor the pandemic and guide interventions. No system existed at the time. The DATCOV system was specially created and moved from vision to preliminary design over a one-week period, and from a sentinel hospital surveillance system covering eight public sector hospitals to a national system for reporting in all public and private hospitals over six months.

2. Leverage technology and ensure data integrity

DATCOV digitised the WHO case report tool to create an online platform for data capture, allowing multiple users in a hospital to capture data. The web platform, which used existing infrastructure that was customised for DATCOV, was key for rapid delivery. A native application was later published, which allowed for data capture directly to the application. This required significantly less connectivity bandwidth and accommodated settings where internet connectivity was less advanced.

The advantages of the platform were that it allowed for (a) data to be submitted by both direct entry or bulk data import, (b) sites to have ownership of their data and easily accessible reports, and (c) easy expansion to include new modules.

While data are shared daily, data protection measures are in place. All patient personal information, health status and treatment, are kept confidential. All data stored in DATCOV are only shared with individuals involved in surveillance with password encryption. A team remains in place to monitor and ensure data quality.

3. Platform and tool: Keeping it simple and appropriate

While the international tools included clinical parameters and diagnostic investigations that could be useful for research studies, DATCOV focused purely on surveillance to guide hospital and public health actions, strategies and policies. DATCOV is designed to capture the minimum required information to allow for the simplest and shortest data entry time. Most fields were tick boxes and dropdowns to allow for little free text. This reduced administrative workload for clinicians in general, with data input remaining feasible during periods of peak hospitalisation.

4. Being responsive, adaptive, flexible and agile

When it was found that some groups had data in existing information systems, DATCOV was modified to accommodate imports into the database, to avoid duplication of data input on two different systems.

DATCOV included the development of additional modules as the need arose, for example, expanding the hospital platform to allow long-term care facilities to report, creating a paediatric registry for COVID-19, follow-up of patients after discharge to determine ongoing symptoms or complications, and capturing 'out of hospital' mortality.

DATCOV was flexible in accommodating additional data fields when they were required. For example, new complications such as Multisystem Inflammatory Syndrome in Children (MIS-C) were added, and data on vaccination were added when the vaccine rollout began.

5. Getting buy-in: Providing data for action

At a local level, convincing busy healthcare workers and data staff to submit data on a daily basis requires simplified systems with a clear rationale. Data input requirements were brief, and summary statistics and downloadable line-list data were available on the platform to inform hospital-level statistics and reporting. This supported stakeholder 'buy-in'.

At a provincial and national level, consistently receiving daily line-lists that were trustworthy was key. The provincial government took ownership of the system because of the quality and timeliness of the data, as well as the capacity to generate reports that they could use for planning. At a national level, the data were useful as they provided real-time analysis and reports.

In the early months of the pandemic, when risk factors for mortality were only available from high-income countries, DATCOV addressed a knowledge gap, providing evidence of risks for mortality of locally prevalent conditions such as HIV and tuberculosis. DATCOV also provided valuable data to monitor hospital admission trends in the country, allowing for hospital resource planning.

DATCOV reports were shared widely with provincial and national stakeholders and also with the public through the NICD website. Media, research organisations, academic institutions, non-governmental and civil society organisations access and utilise the reports on a daily basis. The DATCOV team have also used the data to develop and published papers in peer-reviewed journals.

6. Partnership, collaboration and the role of champions

The NICD has collaborated with many stakeholders in the development and rollout of DATCOV. This includes the national and provincial Departments of Health and Social Development, who are key partners in implementation. The private sector hospital groups saw the value of data harmonisation and shared data with DATCOV.

The NICD collaborated with local research organisations such as the South African Medical Research Council (MRC), the National Institute for Occupational Health (NIOH) and the South African Centre for Epidemiological Modelling and Analysis (SACEMA) to conduct focused analyses of the data. There were also collaborations with international organisations such as the WHO and the International Severe Acute Respiratory and emerging Infections Consortium (ISARIC) through pooled analysis of hospitalisation data and participation in a global 'Long COVID' study. A grant was also obtained from the Bill and Melinda Gates Foundation to use DATCOV to conduct enhanced surveillance for non-communicable diseases, HIV and tuberculosis.

The presence of champions was important for facilitating DATCOV implementation. The NDoH and NICD provided oversight and support through a project team that met bi-weekly to review progress and put strategies in place to support the provinces that were behind. There were direct measures including online meetings with those provinces, data capturers were appointed to support the provinces, and there was formal intervention from the Departmental Director General where required. The provincial COVID-19 'war rooms' were particularly strong partners for motivating and mobilising the DATCOV rollout and the high level of provincial ownership contributed to swift implementation. The success of DATCOV is also attributable to willing clinicians and data capturers, who ensured daily submission of data. Non-governmental organisations bridged resource gaps by providing data capturers at hospitals in contexts where human resources were stretched. The ongoing vigilance of the DATCOV team ensured data quality and sustainability of a reliable national COVID-19 surveillance system.

17.5 CONCLUSION

The efforts during the early and ongoing COVID-19 pandemic served to strengthen routine data systems and provided a simple and feasible complementary hospital-based monitoring system. As South Africa reflects on the COVID-19 pandemic response and looks beyond COVID-19, lessons learned will inform routine surveillance systems for NMCs, and rapid responses to new pathogens.

DATCOV has demonstrated the value of hospital-based surveillance and informs understanding of technology-driven approaches that are clear in purpose, simple to administer and adaptive in the context of changing pandemic circumstances. DATCOV offers lessons for the monitoring of future pandemics that are replicable in hospitals with diverse resources in low- and middle-income settings.

Lessons learned in conducting hospital surveillance for COVID-19

1. Context matters. In LMICs, a simple system with a good fit for technological and human resources can be designed and implemented in the short timeframe necessitated by a rapidly advancing pandemic such as COVID-19.

2. Ownership and buy-in for a new surveillance system are key and are best achieved by ensuring the system provides real-time data to inform actions, strategies and policies with minimal complexity.

3. Implementation relied on stakeholders in provinces who steered rollout and individuals in health facilities who understood the value of reliable timeous data and were willing to participate.

4. Data quality was ensured through a centralised team with diverse skills.

5. Vital and reliable data informed understanding of the progression of the pandemic and provided critical insights into morbidity, mortality, comorbidities, virus variants and at-risk sub-populations.

17.6 SELF-ASSESSMENT QUESTIONS

1. List the key technical requirements for a successful hospital surveillance system to monitor the COVID-19 pandemic in South Africa.

2. Describe some key outcomes of the DATCOV hospital surveillance system during the COVID-19 pandemic in South Africa.

17.7 REFERENCES

Akanbi, M.O., Ocheke, A.N., Agaba, P.A., Daniyam, C.A., Agaba, E.I., Okeke, E.N. and Ukoli, C.O. 2012. Use of electronic health records in sub-Saharan Africa: Progress and challenges. *J Med Trop* 14(1), pp. 1–6. PMID: 25243111; PMCID: PMC4167769. Available at: https://pubmed.ncbi.nlm.nih.gov/25243111/.

Arendse T., Cowper B., Cohen C., et al. SARS-CoV-2 cases reported from long term care facilities (care homes) in South Africa. *COVID-19 Special Public Health Surveillance Bulletin.* July 13, 2021. Available at: https://www.nicd.ac.za/wp-content/uploads/2021/07/COVID-19-Special-Public-Health-Surveillance-Bulletin-July-11th-edition2021-1.pdf.

Dryden M., Mudara C., Vika C., et al. Long COVID in South Africa: Findings from a longitudinal cohort of patients at one month after hospitalisation with SARS-CoV-2, using an ISARIC multi-country protocol. *COVID-19 Special Public Health Surveillance Bulletin.* August 4, 2021. Available at: https://www.nicd.ac.za/wp-content/uploads/2021/08/COVID-19-Special-Public-Health-Surveillance-Bulletin-August-2nd-edition-2021.pdf.

García-Basteiro, A.L., Chaccour, C., Guinovart, C., Llupià, A., Brew J., Trilla, A. and Plasencia, A. 2020. Monitoring the COVID-19 epidemic in the context of widespread local transmission. *Lancet Respir Med* 8(5), pp. 2019–21. doi: https://doi.org/10.1016/S2213-200(20)30162-4.

Jassat W., Cohen C., Tempia C., et al. 2021b. Risk factors for COVID-19-related in-hospital mortality in a high HIV and tuberculosis prevalence setting in South Africa: a cohort study. *The Lancet HIV,* 2021 (8): pp. e554-e567. Available at: https://doi.org/10.1016/S2352-3018(21)00151-X.

Jassat, W., Cohen, C., Tendesayi, K., Kufa, T., Goldstein, S., Masha, M., Cowper, B., Slade, D., Greyling, C., Soorju, S., Kai, R., Walaza, S. and Blumberg, L. 2020. COVID-19 special public health surveillance bulletin. NICD 18(1), pp. 1–15. Available at: https://www.nicd.ac.za/wp-content/uploads/2020/06/COVID-19-Special-Public-Health-Surveillance-Bulletin-10-June-2020-005.pdf.

Jassat W., Mudara C., Ozougwu L., et al. 2021a. Difference in mortality among individuals admitted to hospital with COVID-19 during the first and second waves in South Africa: a cohort study. *The Lancet Global Health,* 2021 (9): pp. e1216-e1225. https://doi.org/10.1016/S2214-109X(21)00289-8.

Katurura, M.C., Cilliers, L., Africa, S., Cilliers, L. and Cilliers, L. 2018. Electronic health record system in the public health care sector of South Africa: A systematic literature review. *African Journal of Primary Health Care & Family Medicine* 10(1), pp. 1–8.

Kufa T., Jassat W., Cohen C., et al. Epidemiology of SARS-CoV-2 infection and SARS-CoV-2 positive hospital admissions among children in South Africa. *Authorea.* September 25, 2021. DOI: 10.22541/au.163255389.97597700/v1).

Masha M., Arendse T., Cohen C., et al. Clinical characteristics, outcomes and epidemiology of pregnant women hospitalised with COVID-19 in South Africa. *COVID-19 Special Public Health Surveillance Bulletin.* March 5, 2021. https://www.nicd.ac.za/wp-content/uploads/2021/07/COVID-19-Special-Public-Health-Surveillance-Bulletin-5-March-2021.pdf.

Naidoo, S. 2012. The South African national health insurance: A revolution in health-care delivery! *J Public Health* 34(1), pp. 149–50.

NICD. 2020a. First case of COVID-19 coronavirus reported in SA. Available at: https://www.nicd.ac.za/first-case-of-covid-19-coronavirus-reported-in-sa/.

NICD. 2020b. Notifiable Medical Conditions. Available at: https://www.nicd.ac.za/nmc-overview/.

NIOH. COVID-19 Hospital Surveillance-Weekly Update on Hospitalized HCWs. https://www.nioh.ac.za/covid-19-occupational-health-surveillance/.

South Africa Government 2020. Disaster Management Act. Available at: <https://www.gov.za/documents/disaster-management-act-declaration-national-state-disaster-covid-19-coronavirus-16-ma>.

Tegally, H., Wilkinson, E., Giovanetti, M., Iranzadeh, A., Fonseca, V., Giandhari, J., et al. 2020. Emergence and rapid spread of a new severe acute respiratory syndrome-related coronavirus 2 (SARS-CoV-2) lineage with multiple spike mutations in South Africa. *medRxiv* 22 Dec. Available at: https://www.medrxiv.org/content/10.1101/2020.12.21.20248640v1.

WHO. 2020. Global COVID-19 Clinical Platform Rapid core case report form (CRF). Available from: https://www.who.int/publications/i/item/WHO-2019-nCoV-Clinical_CRF-2020.4.

CHAPTER 18

MENTAL HEALTH, PSYCHIATRIC DISEASE, AND COVID-19 IN URBAN SOUTH AFRICA

Andrew Wooyoung Kim

Ugasvaree Subramaney

Indhrin Chetty

Shren Chetty

Preethi Jayrajh

Mallorie Govender

Pralene Maharaj

Eddie Eung Sok Pak

18.1 INTRODUCTION

The 2019 coronavirus (COVID-19) pandemic brought unprecedented challenges to the health sector nationwide and internationally. Current discussions in the medical literature on COVID-19 report a wide range of evolving psychiatric presentations resulting from acute infection as well as the unprecedented and widespread societal changes brought by quarantine and other social policies. This chapter discusses the impact of the COVID-19 pandemic on psychiatric morbidity, public mental health, and mental healthcare systems in South Africa. We also provide a case study from an anthropological and epidemiological study of adults living in Soweto during the first six weeks of the South Africa lockdown. Potential solutions for improving mental healthcare, including the use of telemedicine and the need for curriculum change in public mental health for medical students, are also discussed. A greater understanding of the various psychiatric conditions attributed to COVID-19 infection may allow for earlier screening, more effective treatment, greater positive health outcomes, and better prepared health systems to address future pandemics in South Africa.

Societies across the world have exhibited widespread elevations in psychiatric morbidity, increased risk for mental distress and illness, and novel psychopathological presentations among individuals affected by the 2019 coronavirus disease pandemic (COVID-19) (Rogers et al, 2020; Subramaney et al, 2020). The unprecedented societal shifts brought by the pandemic and the subsequent social policies aimed at mitigating the spread of COVID-19, including the countrywide lockdown, are understood to have both short- and long-term impacts on individual psychological risk, mental healthcare systems, and public mental health (Brooks et al, 2020; Sommer and Bakker, 2020).

The South African government responded swiftly yet assertively to COVID-19 by enforcing strict national measures early in the course of the pandemic to prevent its spread. While the country received international praise for its rapid response, others criticized South Africa for its harsh implementation and forceful government sanctions against non-adherent communities, which included militarisation, demolitions of informal settlements, and even cases of reported police brutality. These measures exist against a stark backdrop of existing inequalities in common mental disorders, which likely may be amplified by the new societal realities brought by the COVID-19 pandemic.

Numerous aspects of life under lockdown, including limited physical mobility, emotional distress, and for some, extreme threats to survival, are known risk factors for mental distress and illness (Brooks et al, 2020). Worldwide, studies on the mental health consequences of quarantine and forced confinement have reported increased individual risk for various psychopathologies, including depression, anxiety, post-traumatic stress disorder, and suicide (Rogers et al, 2020). For millions of South Africans, vulnerability to COVID-19 is amplified by other pre-existing conditions, such as a high prevalence of chronic and infectious disease, alarming rates of poverty (55.5%) and unemployment (29%), and an overburdened healthcare system (Docrat et al, 2019; StatsSA 2019a,b).

Research findings from recent coronavirus pandemics (e.g. SARS, MERS) show that worse mental health status before quarantine is a major risk factor for increased psychiatric morbidity after quarantine (Brooks et al, 2020; Rogers et al, 2020). The latest nationally representative estimates show that the prevalence, incidence, and burden of mental illness in South Africa are relatively high: one in three (30.3%) South Africans will be diagnosed with a mental illness, a quarter of all cases (25%) are considered severe, and nearly half of citizens (47.5%) are at risk of developing a psychiatric disorder in their lifetime (Herman et al, 2009). In spite of these conditions, mental healthcare access and usage is severely limited: only 27% of patients with severe mental illnesses receive treatment, 16% of citizens are enrolled in medical aid, and there are only 0.31 psychiatrists per 100,000 uninsured population (Docrat et al, 2019). These severe barriers to care, high rates of mental illness, and the ongoing pandemic pose concerns for the future of public mental health and mental healthcare systems in South Africa, particularly in urban centres where the impacts of the pandemic are pronounced. The limited capacity of government public health initiatives, state funding, and the nascent COVID-19 research agenda highlight the urgent need for additional screening, treatment, and research efforts nationwide.

In this chapter, we discuss the possible impacts of the COVID-19 pandemic on psychiatric morbidity, public mental health, and mental healthcare systems in South Africa.

18.2 OBJECTIVES

We provide the following objectives for this chapter:

- Review neuropsychiatric manifestations, i.e. mental disorders due to direct effects of the agent/s. This will take the form of an analysis of publications linked to SARS, MERS and COVID-19.
- Provide insight into mental disorders due to secondary effects of the pandemic (e.g. lockdown during COVID-19) using a case study based in Soweto.
- Provide an update of the impact of pandemics on: utilisation of mental healthcare services, voluntary and involuntary mental healthcare users, as well as forensic state patients.
- Describe a model of care incorporating telemedicine: highlights and pitfalls.
- Suggest a plan for curriculum change with regard to teaching medical and other students, particularly those in their clinical training years.

18.3 PSYCHIATRIC SEQUELAE OF COVID-19: A BRIEF REVIEW

The rapid, ongoing production of nascent mental health research on COVID-19 has shared vital insights into the possible psychiatric consequences of the pandemic. Drawing on the global literature, we review the existing evidence on the psychiatric sequelae of COVID-19 infection and the secondary impacts of the COVID-19 pandemic. A more comprehensive discussion of this topic can be found in Subramaney et al (2020).

18.3.1 Neuropsychiatric Sequelae

The neuropsychiatric sequelae of infection due to severe acute respiratory syndrome coronavirus 2 (SARS-CoV-2) include a range of mental conditions that are understood to derive from brain or other physiological damage resulting from either direct effects of infection of the central nervous system (CNS) or through indirect mechanisms such as systemic inflammation (Rogers et al, 2020; Troyer, Kohn and Hong, 2020). Researchers have drawn upon studies on two similar strains of coronaviruses, which also caused widespread respiratory disease across the world, for additional insights – SARS and MERS (Brooks et al, 2020; Rogers et al, 2020).

A series of overlapping neuropsychiatric presentations have been reported in past cases of MERS, SARS, and COVID-19. Research suggests that delirium is a common presentation in the acute stage of COVID-19: Early studies show that 20–30% of COVID-19 patients will experience delirium (Rogers et al, 2020). These presentations are much higher in cases of severe illness, where 60–70% of patients have presented with delirium (O'Hanlon and Inouye, 2020). Preliminary evidence on elderly MERS patients also found that delirium is associated with increased mortality risk (Rogers et al, 2020). Recent studies also report acute psychosis among COVID-19 patients with no prior history of psychosis. In one study, patients exhibited presentations of agitation, disorganisation, paranoid ideation, and auditory hallucinations (Ferrando et al, 2020). Among severe COVID-19 patients requiring intensive care unit (ICU) admission, neurocognitive impairment (e.g. dysexecutive syndrome) may be a sustained consequence of COVID-19 (e.g. months to years) after recovery (Rogers et al, 2020). For SARS and MERS, studies have reported extended physical and psychological effects occurring in the post-illness period (i.e. months to years), but it is yet unknown whether this is also the case for COVID-19.

Growing evidence illustrates the role of psychoneuroimmunological pathways in precipitating a wide range of psychiatric and neuropsychiatric conditions due to human immunodeficiency virus (HIV) infection. Similar mechanisms may underlie the neuro/psychiatric presentations of COVID-19. In addition to acute stress from experiencing COVID-19, infection with SARS-CoV-2 may lead to a hyperinflammatory state (Ferrando et al, 2020; Rogers et al, 2020; Troyer, Kohn and Hong, 2020). Even with no infiltration of the virus into the CNS, peripheral cytokines involved in the anti-viral response may give rise to neuropsychiatric effects by precipitating neuroinflammatory responses and/or compromising blood-brain-interface (BBI) integrity, leading to peripheral immune cell transmigration into the CNS and possible disruption of neurotransmission (Troyer, Kohn and Hong, 2020). Overall, the aetiology of the neuropsychiatric manifestations of COVID-19 is likely affected by a variety of factors, including the current state of immune function, direct effects of the viral infection, the degree of physiological compromise (e.g. hypoxia), pre-existing cerebrovascular disease, and the larger psychosocial experience of COVID-19, and the availability and quality of medical interventions.

18.3.2 Anxiety Disorders

Anxiety disorders may range from a wide variety of concerns around contracting or spreading the virus, inability to regulate uncertainty, limited social interactions, unsafe living conditions, and economic fallout, among others (Kim, Nyengerai and Mendenhall, 2020; Rajkumar, 2020). While these symptoms might not constitute an anxiety disorder, they are currently among the most common symptom presentation emerging during the COVID-19 pandemic (Rogers et al, 2020; Sommer and Bakker, 2020). Generalised anxiety disorder is among the most frequently described presentation among COVID-19 patients. A meta-analysis of SARS, MERS, and COVID-19 studies reported anxiety in the post-illness phase up to three years after infection. Health anxiety is another common presentation seen during the pandemic and may result in individuals seeking medical assistance repeatedly, or conversely, avoiding help-seeking behaviour even when unwell (Rajkumar, 2020). Health anxiety may also result in a mistrust of or reluctance toward health authorities (Huang and Zhao, 2020). Panic attacks may also occur as a distinct disorder or in combination with other psychiatric disorders, though panic attack symptoms such as shortness of breath, chills or heat sensations, and chest pain or discomfort may overlap with symptoms of COVID-19 infection.

18.3.3 Post-Traumatic Stress Disorder (PTSD)

Trauma is defined by the Substance Abuse and Mental Health Services Administration (SAMHSA) as 'an event, series of events, or set of circumstances that is experienced by an individual as physically or emotionally harmful or life threatening and that has lasting adverse effects on the individual's functioning and mental, physical, social, emotional, or spiritual well-being' (SAMHSA, 2014). The DSM-5 diagnostic criteria for PTSD sharpens the definition of 'traumatic event' and there are now four symptom clusters (intrusion symptoms, avoidance symptoms, cognitions and mood symptoms and arousal and reactivity symptoms).

Horesh and Brown (2020) argue that the COVID-19 crisis can and should be viewed from the perspective of trauma. There is no doubt that the COVID pandemic can be likened to a stressor that is particularly traumatic in nature, with resultant symptoms that are in keeping with acute stress disorder (ASD) and post-traumatic stress disorder (PTSD). If COVID-19 can be conceptualised as a form of chronic trauma, it is akin to exposure to an event (experiencing or witnessing, confronting/hearing the news of illness or exposure to infection) together with anxiety, fear, avoidance, hyperarousal and hypervigilance at its core and finally impact on functioning. It remains to be seen whether the neurobiological underpinnings of the pandemic are in keeping with that of PTSD due to other trauma exposures, particularly that due to witnessing the death of a loved one, or looking after a loved one with chronic illnesses i.e. the concomitant hormonal changes with alterations in cortisol and aberrations in neurotransmitters and immune markers.

The pandemic may affect individuals at any or all three levels (individual, interpersonal, or collective) (Figure 18.1). At the individual level, for example, one might feel a heightened sense of vulnerability and can re-experience past traumatic experiences. At the interpersonal level, deterioration of relationships might occur. At the collective level, people are constantly exposed to the illnesses of those around them as well as a societal grappling with deaths and other losses (Horesh and Brown, 2020).

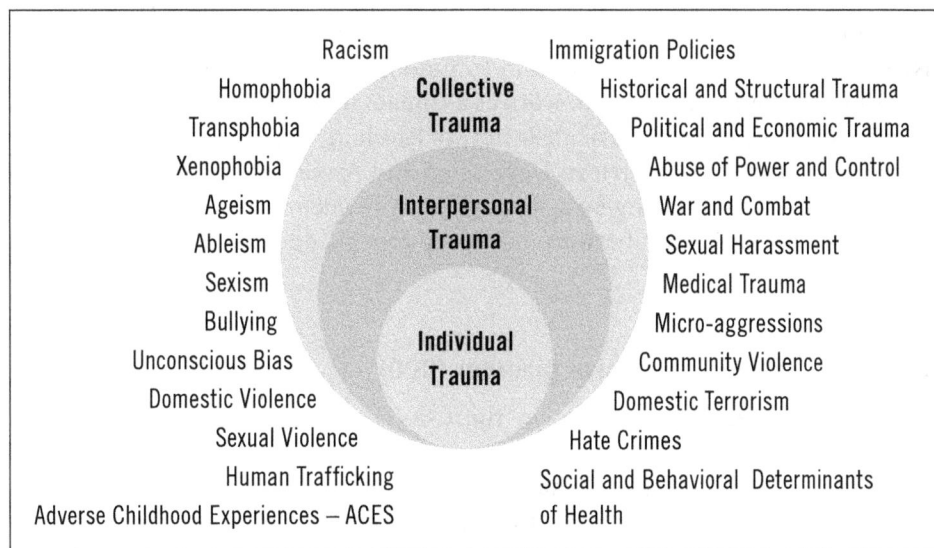

Racism Immigration Policies
Homophobia **Collective** Historical and Structural Trauma
Transphobia **Trauma** Political and Economic Trauma
Xenophobia Abuse of Power and Control
Ageism **Interpersonal** War and Combat
Ableism **Trauma** Sexual Harassment
Sexism Medical Trauma
Bullying Micro-aggressions
Unconscious Bias **Individual** Community Violence
Domestic Violence **Trauma** Domestic Terrorism
Sexual Violence Hate Crimes
Human Trafficking Social and Behavioral Determinants
Adverse Childhood Experiences – ACES of Health

Figure 18.1 Multiple levels and sources of trauma

A bio-psycho-social model on COVID-19 and its impact suggest the following (Horesh and Brown, 2020):

- Biological: age, heightened stress response, coexisting medical and psychiatric comorbidities, increased substance use;
- Psychological: changes in available coping skills, quarantine increasing feelings of anger and confusion, anxiety of contracting the illness, triggering of past traumas;
- Social: housing insecurity, changes to family dynamics, transition to online communication and social media use, loss of social networks and community supports, additional weight of caring for others who are suffering.

Stressful conditions, including unemployment, financial crises and uncertainty, also proffer an opportunity for a cycle of violence to be perpetuated. Additionally, trauma due to gender-based violence and cases of child abuse also warrant attention and intervention as those sectors of the community involving women and children may not have had an opportunity to report and order urgent help. Safe places should be provided for individuals who have experienced violence or those who likely will be exposed to domestic violence (Duan et al, 2020).

At a societal level, it is necessary to enhance our mental health to overcome challenges resulting from the outbreak of the COVID-19 pandemic. It was reported that step-by-step care may be a helpful procedure if applied at the proper time (Winsper et al, 2013). In addition, it is essential to train specific groups to provide urgent psychological first aid and social support (Liu et al, 2020). It is also important to create a reliable and commonplace platform to provide online psychological counselling and to work as a contact tool with the supportive team. Societies such as the South African Society of Psychiatrists (SASOP) and advocacy groups such as the South African Depression and Anxiety Group (SADAG) have been instrumental in setting up a support network such as this. Networking and enhanced communication between advocacy groups, doctors, psychologists and social workers is key.

18.3.4 Obsessive Compulsive Disorder (OCD)

Another prominent presentation in the COVID-19 environment is obsessive compulsive disorder. Numerous countries (e.g. China, India, Italy, United Kingdom, United States, etc.) have shown a recent increase in outpatients presenting with OCD symptoms, with exacerbation of symptoms such as hoarding and washing compulsions in already diagnosed OCD patients (Banerjee, 2020; Wang et al, 2020). Lockdown measures also led to panic buying and hoarding items such as hygiene products, flu medication, and groceries (Banerjee, 2020). Patients may struggle to determine what constitutes excessive behaviour under these extraordinary circumstances and normalise their compulsions as a precautionary response to the global pandemic. Proper hand-washing techniques recommended may also reinforce ritualistic behaviours, another clinical feature of OCD. The influx of information from TV, newspapers and social media sites regarding the virus can add to obsessions about contamination (Wang et al, 2020). During previous epidemics such as SARS, MERS and influenza, researchers reported a worsening of OCD in patients up to one year later (Wang et al, 2020).

18.3.5 Mood Disorders

COVID-19 infection and the secondary effects of the pandemic likely place many at risk for a range of mood disorders. Past research shows that seropositivity for viral illnesses linked to influenza A & B and coronaviruses were associated with a history of mood disorders, including depressive disorders and suicide attempts (Okusaga et al, 2011). One cross-sectional survey conducted in China during the COVID-19 outbreak found that 20.1% of individuals reported depressive symptoms and 18.2% reported sleep disturbances (Huang and Zhao, 2020). As noted with the HIV/AIDS epidemic in South Africa, depression can increase the risk of acquiring the virus, and the presence of mental illnesses can also be a stand-alone risk factor for acquiring HIV/AIDS (Joska, Stein and Grant, 2014). It has been hypothesised that coronaviruses typically invade the nervous system via the olfactory nerve. Thus, mood disorders can result directly from the virus, or secondarily through the resulting immunological response (Brietzke et al, 2020; Regger, Stanley and Joiner, 2020). In persons with pre-existing mood disorders, infection with COVID-19 may result in a relapse of symptoms.

Patients with mood disorders often display cognitive changes which might affect their ability to rationalise the recommended measures of maintaining social distancing, regular washing of hands and surfaces, and the use of a facemask. Symptoms of acute mania include elevated mood, impulsivity, increased goal-directed activity and often, psychosis (APA, 2013). Acutely manic patients might be unable to appreciate the importance of these preventative measures, and therefore may be at higher risk of contracting and spreading the virus.

The numerous and ongoing psychosocial consequences of the pandemic may also result in the relapse of depressive disorders, bipolar disorder and suicidality (Regger, Stanley and Joiner, 2020), particularly due to the widespread economic shocks of the lockdown. The United Nations Development Programme has estimated an income loss of more than $220 billion in developing countries such as South Africa due to the pandemic (UNDP, 2020). Recessions inevitably lead to job losses, and unemployment is an independent risk factor for the development of depressive disorders. A systematic review found a positive association between recession and higher suicide rates (Oyesanya, Lopez-Morinigo and Dutta, 2015) with increases in global suicide rates during the 2008 recession of 20–30% (Nordt et al, 2015).

Social isolation is also a risk factor for depressive disorders. Quarantine and social distancing measures, which limit social interactions and communal gatherings during lockdown, have removed vital social support systems for many individuals. The lockdown also poses major barriers to accessing care. Some clinics, including in South Africa, are only allowing the patient to enter healthcare facilities, which is challenging in a discipline where collateral information is often imperative to assessing a patient's progress. Restrictions on the availability of transport may also lead to decreased follow-up at clinics, non-adherence and subsequent relapses.

18.3.6 Psychotic Disorders

It has been postulated that prenatal exposure to a virus increases risk of developing schizophrenia later in life. Data from the aftermath of the Spanish influenza of 1918 reported an association between exposure to general respiratory viruses such as influenza and subsequent psychotic episodes later in life (Mednick et al, 1988; Vlessides, 2020). The response of immunoglobulin G was investigated against four human coronavirus strains that were prevalent at the time. Evidence showed that in approximately 90% of adults diagnosed with psychosis, elevated levels of antibodies to one or more viruses was found. Pandemics like the Spanish flu demonstrated that these viruses can have a more immediate effect, resulting in cases of acute psychosis soon after or at the time of infection. Further research is required as it remains unclear whether this is the direct effects of the virus on the brain, systemic inflammation due to infection, or a post-viral immune activation (Vlessides, 2020).

Conditions of psychosocial stress and trauma during the pandemic may precipitate, exacerbate, or influence the nature of the psychotic symptoms (Fischer et al, 2020; Luming, 2020). Patients presenting with psychosomatic delusions may experience intense paranoia (Luming, 2020). In one case, a 38-year-old married woman with secondary level education, good premorbid functioning, and no prior psychiatric history believed she was potentially infected with the SARS-CoV-2 virus after a visit to her dentist (who had recently vacationed in France and was not donning a mask). Within four days, she became anxious with malaise and fever, developed command auditory hallucinations to go to multiple health centres for testing and began to feel 'an evil demonic force which would take her soul in order to possess her'. She also had visual hallucinations of shadows, delusions of reference and a formal thought disorder. The voice ultimately ordered her to kill her family. She was diagnosed with an acute psychotic disorder and was treated effectively with antipsychotic treatment (Huarcaya-Victoria, Herrera and Castillo, 2020). Finally, media coverage during pandemics or crises can also unduly influence psychotic manifestations (Fischer et al, 2020). Difficulties in distinguishing 'normal paranoia' around the illness and psychosis is best managed by a mental healthcare practitioner.

18.3.7 Children and Mental Health

Children's mental health has been overshadowed by the drastic and necessary measures taken to curb the spread of infection. The first onset of mental disorders typically occurs in childhood or adolescence (Kessler et al, 2007). In a survey conducted on primary school children in Hubei Province in China to evaluate the impact of home confinement on the mental health of children, increased rates of depressive and anxiety symptoms were found, and the authors concluded that 'serious infectious diseases may influence the mental health of children as other traumatic experiences do' (Xie et al, 2020). The direct impact on a child may be related to anxiety and uncertainty about an unfamiliar infectious condition, contraction of the virus (with the potential for self-isolation, quarantine in hospital, and separation from family), having vulnerabilities to contracting the illness (e.g. being immunocompromised or respiratory disease), or having a loved one experience or die from COVID-19 (Pfefferbaum and North 2020).

Social interactions are an important component of a child's emotional development and capacity for social competence (AAP, 2020). School closure has resulted in academic and social losses, but in South Africa, there are further challenges due to limited access to online education, malnutrition (with the suspension of school feeding programmes), and the lack of provision of school-based therapeutic interventions for children with disabilities (e.g. occupational therapy). The implementation of home confinement has also resulted in social isolation, school closure, play restrictions and a major lifestyle and routine adjustment, and parents staying at home may not always translate into more child-focused interactions. Additionally, lockdown restrictions limit the potential psychological benefits effects of exercise and physical activity for children. Finally, many South African children live in overcrowded, confined spaces and do not have access to private outdoor areas. Co-parenting, custody arrangements, and movement of children between households during lockdown might also lead to added stress in children.

18.3.8 Healthcare Workers

Healthcare workers are employed in environments that present them with often unique and hazardous challenges, many of which are encountered daily and seen as an inherent part of work responsibilities. The COVID-19 pandemic introduced additional work hazards in the healthcare environment (AAP, 2020). Globally, various difficulties have been exacerbated due to the pandemic and newer challenges have emerged. These include the requirement for much stricter biosecurity measures, the constant risk of contracting the disease, increased workloads, concerns about putting family members at risk and the stigma faced by healthcare workers (Rogers et al, 2020). The World Health Organisation (WHO) has acknowledged an increased risk of anxiety amongst healthcare workers and a possible increase in burnout and PTSD (Cullen, Gulati and Kelly, 2020; WHO, 2020). Healthcare workers have also been faced with significant shortages of personal protective equipment, the lack of specific treatments, constant media coverage and a sense of not being supported adequately. Additionally, reasons for psychological distress include fears of contracting the virus, passing on the virus to families, increased patient load, and staff shortages (Lai et al, 2020; Xiong and Peng, 2020).

One cross-sectional study of healthcare workers in multiple hospitals in China assessed the mental health outcomes and associated factors among healthcare workers who were involved in managing COVID-19 patients (Lai et al, 2020). 50.4% of participants reported symptoms of depression, 44.6% anxiety, 34.0% insomnia and 71.5% distress. Symptoms were more severe across all measurements among nurses, women, frontline workers and those working in Wuhan, the epicentre of the epidemic. There have also been reports of medical personnel succumbing to suicide during the COVID-pandemic. Even during non-pandemic circumstances, physicians and healthcare workers face elevated risks for suicide (Duthell et al, 2019).

The COVID-19 pandemic and the severe constraints on resources have highlighted certain serious ethical dilemmas faced by frontline workers (Gostin, Friedman and Wetter, 2020; Ross, 2018). Specific interventions designed to meet the concerns and challenges faced by healthcare workers during the pandemic must include the availability and accessibility of mental health services to healthcare workers within the workplace to enable early detection and management of mental health issues.

18.4 CASE STUDY: EXAMINING THE MENTAL HEALTH IMPACTS OF COVID-19 CONDITIONS DURING THE FIRST SIX WEEKS OF THE NATIONAL LOCKDOWN IN SOWETO

Soon after the South African lockdown, the first author and colleagues (Kim et al, 2020a,b) quickly shifted an existing study to investigate the mental health impacts of the COVID-19 pandemic among adults residing in Soweto, a major township southwest of Johannesburg which houses communities with high reported rates of comorbidities such as diabetes, hypertension, and HIV. Using a community-based epidemiological surveillance study, the study team based out of Chris Hani Baragwanath Academic Hospital combined pre-existing data on health behaviours, disease status, and social environments with telephonic survey data on perceptions of COVID-19 and mental illness risk to characterise experiences during lockdown, understandings of the novel coronavirus, and the mental health impacts of the pandemic.

In a sample of 221 adults, a higher perceived risk of COVID-19 infection predicted greater depressive symptoms ($p < 0.001$; Figure 18.2), particularly among adults with histories of childhood trauma, though this effect was marginally significant ($p = 0.063$; Figure 18.3). Greater knowledge of COVID-19 prevention and transmission was also associated with a lower perceived risk of depression but higher depressive symptoms. While a large majority of participants reported that experiences of the COVID-19 pandemic did not affect their mental health (or 'mind'), 10–20% of participants reported potent experiences of anxiety, fear, and 'thinking too much' as a result of the pandemic. These concerns during the lockdown were driven and exacerbated by the inability to care for themselves and their families, crippling economic struggles, personal vulnerability due to illness, the invisible nature of COVID-19 transmission, and a lack of awareness of the disease. These results highlight the compounding effects of past traumatic histories and recent stress exposures on exacerbating the severity of depressive symptoms among adults living in an urban South African context.

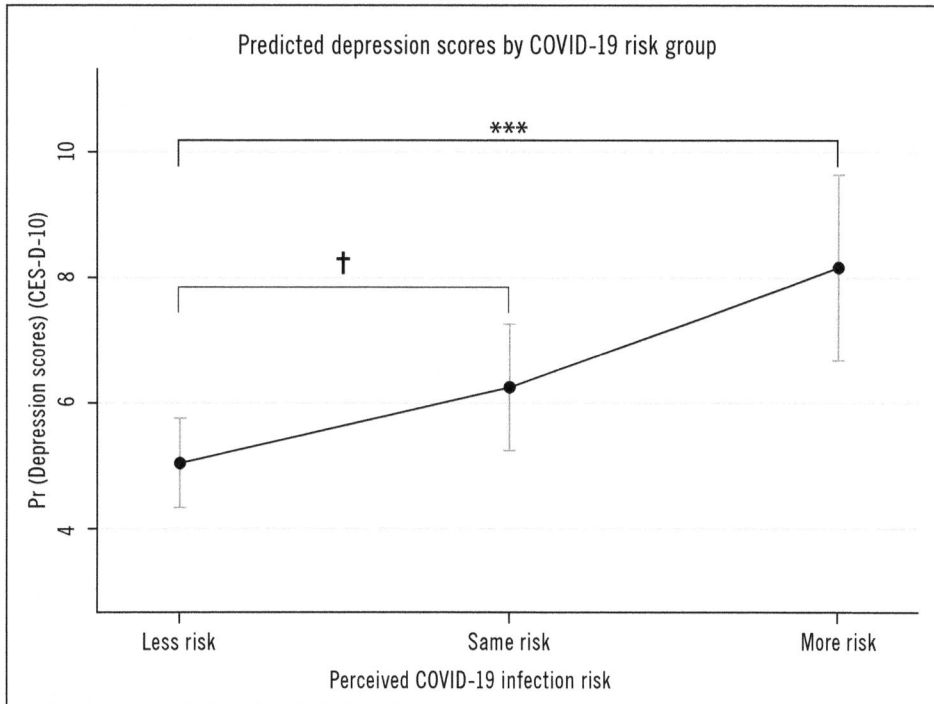

Figure 18.2 Predicted depression scores by perceived COVID-19 risk group

Note: Greater perceived risk of COVID-19 infection corresponds with greater depression symptomatology in adults living in Soweto. The effect of being in the 'More risk' group is highly significant ($p = <0.001$) relative to being at 'Less risk', while the effect of perceiving that one is at the 'Same risk' of COVID-19 infection relative to other individuals living in Soweto on depression symptoms is marginally significant ($p = 0.088$). The respective predicted CES-D-10 scores for each group are as provided:

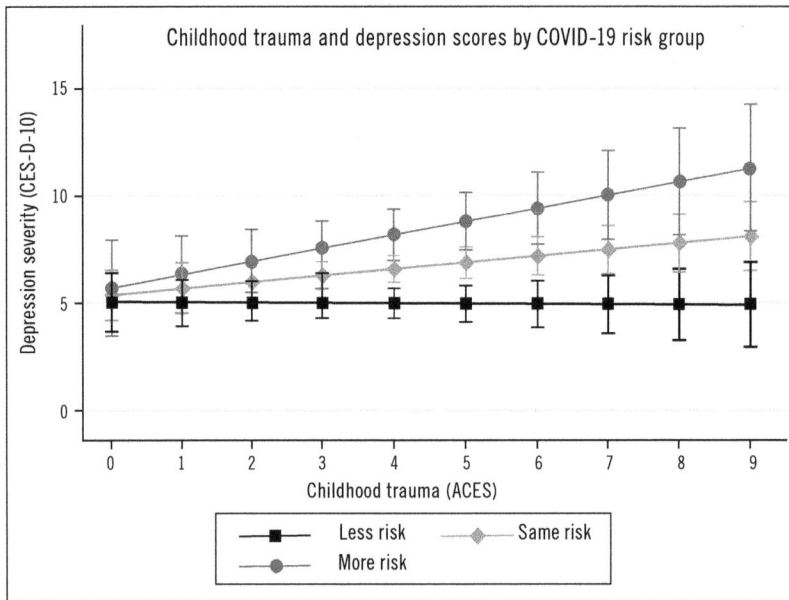

Figure 18.3 Childhood trauma (ACES) and Depression scores (CESD) by COVID-19 risk group

Note: Greater childhood trauma (ACES) potentiates the positive relationship between greater perceived COVID-19 risk and the severity of depressive symptomatology. The effect of the interaction between childhood trauma and perceived COVID-19 risk on depression is marginally significant ($F[1, 208] = 3.51$, $p = 0.0625$).

18.5 IMPACT OF COVID-19 ON THE UTILISATION OF MENTAL HEALTH SERVICES

Utilisation of mental healthcare services at specialised psychiatric hospitals are also impacted severely during pandemics of this nature. For example, in Southern Gauteng, two specialised hospitals made the decision to close certain services (e.g. eating disorders, psychotherapy and court-ordered forensic services) in preparation for the expected increase in COVID-19 admissions and additional resources needed to treat COVID-19 patients. Requirements of the Mental Health Care Act 17 of 2002 regarding admission of involuntary and assisted mental healthcare users (MHCUs), as well as forensic state patients for observation under the Criminal Procedures Act, create tremendous pressure for emergency medicine departments and units dealing with acute psychiatric admissions. Such individuals cannot be referred for further treatment meaning that such facilities may be inundated as a result of COVID-19.

Pre- and post-lockdown, admission and discharge data at Sterkfontein Psychiatric Hospital indicate that for three months prior to lockdown (before 26 March 2020), the hospital admitted 92 patients to the general psychiatry wards and up to 26 forensic patients per month for a 30-day observation. Following the lockdown (for the period 26 March to 15 July) and exposure to COVID-19 cases (and including the death of a nurse due to covid-19), this decreased to 82 admissions and none for forensic observation. While many MHCUs expressed fear of leaving their homes, many also experienced increased anxiety for their health which might have led to an increase in admissions at acute units.

The need for mental healthcare services during lockdown is further noted in an online survey conducted by the South African Depression and Anxiety Group. Findings were that 65% of people felt stressed or very stressed about the imposed lockdown (SADAG, 2020). The main challenges faced during the lockdown included: anxiety and panic (55%), financial stress and pressure (46%), depression (40%), poor family relations (30%), feelings of suicide (12%), and substance abuse (6%).

18.6 SOLUTIONS FOR PUBLIC MENTAL HEALTH

18.6.1 Telemedicine: Highlights and Pitfalls

Severe barriers to mental healthcare amidst high rates of mental illness and COVID-19 necessitate additional emergency psychological resources and accessible, long-term services. Widespread evidence highlights the therapeutic effectiveness and accessibility of phone-based counselling, particularly during public health crises and healthcare restricted settings (Sood et al, 2007). Telemedicine (i.e. telehealth), or the use of telecommunications to deliver care outside of healthcare facilities, are critical resources for high-risk and hard-to-access communities during public health emergencies. Numerous telehealth psychological interventions worldwide have shown to be cost-efficient, lead to sustained, decreased mental illness risk, and improve mental well-being, particularly public health emergencies (Bashshur et al, 2016; Yellowlees et al, 2008). More than 96% of households have access to a cellphone or landline based on StatsSA's 2018 General Household Survey (StatsSA, 2019c). Additionally, low costs, convenience, and privacy have made telemedicine a prioritised mode of healthcare delivery in South Africa (Botha and Booi, 2016). The lack of national-level mental health research infrastructures, however, limits immediate studies on the mental health impacts of COVID-19 and the evaluation of telemedicine interventions to improve mental well-being.

18.6.2 Adapting Medical Education and Curriculum during COVID-19

COVID-19 has also brought challenges to the teaching and training of both undergraduate and postgraduate students at universities, particularly medical students. This has resulted in massive changes to the curricula as well as the assessment process. Online teaching content, with videos, links to articles as well as presentations with voice over PowerPoint were swiftly made available in place of classroom lectures. Many universities also provided funding for data and laptops to needy students in certain cases. Clinical students who returned to the hospitals were very soon caught up in the workspace of exposure to patients with the virus. In some instances, they served as sources of infection within the clinical environment as numbers of cases soared in the community.

The Professional and Ethics Standard Committee (PESC) of the Faculty of Health Sciences at the University of the Witwatersrand in Johannesburg embodied the essence of the students' role in the pandemic in a PESC notice entitled 'Student practitioners in the COVID-19 crisis: Faculty and Student Responsibilities and the Duty of Care' (19 June 2020):

> The committee notes that there are personal and professional ethical dilemmas faced by both the faculty leadership and the student practitioner body in the current crisis situation. It is acknowledged that it is in everyone's interests for the academic programme to be disrupted as little as possible; it is also acknowledged that students may be anxious about the clinical environment while the threat of COVID-19 infection remains high. Furthermore, with inequalities in South African society students are not all affected in the same way. Those from more privileged socio-economic backgrounds are at lesser risk because they have access to safer transport, can maintain social distancing more easily, and have peace of mind in knowing that they and their loved ones are guaranteed healthcare. The extreme differences in students' contextual realities must be taken into account in all decisions regarding the resumption of the academic programme (Wits PESC, 2020:1).

Due to time lost from the lockdown, clinical blocks were shortened in length and clinical teachers experienced an increasing amount of pressure to manage the academic setting. Clinical assessments methods also changed from using patients to virtual and paper-based material. Ongoing discussions and regular meetings held to discuss the implementation, as well as provide ongoing support to students led to another level of stress and anxiety. Many students embraced the challenge and quickly became a part of the solution, with non-medical students volunteering and some medical students in the non-clinical years assisting with screening at hospital sites.

These challenges become in and of themselves new learning material. Novel teaching approaches with different ways of thinking have become the norm. Certain training, e.g. psychotherapy training for psychiatry registrars underwent radical changes, with the use of telemedicine and virtual consultations. For this, both patients and registrars need to have access to confidential, reliable technology, thus reaching communities in need are often a challenge. Ethical issues of consent and managing high-risk individuals in this manner warrant detailed discussion. Indeed, psychotherapy (and any other modality of postgraduate training) supervision may be done using virtual spaces via Skype, Zoom, Microsoft teams, etc.

Upon return to the university, students were naturally anxious for themselves and their loved ones. A recent University of Washington study, that considered student and trainee responses to the COVID-19 pandemic, found high levels of anxiety amongst students, including fear for their own safety and that of those closest to them (Gallagher and Schleyer, 2020). Recognition of this by faculty and incorporating it into the teaching and training framework was vitally important. What was emphasised was the recognition and value of their commitment, as well as the benefits afforded by the new context and clinical environment, e.g. the unique learning opportunities, financial benefits, the saving of the academic year and the personal satisfaction of being part of the efforts to provide healthcare and save lives in the face of the pandemic.

Students that fell behind in their studies because of not being able to return to the clinical context, infected students who fell behind in their studies while under quarantine, and who were not able to return to the clinical platform until they had recovered as well as the provision of support for students who were unable to access to online learning when this was rolled-out were not disadvantaged. Support was also provided for students who experienced stress or trauma as a result of working in the healthcare context in this crisis.

Most importantly, reform for the curriculum change in both undergraduate and postgraduate teaching platforms is needed, internationally and for Africa, unique to our context. Mental health modules should include public mental health perspectives of pandemics and mental health. This would include all aspects, such as the aetiology, mode of presentation and management of the various neuropsychiatric presentations of the viral outbreak, responses of known mental healthcare users to outbreaks, the appropriate use of telemedicine in times of need, policies and frameworks of management for patients and their families with specific reference to risk to contract the infection, asymptomatic MHCUs, those with mild illness, moderate to severe illness and critically ill. The opportunities to manage stigma in mental health, managing traumatic stress, loss and bereavement are endless. Online curricula such as the medical student COVID-19 curriculum developed by Harvard University (https://curriculum.covidstudentresponse.org) includes a module on mental health in the time of COVID-19, with aspects of the biopsychosocial framework, special considerations for at-risk populations, and evolving clinical practices in mental healthcare.

18.7 CONCLUSION

In this chapter, we review the mounting evidence accrued both locally and globally that highlights the widespread mental health impacts of both direct COVID-19 infection as well as the secondary impacts of the pandemic and its associated social policies. We illustrate these effects on public mental health in a case study from the first empirical study of the mental health impacts of the pandemic in South Africa, and also provide a snapshot of the utilisation of mental healthcare services of psychiatric facilities in Gauteng Province. Finally, we describe two potential solutions – telepsychiatry and adaptations to medical education and curricula – to mitigate the adverse consequences on public mental health and bolster the educational capacity of our country's future frontline healthcare workers. As the course of the pandemic continues worldwide, we offer these reflections to help researchers, practitioners, and policymakers address the ongoing mental health impacts of the COVID-19 pandemic and strengthen future responses to public health emergencies and disease pandemics.

18.8 SELF-ASSESSMENT QUESTIONS

1. What are the common neuropsychiatric manifestations of COVID-19?
2. What important public mental health solutions can one consider when managing pandemics?

18.9 REFERENCES

American Psychiatric Association. 2013. Diagnostic and Statistical Manual of Mental Disorders. 5 ed. Arlington (VA): American Psychiatric Publishing.

Banerjee, D. 2020. The other side of COVID-19: Impact on obsessive compulsive disorder (OCD) and hoarding. *Psychiatry Research*, p. 288.

Bashshur, R.L., Shannon, G.W., Bashshur, N. and Yellowlees, P.M. 2016. The empirical evidence for telemedicine interventions in mental disorders. *Telemedicine and e-Health* 22(2), pp. 87–113.

Botha, A. and Booi, V. 2016, May. mHealth implementation in South Africa. In 2016 IST-Africa Week Conference, IEEE (May), pp. 1–13.

Brietzke, E., Magee, T., Freire, R.C.R., Gomes, F.A. and Miley. R. 2020. Three insights on psychoneuroimmunology of mood disorders to be taken from the COVID-19 pandemic. *Brain, Behavior, & Immunity – Health*, p. 5.

Cao, W., Fang, Z., Hou, G., Han, M., Xu, X., Dong, J. and Zheng, J. 2020. The psychological impact of the COVID-19 epidemic on college students in China. *Psychiatry research*, p. 112934.

China Global Television Network. 2020. Why are COVID-19 doctors committing suicide? Available at: https://newsus.cgtn.com/news/2020-04-29/Why-are-COVID-19-doctors-committing-suicide--Q4yi8yhYB2/index.html.

Cullen, W., Gulati, G. and Kelly, B. 2020. Mental health in the COVID-19 pandemic. *QJM: An International Journal of Medicine* 113, pp. 311–2.

Docrat, S., Besada, D., Cleary, S., Daviaud, E. and Lund, C. 2019. Mental health system costs, resources and constraints in South Africa: a national survey. *Health Policy and Planning* 34(9), pp. 706–719.

Duan, L. and Zhu, G. 2020. Psychological interventions for people affected by the COVID-19 epidemic. *The Lancet Psychiatry* 7(4), pp. 300–302.

Duthell, F., Aubert, C., Pereira, B., Dambrun, M., Moustafa, F. and Mermillod, M. 2019. Suicide among physicians and health care workers: a systematic review and meta-analysis. *PloS ONE* 14(12).

Professional and Ethical Standards Committee, Faculty of Health Sciences, University of the Witwatersrand. 2020. Student practitioners in the Covid-19 crisis: Faculty and student responsibilities and the duty of care.

Ferrando, S.J., Klepacz, L., Lynch, S., Tavakkoli, M., Dornbush, R., Baharani, R., Smolin, Y. and Bartell, A. 2020. COVID-19 psychosis: a potential new neuropsychiatric condition triggered by novel coronavirus infection and the inflammatory response? *Psychosomatics* 61(5), pp. 551–555.

Fischer, M., Coogan, A.N., Faltraco, F. and Thome, J., 2020. COVID-19 paranoia in a patient suffering from schizophrenic psychosis–a case report. *Psychiatry Research* 288, p. 113001.

Galea, S., Merchant, R. M. and Lurie, N. 2020. The mental health consequences of COVID-19 and physical distancing: the need for prevention and early intervention. *JAMA Internal Medicine* 180(6), pp. 817–818.

Gallagher, T.H. and Schleyer, A.M. 2020. "We Signed Up for This!"—student and trainee responses to the COVID-19 pandemic. *New England Journal of Medicine*.

Gostin, L.O., Friedman, E.A. and Wetter, S.A. 2020. Responding to COVID-19: how to navigate a public health emergency legally and ethically. Wiley Online Library. Available at: https://onlinelibrary.wiley.com/doi/10.10.1002/hast.1090.

Guidance on providing pediatric well-care during COVID-19. 2020. *American Academy of Pediatrics*. Available at: https://services.aap.org/en/pages/2019-novel-coronavirus-covid-19-infections/guidance-on-providing-pediatric-well-care-during-covid-19/.

Herman, A.A., Stein, D.J., Seedat, S., Heeringa, S.G., Moomal, H. and Williams, D.R. 2009. The South African Stress and Health (SASH) study: 12-month and lifetime prevalence of common mental disorders. *South African Medical Journal* 99(5).

Horesh, D. and Brown, A.D. 2020. Traumatic stress in the age of COVID-19: A call to close critical gaps and adapt to new realities. *Psychological Trauma: Theory, Research, Practice, and Policy* 12(4).

Huang, Y. and Zhao, N. 2020. Generalized anxiety disorder, depressive symptoms and sleep quality during COVID-19 outbreak in China: a web-based cross-sectional survey. *Psychiatry Research*, p. 112954.

Huarcaya-Victoria, J., Herrera, D. and Castillo, C. 2020. Psychosis in a patient with anxiety related to COVID-19: A case report. *Elsevier Psychiatry Research.* 29 Apr. 289, p. 113052.

Joska, J.A., Stein, D.J. and Grant, I. 2014. HIV and Psychiatry. 1 ed. London, UK: John Wiley & Sons Limited, p. 84.

Kessler, R.C., Amminger, G.P., Aguilar-Gaxiola, S., Alonso, J., Lee, S. and Ustun, T.B. 2007. Age of onset of mental disorders: a review of recent literature. *Current opinion in psychiatry* 20(4), p. 359.

Kim, A.W., Nyengerai, T. and Mendenhall, E. 2020. Evaluating the mental health impacts of the COVID-19 pandemic: perceived risk of COVID-19 infection and childhood trauma predict adult depressive symptoms in urban South Africa. *Psychological Medicine*, pp. 1–13.

Kim, A.W., Burgess, R., Chiwandire, N., Kwinda, Z., Tsai, A.C., Norris, S.A. and Mendenhall, E. 2020. Perceptions, understandings, and impacts of the COVID-19 pandemic in urban South Africa. The South African Journal of Psychiatry: SAJP: the Journal of the Society of Psychiatrists of South Africa. 2021;27.

Lai, J., Ma, S., Wang, Y., Cai, Z., Hu, J., Wei, N., Wu, J., Du, H., Chen, T., Li, R., Tan, H., Kang, L., Yao, L., Huang, M., Wang, H., Wang, G., Liu, Z. and Hu, S. 2020. Factors associated with mental health outcomes among health care workers exposed to coronavirus disease 2019. *JAMA Network Open* 3(3).

Lewis-O'Connor, A., Warren, A., Lee, J.V., Levy-Carrick, N., Grossman, S., Chadwick, M., Stoklosa, H. and Rittenberg, E. 2019. The state of the science on trauma inquiry. *Women's Health* 15, p.1745506519861234.

Liu, S., Yang, L., Zhang, C., Xiang, Y. T., Liu, Z., Hu, S. and Zhang, B. 2020. Online mental health services in China during the COVID-19 outbreak. *The Lancet Psychiatry* 7(4), pp. e17–e18.

Luming, L. Challenges and priorities in responding to COVID-19 in inpatient psychiatry. 2020. *American Psychiatric Association.* Last Updated 23 April 2020. Available at: https://ps.psychiatryonline.org/doi/10.1176/appi.ps.202000166.

Mednick, S.A., Machon, R.A., Huttunen, M.O. and Bonett, D. 1988. Adult schizophrenia following prenatal exposure to an influenza epidemic. *Archives of General Psychiatry* 45(2), pp. 189–92.

National Alliance on Mental Illness. 2020. Mental health facts. Available at: https://www.nami.org/NAMI/media/NAMI-Media/Infographics/Children-MH-Facts-NAMI.pdf.

Nordt, C., Warnke, I., Seifritz, E. and Kawohl, W. 2015. Modelling suicide and unemployment: a longitudinal analysis covering 63 countries. *The Lancet Psychiatry* 2(3), pp. 239–45.

O'Hanlon, S. and Inouye S.K. 2020. Delirium: a missing piece in the COVID-19 pandemic puzzle. *Age & Ageing*, pp. 1–2. doi: 10.1093/ageing/afaa094.

Okusaga, O., Yolken, R.H., Langenberg, P., Lapidus, M., Arling, T.A., Dickerson, F.B., Scrandis, D.A., Severance, E., Cabassa, J.A., Balis, T. and Postolache, T.T. 2011. Association of seropositivity for influenza and coronaviruses with history of mood disorders and suicide attempts. *Journal of Affective Disorders* 130(1–2), pp. 220–225.

Oyesanya, M., Lopez-Morinigo, J., Dutta, R. 2015. Systematic review of suicide in economic recession. *World Journal of Psychiatry* 5(2), pp. 243–54.

Pfefferbaum, B. and North, C.S. 2020. Mental health and the Covid-19 pandemic. *The New England Journal of Medicine* 383(6), pp. 510–512.

Rajkumar, R.P. 2020. COVID-19 and mental health: A review of the existing literature. *Asian Journal of Psychiatry*, p. 102066.

Regger, M.A., Stanley, I.H. and Joiner, T.E. 2020. Suicide mortality and coronavirus disease 2019 a perfect storm? *JAMA Psychiatry*. doi: 10.1001/jamapsychiatry.2020.1060.

Rogers, J.P., Chesney, E., Oliver, D., Pollak, T.A., McGuire, P., Fusar-Poli, P., Zandi, M.S., Lewis, G. and David, A.S. 2020. Psychiatric and neuropsychiatric presentations associated with severe coronavirus infections: a systematic review and meta-analysis with comparison to the COVID-19 pandemic. *The Lancet Psychiatry* 7(7), pp. 611–627.

Ross, F. 2018. The cost of ignoring our doctors' mental health. *USA Mental Health First Aid*. Available at: www.mentalhealthfirstaid.org/external/2018/02/cost-ignoring-doctors-mental-health/.

Sommer, I.E. and Bakker, P.R. 2020. What can psychiatrists learn from SARS and MERS outbreaks? *The Lancet Psychiatry* 7(7), pp. 565–566.

Sood, S., Mbarika, V., Jugoo, S., Dookhy, R., Doarn, C.R., Prakash, N. and Merrell, R.C. 2007. What is telemedicine? A collection of 104 peer-reviewed perspectives and theoretical underpinnings. *Telemedicine and e-Health* 13(5), pp. 573–590.

South African Depression and Anxiety Group. 2020. SADAG's online survey findings on COVID-19 and mental health (21 April 2020). Available at: http://www.sadag.org/index.php?option=com_content&view=article&id=3092:sadag-s-online-survey-findings-on-covid-19-and-mental-health-21-april-2020&catid=149:press-releases&Itemid=226.

StatsSA. 2019a. Five facts about poverty in South Africa, April. Available at: http://www.statssa.gov.za/?p=12075.

StatsSA. 2019b. Unemployment rises slightly in third quarter of 2019, October Available at: http://www.statssa.gov.za/?p=12689.

StatsSA. 2019. General household survey.

Subramaney, U., Kim, A.W., Chetty, I., Chetty, S., Jayrajh, P., Govender, M., Maharaj, P. and Pak, E. 2020. Coronavirus disease 2019 (COVID-19) and psychiatric sequelae in South Africa: Anxiety and beyond. *Wits Journal of Clinical Medicine* 2(2), pp. 115–122.

Troyer, E.A., Kohn, J.N. and Hong, S. 2020. Are we facing a crashing wave of neuropsychiatric sequelae of COVID-19? Neuropsychiatric symptoms and potential immunologic mechanisms. *Brain, behavior, and immunity* 87, pp. 34–39.

United Nations Development Programme. 2020. COVID-19: Looming crisis in developing countries threatens to devastate economies and ramp up inequality. Available at: https://www.undp.org/content/undp/en/home/news-centre/news/2020/COVID19_Crisis_in_developing_countries_threatens_devastate_economies.html.

Varatharaj, A., Thomas, N., Ellul, M.A., Davies, N.W., Pollak, T.A., Tenorio, E.L., Sultan, M., Easton, A., Breen, G., Zandi, M. and Coles, J.P. 2020. Neurological and neuropsychiatric complications of COVID-19 in 153 patients: a UK-wide surveillance study. *The Lancet Psychiatry* 7(10), pp. 875–882.

Vlessides, M. 2020. COVID-19 and Psychosis: is there a link? *Medscape*. Available at: https://wwww.medscape.com/viewarticle/930224.

Wang, C., Pan, R., Wan, X., Tan, Y., Xu, L., Ho, C.S. and Ho, R.C. 2020. Immediate psychological responses and associated factors during the initial stage of the 2019 coronavirus disease (COVID-19) epidemic among the general population in China. *International journal of environmental research and public health* 17(5), p. 1729.

Winsper, C., Singh, S.P., Marwaha, S., Amos, T., Lester, H., Everard, L., Jones, P., Fowler, D., Marshall, M., Lewis, S. and Sharma, V. 2013. Pathways to violent behavior during first-episode psychosis: a report from the UK National EDEN Study. *JAMA psychiatry* 70(12), pp. 1287–1293.

Wits Professional and Ethics Standard Committee. 2020. Student practitioners in the COVID-19 crisis: Faculty and student responsibilities and the duty of care. 19 June 2020.

World Health Organization. 2020. WHO Timeline – COVID-19. Available at: https://www.who.int/news-room/detail/27-04-2020-who-timeline---covid-19.

Xiang, Y.T., Yang, Y., Li, W., Zhang, L., Zhang, Q., Cheung, T. and Ng, C.H. 2020. Timely mental health care for the 2019 novel coronavirus outbreak is urgently needed. *The Lancet Psychiatry* 7(3), pp. 228–229.

Xie, X., Xue, Q., Zhou, Y., Zhu, K., Liu, Q., Zhang, J. and Song, R. 2020. Mental health status among children in home confinement during the coronavirus disease 2019 outbreak in Hubei Province, China. *JAMA pediatrics* 174(9), pp. 898–900.

Xiong, Y. and Peng, L. 2020. Focusing on health-care providers' experiences in the COVID-19 crisis. *The Lancet Global Health.* doi: https://doi.org/10.1016/S2214-109X(20)30214-X.

Yang, Y., Li, W., Zhang, Q., Zhang, L., Cheung, T. and Xiang, Y.T. 2020. Mental health services for older adults in China during the COVID-19 outbreak. *Lancet Psychiatry* 7(4), p. e19.

Yellowlees, P., Burke, M.M., Marks, S.L., Hilty, D.M. and Shore, J.H. 2008. Emergency telepsychiatry. *Journal of telemedicine and telecare* 14(6), pp. 277–81.

Zhou, J., Liu, L., Xue, P., Yang, X. and Tang, X. 2020. Mental health response to the COVID-19 outbreak in China. American Psychiatric Association. Last Updated: 7 May 2020. Available at: https://ajp.psychiatryonline.org/doi/10.1176/appi.ajp.2020.20030304.

CHAPTER 19

PANDEMICS AND PRIMARY HEALTHCARE

Richard Cooke

19.1 INTRODUCTION

Forty years after Alma Ata, primary healthcare (PHC) remains the necessary foundation for health-related sustainable development goals and universal health coverage (WHO and UNICEF, 2018). Described as the 'whole of society approach' to health, a strong primary healthcare sector is more important than ever.

The COVID-19 pandemic arrived in South Africa as wide-spread improvement in the country's primary healthcare outcomes remains elusive (South African National Department of Health, Statistics South Africa, 2017), with the exception of Human Immunodeficiency Virus (HIV)-related indicators (South African National AIDS Council, 2017). As COVID-19 exposes both the strengths and weaknesses of any health system, turning the lens on provision of and access to PHC services in the face of a pandemic, is of key interest.

This chapter examines PHC provision, when viewed from the perspective of the South African response to the COVID-19 pandemic. The costs of COVID (direct, indirect/hidden and delayed) are considered, particularly for how they are relevant to PHC. The inadequacies and inequities associated with the actual delivery of and access to PHC are also noted, especially as laid bare by the pandemic.

This chapter describes practical approaches to readying and implementing COVID-19 responses in primary healthcare facilities. A section includes discussion of the purpose and operations of a temporary field hospital, including interrogation of the value such facilities add, in the context of the health system as a whole.

In contrast to the structural weaknesses in PHC accentuated by a disruptive pandemic, the sector may respond with necessary innovations. This chapter draws on systems thinking and complexity theory to propose novel ideas in the PHC-based response to the COVID-19 pandemic.

19.2 OBJECTIVES

The objectives of this chapter are to:

- Identify the spectrum of PHC-related costs caused by a pandemic, including direct, indirect/hidden and delayed costs.
- Highlight how a pandemic affects access to quality PHC, in the context of significant inequities in a health system.
- Describe the approach to readying a PHC facility for a pandemic response.
- Detail the operations and value of a temporary field hospital set up to assist in a COVID-19 response.
- Propose innovations to a pandemic PHC response, involving motivational behaviour, disease prevention and the allocation of human resources for health.

19.3 THE COST OF COVID-19 TO PRIMARY HEALTHCARE

Over and above the more obvious direct health-related costs of COVID-19 to individuals and communities, hidden/indirect and delayed costs paint a fuller picture of the situation. The reality is that the virus alone is not directly responsible for the overall negative impact of a pandemic.

19.3.1 The Direct Costs of COVID-19

Projections of the course of the pandemic in low/middle-income countries cast a dire picture early in the pandemic (Walker et al, 2020). At the end of May 2021, recorded COVID-19 deaths were about 950 per million population (World Health Organisation, 2012a). In South Africa, the country's recorded excess mortality at the time was roughly three times higher (South African Medical Research Council, 2021), indicating that the official statistics underestimated the number of infected people.

COVID-19 death is associated with increasing age, diabetes, hypertension and chronic kidney disease (Boulle et al, 2020). In communities with high rates of obesity and associated comorbidities the vulnerable are even more at risk. In South Africa, for example, 31% of men and 64% of women fall into the overweight or obese categories (Body Mass Index, BMI 25 kg/m^2 or more) (Shisana et al, 2013).

19.3.2 The Indirect/Hidden COVID-19 Cost to Primary Healthcare

As opposed to the direct cost of COVID-19 in the form of morbidity and mortality, some important but indirect (and often hidden) costs of COVID-19 are associated with reduced access to healthcare to meet essential needs, as well as with the specific impact of COVID-19 regulations on livelihoods.

19.3.2.1 COVID-19 and access to primary healthcare

Good quality primary healthcare is defined as first contact care, focusing on continuity of care, amongst other attributes (Starfield, Shi and Macinko, 2005). Decreased access to essential care at primary healthcare level has been a significant consequence of the COVID-19 pandemic.

Penchansky and Thomas (1981) developed a framework to describe the different dimensions of access to care. Descriptors of the dimensions help with a general understanding (Wyszewianski, 2002; Shengelia, Murray and Adams, 2003). However, consideration of these dimensions in the context of a pandemic, allows for a deeper understanding of its impact on primary healthcare.

Table 19.1 PHC access in a pandemic

Access to care	Description	COVID-19 pandemic reality
Accessibility	Distance to, and how easily the client can reach provider's location	Limited/no public transport
Affordability	How the provider's charges relate to the client's ability and willingness to pay for services	Less disposable income and medical cover due to job losses in weak economy
Accommodation	The extent to which the provider's operation is organised to meet the client's constraints and preferences	Fear/anxiety in communities of infection risk, despite PHC facility readiness
Availability	The extent to which the provider has the requisite resources (personnel and technology), to meet client's needs	Closure of facilities, absent/ill healthcare workers
Acceptability	The extent to which the client and provider are comfortable with age, sex, social class, and ethnicity, as well as the diagnosis/type of coverage	Inequities in access to care facing disadvantaged communities (poor, women, disabled persons, migrants)

Given the focus on the treatment of acute and emergency cases, ongoing control of chronic conditions, including mental health, is difficult. The mentally ill and unwell are especially compromised, as the pandemic-related social isolation is itself a precipitating factor in the development of mental illness.

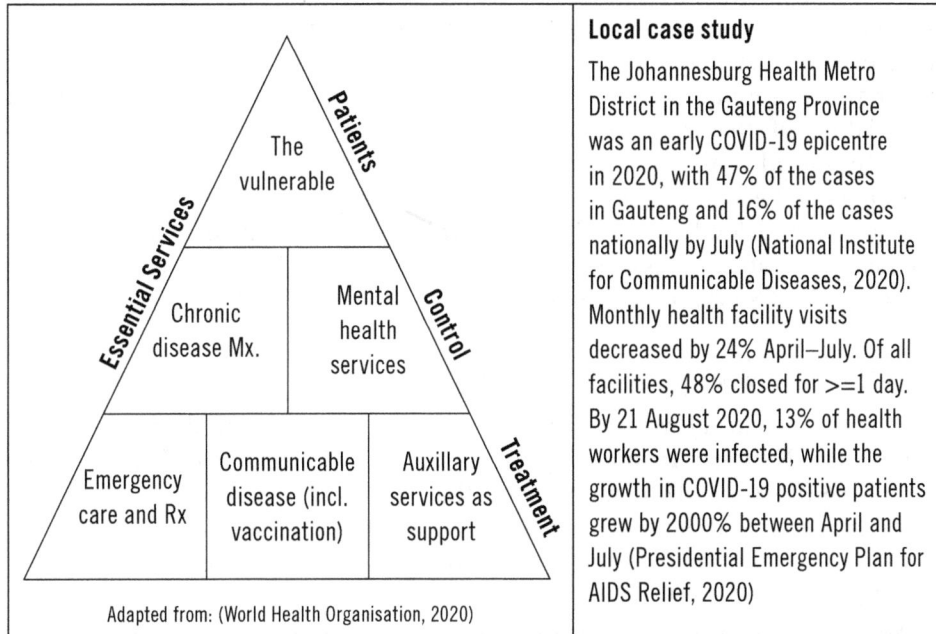

Local case study

The Johannesburg Health Metro District in the Gauteng Province was an early COVID-19 epicentre in 2020, with 47% of the cases in Gauteng and 16% of the cases nationally by July (National Institute for Communicable Diseases, 2020). Monthly health facility visits decreased by 24% April–July. Of all facilities, 48% closed for >=1 day. By 21 August 2020, 13% of health workers were infected, while the growth in COVID-19 positive patients grew by 2000% between April and July (Presidential Emergency Plan for AIDS Relief, 2020)

Adapted from: (World Health Organisation, 2020)

Figure 19.1 PHC Services in a pandemic: Essential and vulnerable

19.3.2.2 Lockdowns and primary healthcare

Reducing transmission requires fewer interactions between humans for protracted periods. To this end, a 'lockdown' introduces various measures, including travel bans, the introduction of curfews, and limitations on the number and size of gatherings indoors and outdoors (e.g. religious, educational and social gatherings). Closure of non-essential services and businesses also reduces both the number and length of interactions. Implemented to different degrees ('levels'), a lockdown reduces the direct medical 'cost' of COVID-19, in the form of the mortality and morbidity associated with the pandemic.

Lockdowns do not necessarily reduce the prevalence of infections overall; instead serve to 'flatten the curve', so reducing spikes in infection rates, allowing health services not to be overwhelmed.

Because of the relative ease of transmission of the virus, as well as the uncertainty and novelty of the COVID-19 pandemic, a broad, blunt approach was required at the outset, to influence the behaviour of all sectors of society. In South Africa, a country-wide lockdown was implemented at an early stage, compared to international trends. Epidemiologically, government did not have reason to roll out selective lockdown measures for certain communities or regions, other than at a provincial level. Due to South Africa's unequal society, such an approach would have been morally and politically unpalatable.

Notwithstanding its value in preventing transmissions, a lockdown restricts human rights. This restriction must be subject to close scrutiny to determine if it upholds the *Siracusa Principles*, a consensus on the conditions under which limitations on civil and political rights are acceptable (American Association of the International Commission of Jurists, 1985). Many legal constitutions also allow for limitations of certain rights. For example, under section 36 of the South African Constitution, the right to freedom of movement, health care and food may be limited through enforcement of a lockdown, as deemed reasonable, necessary and proportional to its purpose (Constitution of the Republic of South Africa, 1996).

19.3.2.3 The weak economy and PHC

Economic and social well-being are well-recognised social determinants of health. The National Income Dynamics Study – Coronavirus Rapid Mobile Survey (NIDS-CRAM) demonstrates that over 2.2 million jobs were lost between March and September 2020 in South Africa (Spaull et al, 2020). This is similar in magnitude to the number of jobs created in the country during the 10 years to end 2019.

NIDS–CRAM has shown that poorer workers suffered more job losses than the richest in the COVID-10 pandemic (Spaull et al, 2020). Similarly, informal workers felt the impact more than those in the formal sectors. Women and especially women of colour suffered more job losses than men did, not least because twice the number of women compared to men (roughly 3.4 million women versus 1.7 million men) indicated that looking after children during the pandemic prevented them from going to work, or made working very difficult. While the COVID-19 Social Relief of Distress grant of R350, as well as the increase in other South African grants assisted in the short term, these are only temporary measures.

19.3.3 The Delayed COVID-19 Cost to Primary Healthcare

Delayed costs may be otherwise described as the unanticipated costs that reveal the full extent of a pandemic over time. Models estimate that COVID-19-related disruptions to essential services lasting up to 12 months could lead to as many as 2.3 million additional deaths in children under the age of five in low- and middle-income countries (Roberton et al, 2020). International examples also demonstrated a reduction in both in-person visits (such as well-child visits, Papanicolaou testing, and haemoglobin A1c testing) and visits related to preventative and chronic illness to community health centres in the United States (Heintzman et al, 2020).

While the full impact by any projections are impossible to fully quantify, models predict that worldwide deaths due to HIV, tuberculosis, and malaria over the next five years will increase by up to 10%, 20%, and 36%, respectively, due to the COVID-19 pandemic (Hogan et al, 2020).

Logic suggests that interruptions to antiretroviral therapy (ARVs) would be significant, which could occur during a period of high health system demand. However, a recent South African study found that follow-up for ARV collection at 65 clinics in KwaZulu-Natal was well maintained through 2020 (Dorward et al, 2021). Yet, both the testing and ARV start numbers decreased. These findings suggest that those with pre-existing access to chronic care are less impacted than individuals still to be diagnosed and started on treatment.

For tuberculosis (TB), the greatest impact would likely be from reductions in timely diagnosis and initiation of treatment in newly diagnosed cases, caused by prolonged periods of COVID-19 suppression interventions. The greatest impact on the malaria burden could be due to the interruption of planned net campaigns. These disruptions could lead to a loss of life-years lived over the next five years that is of the same order as the impact from the COVID-19 pandemic in places with a high burden of malaria, HIV and TB (Hogan et al, 2020).

A recent estimate suggests that if the COVID-19 pandemic led to a reduction of 25% in expected TB detection for three months – which is a realistic possibility given the levels of disruption in TB services being observed in multiple countries – that a 13% increase in TB deaths can be expected. This would bring the level of TB mortality back to those observed five years ago. This translated means that between 2020 and 2025, an additional 1.4 million TB deaths could occur as a consequence of the COVID-19 pandemic (Roberton et al, 2020).

In terms of mental health, a review of 28 articles from seven countries (Rajkumar, 2020), an Italian study early on in the global pandemic (Delmastro and Zamariola, 2020), and a more qualitative local South African study (Human Sciences Research Council, 2020) provide evidence of a significant increase in anxiety, depression and other mental health disorders, due to the pandemic.

The longer-term health of children is also compromised. Only 25% of respondents in the NIDS-CRAMS survey indicated that a child received a school meal in the previous seven days compared to 80% pre-COVID.

The distinction between indirect or hidden and delayed costs is somewhat arbitrary; these costs may overlap. Many of the effects on the health and welfare of individuals facing a weak economy, for example, may only manifest in the long term. Mental health may deteriorate over time, for example, or a family living close to the breadline may cope for a protracted period, before chronic health problems surface. The state of the economy influences many different social determinants of health.

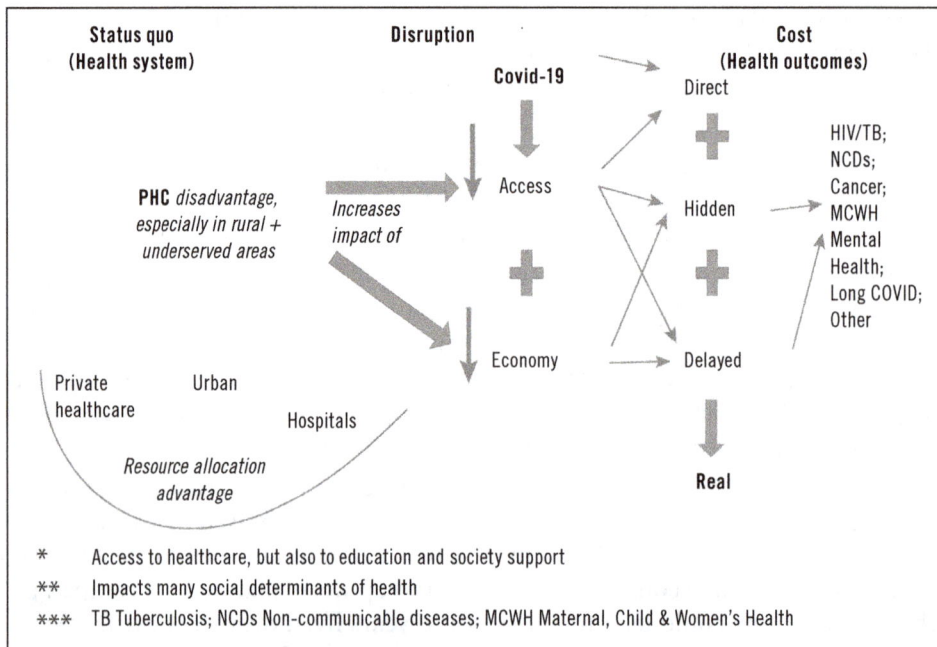

Figure 19.2 The cost of COVID-19

19.4 PHC FACILITY READINESS

Each country may adopt different approaches to designate and support essential services during a pandemic. Generally, however, identification of infected and symptomatic individuals is critical; a process that ironically brings these individuals in contact with the health service, and therefore in contact with other people who may be vulnerable to contract the disease. A balanced and structured approach to primary healthcare services is required to keep staff and patients safe, while allowing normal healthcare services to continue as best possible, but diagnosing and treating COVID-19 patients efficiently and effectively.

A PHC facility readiness programme in Johannesburg, South Africa, identified 10 essential components to set up a facility (Wilkinson et al, 2020) which when combined with the use of personal protective equipment, minimise the risk of the spread of infection to patients and healthcare workers (HCWs). Patients need to use a single point of entry to the premises, after which each attends the sanitation station. After a first screening, the patients with symptoms of COVID-19 visit a 2nd screening and management station, followed by a visit to an HIV testing station and a specialised clinical service station if required. Testing for COVID-19 and TB then completes the visit in **five** steps for these symptomatic patients, who will leave by a separate exit to other patients. The patients without COVID-19 symptoms attend the sanitation station before accessing the routine primary healthcare services of the clinic.

A clinic operating during a pandemic has **four** main purposes. First, to protect patients from COVID-19 infection, to protect healthcare workers from infection, to allow health facilities to continue to deliver health services and to facilitate COVID-19 testing, referral and management.

Flow of patients and staff is critical to ensure as little interaction between symptom-positive and symptom-negative patients as possible. There should be as few service points as possible, and patients need to spend as little time as possible at the facility.

Setting up **three** zones in the facility, clearly labelled based on a system of coloured markings, helps to manage the flow of patients and healthcare workers.

Table 19.2 Managing PHC patient flow in a pandemic

Patient flow	Zoning	COVID-19 risk
	Yellow (outside entrance)	Indeterminate
	Orange (tents/prefab)	High-risk (symptom +ve)
	Blue (clinic)	Low(er)-risk (symptom −ve)
Orange zone: COVID-19 high-risk zone for symptom positive patients	**Tasks**	
	Assess severity of the symptoms, and manage/refer accordingly	
	Determine need for COVID-19 testing using current Patient- Under-Investigation (PUI) definition	
	Provide counselling on home isolation and patient information leaflet	
	Establish HIV status to determine TB risk (test both)	
	Address reason for clinic attendance	

Preparation of facilities needs resources; allocating each to one of **two** groups (priority and non-priority) in the sub-district/district allows the prioritising of the bigger PHC facilities in the catchment area according to agreed criteria (e.g. larger facilities may be targeted first). This is helpful from a project management perspective.

No health facility operates in isolation. Strengthening the referral systems (both up and down) increases efficiencies and effectiveness of the service in a pandemic. Liaising with the community to educate them about the preparedness of the clinics is also vital to the project's success. All stakeholders therefore engage together collaboratively, operating as **one** single health system.

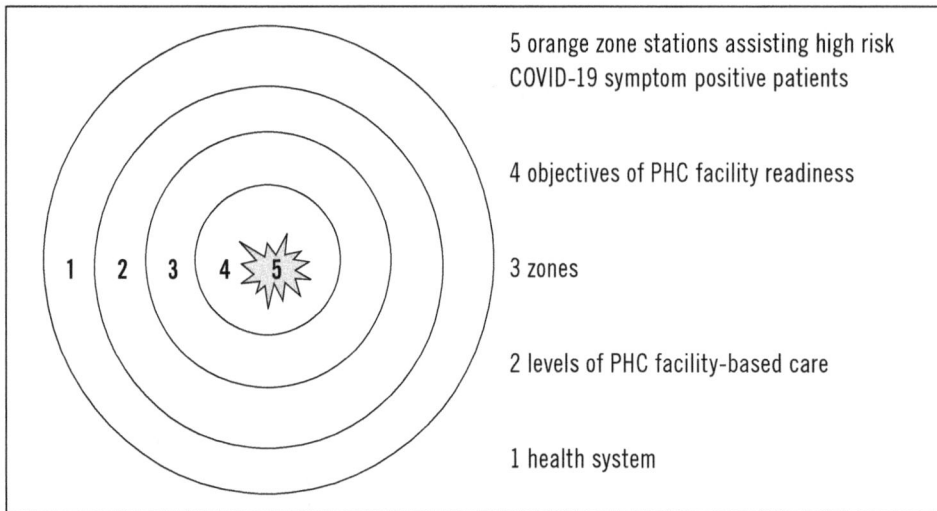

Figure 19.3 Memory aid: Preparation of PHC facilities

19.4.1   The Doctor-Patient Consultation During a Pandemic

The family medicine discipline, itself linked strongly to primary healthcare, promotes the practice of patient-centred care, as ethically mandatory, and often helpful in improving health outcomes, both related to the clinical picture and to patient satisfaction (Rathert, Wyrwich and Boren, 2013).

The COVID-19 pandemic has accentuated a very common, but often unrecognised reality; the respective agendas' of provider and the ambulatory patient often differ. On the one hand, there is an urgency and focus required to manage a pandemic. In the previous example of COVID-19 facility readiness, patients are often bluntly 'zoned' into homogenous groups, differing only if they have symptoms suggestive of COVID-19. Conversely, many symptom-positive patients have attended the clinic with a different primary healthcare need. While prioritising the investigation and management of their presenting symptoms, such patients receive assistance as comprehensively and practically as possible. This includes requesting a blue zone healthcare worker visit an orange zone patient to address individual patients' needs. Anecdotal evidence suggests this approach builds collaboration and satisfaction, and promotes access to care.

19.5   TEMPORARY FIELD FACILITIES 'FIELD HOSPITALS'

Dealing with a pandemic places severe pressure on service delivery. Temporary field healthcare facilities are set up to allow the health system to cope during periods of peak demand associated with pandemics.

Home isolation is an important alternative to hospital isolation in such field facilities, but is often psychologically or practically difficult for patients. The original COVID-19 pandemic field hospitals, the Fangcang shelter hospitals in Wuhan, China, were developed with this in mind (Chen et al, 2020).

Field hospitals are also set up to provide higher levels of medical care. Key to providing this functionality is the availability of skilled human resources, equipment and support services to run the services. A field hospital is often a simple structure (e.g. a big exhibition hall), limited with respect to the dedicated space available for different services, e.g. radiology or laboratory. Mobile point-of-care investigations are required, supported by agile and frequent courier systems to and from more established facilities.

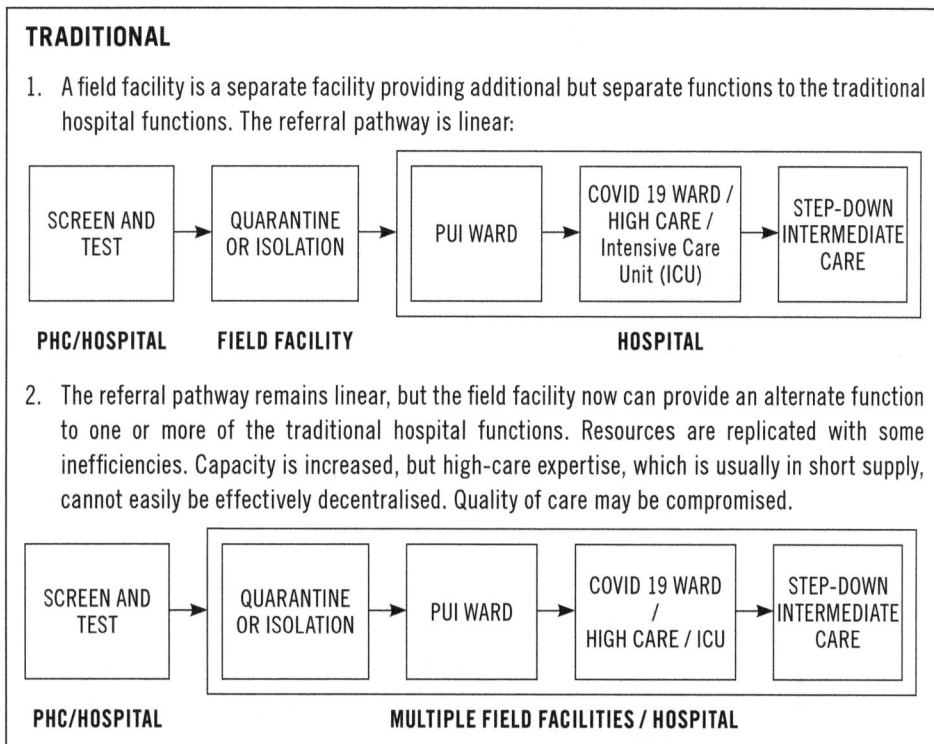

TRADITIONAL

1. A field facility is a separate facility providing additional but separate functions to the traditional hospital functions. The referral pathway is linear:

SCREEN AND TEST → QUARANTINE OR ISOLATION → PUI WARD → COVID 19 WARD / HIGH CARE / Intensive Care Unit (ICU) → STEP-DOWN INTERMEDIATE CARE

PHC/HOSPITAL **FIELD FACILITY** **HOSPITAL**

2. The referral pathway remains linear, but the field facility now can provide an alternate function to one or more of the traditional hospital functions. Resources are replicated with some inefficiencies. Capacity is increased, but high-care expertise, which is usually in short supply, cannot easily be effectively decentralised. Quality of care may be compromised.

SCREEN AND TEST → QUARANTINE OR ISOLATION → PUI WARD → COVID 19 WARD / HIGH CARE / ICU → STEP-DOWN INTERMEDIATE CARE

PHC/HOSPITAL **MULTIPLE FIELD FACILITIES / HOSPITAL**

ALTERNATIVE

3. Hospitals are relieved of the lower care functions of isolation and step-down, intermediate care. Additional resources capacitate the high-care/ICU services at tertiary hospitals. Referral is now a circular pathway, as Quarantine & Isolation (Q&I) and step-down intermediate care are combined in one field hospital. This improves the clinical governance of patients in the district-based field hospital(s).

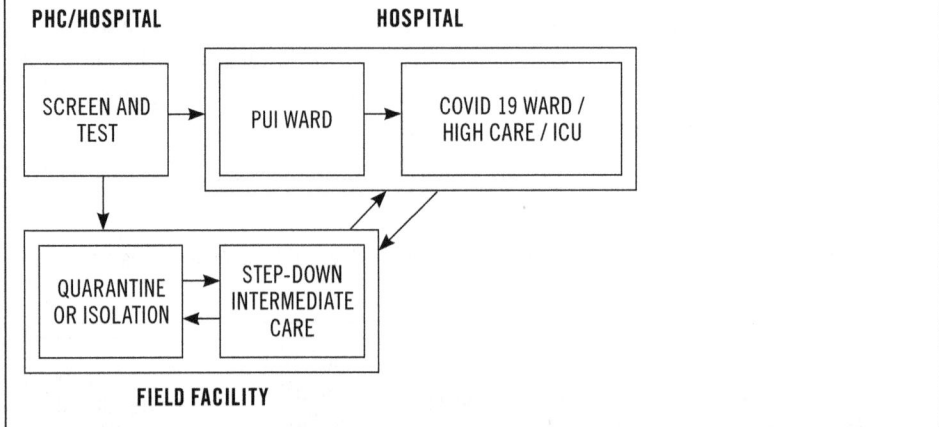

Figure 19.4 The 'system fit' of temporary health facilities in a pandemic

Patients favoured for a field hospital are (i) step-down, and/or (ii) stable, on a predictable, improving trend, and/or (iii) higher-acuity exceptions where risk is mitigated.

Converted from a series of exhibition halls, the Nasrec field hospital opened in April 2020 as a bespoke 500-bed isolation and quarantine site to accommodate those who could not self-isolate or quarantine at home. It was later expanded to include 1 000 beds for 'priority 3 patients' informed by projected infection peak numbers anticipated for August 2020. Since opening, 1 658 patients were admitted to the field hospital: 1 254 clients were admitted for isolation, 117 for quarantine and 287 as priority 3 'oxygen bed' patients. Other than management of the COVID-19-specific clinical picture as a continuation the hospital care, patient services included:

- Diabetic management: Introduction of tight sugar control with twice-daily insulin, empowering patients to self-manage. An external service provider assisted with telephonic support for three months post-discharge.

- Family liaison service: A dedicated support service connecting with a patient's family from NASREC admission date, to ensure safe discharge with a fully informed patient and family.

- Therapeutic services: Occupational health and physiotherapy services, in individual and group sessions.

- Mental health services: Provision of psychological first aid by clinicians at Nasrec, and a psychologist to run individual/group sessions.

The Nasrec Field Hospital was decommissioned on 28 February 2021, in favour of utilising existing government health infrastructure.

Figure 19.5 Local case study: Nasrec Field Hospital

The value-add of any healthcare service should be measured by the quality of care provided to patients. The table below considers a different aspect of care, in consideration of the benefits and limitations of a field hospital, within the context of the health system.

Table 19.3 The value-add of a field hospital

ASPECT OF CARE	BENEFIT	RATIONALE
Continuity	Significant	Operates as an auxiliary service, whether or not operating separately to a parent. Provides capacity to continue lower-acuity care under less time pressures, by transfer from regional/tertiary COVID wards. May also facilitate on-referral from PHC to secondary/tertiary, through temporary admission, in select circumstances.

➡

ASPECT OF CARE	BENEFIT	RATIONALE
Efficiency	Limited	All systems (HR, clinical equip/tech, laundry, catering, waste removal, etc.) have to be resourced/financed. Services need to be dedicated and therefore duplicated. Services come online iteratively, not all at once. Improved bed utilisation rate (BUR) and average length of stay (ALOS) at referral facility, but cost/benefit ratios will not necessarily be improved for the system overall.
Effectiveness	Limited/ Significant	Assists in freeing up beds, therefore helps manage demand for (and outcomes of) higher acuity care at referral (transfer) facility. If the benchmark is mortality, then only directly effective if replicating high-care/ICU care to cope with unpredictable demand. Otherwise, it will assist in allowing compartmentalising levels of care (clinical management matches level of care) for better outcomes overall. Unplanned readmissions will likely be reduced, if geographically close to 'parent' facility.
Integration	Significant	Facilitates better preparation for back-referral to PHC/ DHS. Allows for a holistic approach to mental health interventions, family liaison project, patient rehabilitation programme, patient education and chronic disease management before discharge.
Agility	Significant	Provides clinicians with the necessary agility to respond to patients' clinical progression (improvement/deterioration) with up/down referral. Favours the lower-acuity patient, and/ or patient with more certain prognosis (e.g. step-down vs patients under investigation (PUIs)). Helped if geographically close to parent/referring facilities.
Overall		The aim of a field hospital is to complement, rather than substitute, other services as interdependent components within the health system. Does not simply add value to a measure of the extra beds the facility houses. The benefits are selective, and conditional on a working partnership with the 'parent' facility/facilities. A field hospital cannot substitute for, nor simply duplicate COVID-related capacity of a regional/tertiary/quaternary service. The sustainability required of a field hospital to offer COVID-related services requires timely and careful review, dependent on the progression of the pandemic, and the relative needs of other under-resourced healthcare services. On closing or scaling back between 'pandemic waves', the possibility of wasted resources on a white elephant must be balanced with the challenges of an agile response when needed.

19.6 INNOVATIONS IN COVID-19 RESPONSES

Systems thinking involves the study of systems as a whole with specific analysis of all interrelated parts (Waters Foundation, 2018). Viewing a pandemic from multiple perspectives is key to understanding the gaps and bringing about solutions to manage the crisis. This is arguably most applicable for primary healthcare, as a complex and multi-dimensional system.

Complexity science expands on the reductionistic framework by not only understanding the parts that contribute to the whole but by understanding how each part interacts with all the other parts (Turner and Baker, 2019). Such an understanding promotes innovation, so countering the impacts of a pandemic.

19.6.1 Innovations in Education/Messages Regarding Adherence to COVID-19 Regulations

In public health messaging during a pandemic, promoting the individual choice of the patient is key to patient-centeredness and improved patient satisfaction. Messages focusing on the prevention of disease are attractive to recipients, implying negative consequences can be avoided.

Levels of prevention of disease, namely primordial, primary, secondary, tertiary and quaternary levels are well-described (Baumann and Karel, 2013). COVID-19- related interventions may be compared at each level of prevention, considered for each of the intervention target (individual vs. community), severity of illness, degree of medical intervention and – critically – individual choice. While primordial prevention measures are implemented by the state, primary prevention is the current focus for influencing individuals' behaviour in a viral pandemic. Vaccination is a key primary prevention measure, and is once-off (disregarding vaccination boosters). Other primary prevention measures (social distancing, hand hygiene, wearing facemasks) are difficult to promote successfully, especially in the face of significant COVID-19 fatigue. Secondary prevention involves screening for asymptomatic illness (for example, oxygen saturation levels); tertiary prevention is more serious still. Considering the consequences, the reality is that each level is more serious and difficult to manage than the former, with the exception of the primary prevention.

Adopting an empathetic and respectful approach is critical; the client still has autonomy of choice in the provider-patient relationship. The appeal of this measure of individual choice early pre-diagnosis is significant. Once past the primary prevention measures in the progression of illness, the patient autonomy reduces, as the provider necessarily takes on the greater share of the decision-making around the illness. The diagram below captures the limited opportunity for personal choice, in the face of government regulations initially, followed by the possibility of increasing acuity once the diagnosis is made.

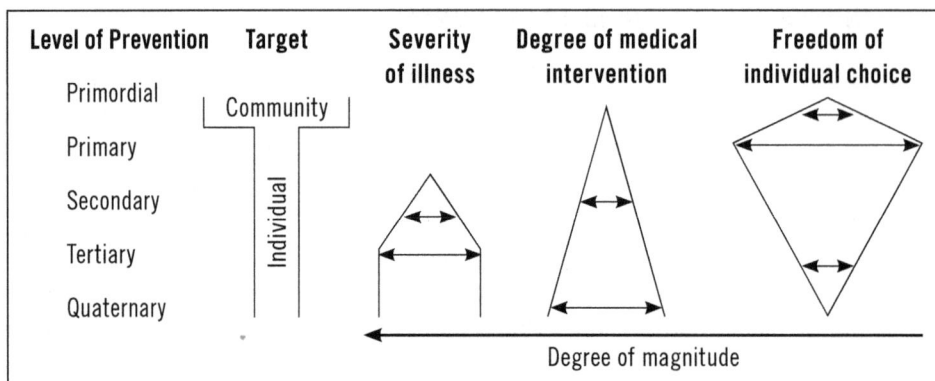

Figure 19.6 Human behaviour in a pandemic: Framing choice and consequence

19.6.2 Innovations in Human Resources

A pandemic forces resource allocation to be based on need. The South Korean response to the COVID-19 pandemic provides an interesting case study of a rapid response by deploying 'public health doctors', who were doing community service in lieu of mandatory military service (Choi, 2020).

South African health managers should consider more efficient and cost-effective human resourcing solutions as demand on the system outstrips the capacity to respond. Well-researched but poorly implemented interventions are now gaining traction:

- The importance of a multidisciplinary team is typically undervalued, but well established as an effective tool; task shifting and sharing must be a priority (World Health Organization, 2008).
- The cost-effectiveness of mid-level healthcare workers, such as clinical associates, especially in district settings, is well-established (Tshabalala et al, 2019).
- Healthcare workers eligible for mandatory service, such as community service in South Africa, must be allocated and funded on the basis of need and equity, based on objectively verifiable indicators such as the deprivation index or vacancy rates by district (Reid, 2018), or COVID-19 pressure on service delivery.

19.6.3 Innovation in Infection Prevention and Control

In an effort to reduce COVID-19 transmission amongst South African healthcare workers in PHC, managers differentiated between low-risk and high-risk clinical settings. As the pandemic evolved, low-risk transmission settings became high-risk as the number of infected persons grew. The approach to personal protective equipment (PPE) changed to focus on the appropriate equipment for the type of clinical engagement, irrespective of the type of clinical setting.

19.6.4 **Innovation in Vaccination Strategies**

Vaccination is a key primary healthcare intervention, affording recipients proven protection against serious COVID-19 illness, hospitalisation and death. Vaccinating as many of the population as quickly as possible is critical, beginning with the more vulnerable groups. The Johannesburg Metro Health District vaccination strategy is informed by identifying 'touch points', for when community members do and do not interact with the health system. A vaccination action plan follows, aided for the simplicity of a come-2-us vs go-2-you (us = provider) approach.

Table 19.4 Come-2-us vs go-2-you approach

COME- 2-US Ordinarily many/regular touchpoints		GO-2-YOU Ordinarily few/irregular touchpoints
Health Facilities		Congregate (old age homes)
Non-medical sites		Fixed (migrants)
Special (site-relevant) – Mobility + Convenience (Drive thru) – Promotion by activists/sector leaders – Queue priority criteria – Conducive to volunteer programme – Catering/Med waste/Security separate		Special (vaccinee-relevant) – Mobility (e.g. frail care/wards) – Remote (e.g. rural) – Equity (e.g. migrants)
Larger sites 1) Waiting area 2) Screening 3) Covid testing and mx 4) Registration 5) Verification	6) Count & Label 7) Queue & Educ. 8) Vaccination 9) Pharmacy 10) Observation 11) Resuscitation 12) ICT	**Smaller mobile vaccination teams** 1) Transport 2) Cooler box 3) Vaccines (prefer 1 dose regimen) 4) Tablet + Data+ paper back/up 5) PPE 6) Map app + partner

19.7 CONCLUSION

Pandemics are catastrophes that cause untold losses to the health of individuals, families and communities. The full impact of COVID-19 will not be known for years to come. The consequences of this pandemic for PHC, as the 'front door of the health care system' (World Health Organisation, 2021b) distinguish this sector as both vulnerable yet critically important. This chapter has covered some of the unfortunate PHC realities laid bare by the pandemic, but has also detailed pragmatic approaches to delivering PHC, supported by some innovative and systems-oriented thinking.

While COVID-19 is a global crisis, the status quo has been disrupted; perhaps the aspirations of primary healthcare as the key to securing improved health for individuals, families and communities, may still be realised in South Africa and beyond.

19.8 SELF-ASSESSMENT QUESTIONS

1. In what ways does a COVID-19 pandemic directly and indirectly affect access to primary healthcare services?
2. Explain what is meant by the phrases 'agility of response' and 'continuity of care' with respect to the value that a field hospital may provide to a COVID-19 referral hospital.

19.9 REFERENCES

American Association of the International Commission of Jurists (1985) 'Siracusa Principles', in, p. 25.

Baumann, L.C. and Karel, A. 2013. Prevention: Primary, Secondary, Tertiary. In M.D. Gellman and J.R. Turner (Eds) *Encyclopedia of Behavioral Medicine*. New York, NY: Springer New York, pp. 1532–1534. doi:10.1007/978-1-4419-1005-9_135.

Boulle, A., et al. 2020. Risk factors for COVID-19 death in a population cohort study from the Western Cape Province, South Africa. *Clinical Infectious Diseases* [Preprint]. doi:10.1093/cid/ciaa1198.

Chen, S., et al. 2020. Fangcang shelter hospitals: a novel concept for responding to public health emergencies. *The Lancet* 395(10232), pp. 1305–1314. doi:10.1016/S0140-6736(20)30744-3.

Choi, S. 2020. A Hidden Key to COVID-19 Management in Korea: Public Health Doctors. *Journal of Preventive Medicine and Public Health* 53(3), pp. 175–177. doi:10.3961/jpmph.20.105.

Constitution of the Republic of South Africa [No. 108 of 1996] (1996), (38), p. 107.

Delmastro, M. and Zamariola, G. 2020. Depressive symptoms in response to COVID-19 and lockdown: a cross-sectional study on the Italian population. *Scientific Reports* 10(1), p. 22457. doi:10.1038/s41598-020-79850-6.

Heintzman, J., et al. 2020. SARS-CoV-2 Testing and Changes in Primary Care Services in a Multistate Network of Community Health Centers During the COVID-19 Pandemic. *JAMA* 324(14), p. 1459. doi:10.1001/jama.2020.15891.

Hogan, A.B., et al. 2020. Potential impact of the COVID-19 pandemic on HIV, tuberculosis, and malaria in low-income and middle-income countries: a modelling study. *The Lancet. Global Health* 8(9), pp. e1132–e1141. doi:10.1016/S2214-109X(20)30288-6.

Human Sciences Research Council. 2020. Remember our mental health during the lockdown: the voices behind the numbers. Available at: http://www.hsrc.ac.za/en/research-outputs/view/10653.

Penchansky, R. and Thomas, J.W. 1981. The concept of access: definition and relationship to consumer satisfaction. *Medical Care* 19(2), pp. 127–140. doi:10.1097/00005650-198102000-00001.

Presidential Emergency Plan for AIDS Relief. 2020. PEPFAR Jhb Metro Report COVID-19 Report.

Rathert, C., Wyrwich, M.D. and Boren, S.A. 2013. Patient-centered care and outcomes: a systematic review of the literature. *Medical care research and review: MCRR* 70(4), pp. 351–379. doi:10.1177/1077558712465774.

Reid, S. 2018. South Africa: what have we learnt? *South African Health Review*, p. 10.

Roberton, T., et al. 2020. Early estimates of the indirect effects of the COVID-19 pandemic on maternal and child mortality in low-income and middle-income countries: a modelling study. *The Lancet. Global Health* 8(7), pp. e901–e908. doi:10.1016/S2214-109X(20)30229-1.

Shengelia, B., Murray, C.J.L., Adams, O.B. Beyond access and utilization: defining and measuring health system coverage. In Health System Performance Assessment. Debates, methods and empiricism. edited by Murray CJL, Evans DB. Geneva: World Health Organisation: 2003:221-234.

Shisana, et al. 2013. South African National Health and Nutrition Examination Survey (SANHANES-1). HSRC Press.

South African National AIDS Council. 2017. National Strategic Plan on HIV, TB and STIs 2017–2022. Pretoria: SANAC; 2017.

South African National Department of Health, Statistics South Africa. 2017. South African Demographic and Health Survey 2016: Key Indicators Report.

Spaull, et al. 2020. *NIDS-CRAM-Wave2-Synthesis Report*.

Tshabalala, Z., et al. 2019. Clinical associates in South Africa: optimising their contribution to the health system, p. 10.

Turner, J.R. and Baker, R.M. 2019. Complexity Theory: An Overview with Potential Applications for the Social Sciences. *Systems* 7(1), p. 4. doi:10.3390/systems7010004.

Walker, P.G.T., et al. 2020. The impact of COVID-19 and strategies for mitigation and suppression in low- and middle-income countries. *Science*, p. eabc0035. doi:10.1126/science.abc0035.

Waters Foundation. 2018. What is Systems thinking?, Waters Center for systems thinking. Available at: https://www.watersfoundation.org/systems-thinking-tools-and-strategies/what-is-systems-thinking/.

WHO and UNICEF. 2018. A vision for Primary Health Care in the 21st Century. Towards universal health coverage and the sustainable development goals.

Wilkinson, L.S., et al. 2020. Preparing healthcare facilities to operate safely and effectively during the COVID-19 pandemic: The missing piece in the puzzle. *South African Medical Journal = Suid-Afrikaanse Tydskrif Vir Geneeskunde* 110(9), pp. 835–836. doi:10.7196/SAMJ.2020.v110i9.150.

World Health Organization. 2008. Task shifting: global recommendations and guidelines. Available at: https://www.who.int/workforcealliance/knowledge/resources/taskshifting_guidelines/en/.

World Health Organization. 2020. Maintaining essential health services: operational guidance for the COVID-19 context Interim Guidance. Available at: https://www.who.int/publications-detail-redirect/WHO-2019-nCoV-essential-health-services-2020.1.

World Health Organization. 2021a. COVID-19 Weekly Epidemiological Update. Edition 42.

World Health Organization. 2021b. Primary Health Care Fact Sheet. Fact Sheet. Available at: https://www.who.int/news-room/fact-sheets/detail/primary-health-care.

Wyszewianski, L., 2002. Access to care: Remembering old lessons. Health Services Research, 37(6), p.1441. Available at: https://www.ncbi.nlm.nih.gov/pmc/articles/PMC1464050/pdf/hesr_edit.pdf.

CHAPTER 20

PANDEMICS AND CRITICAL CARE

Mervyn Mer

Nathan D. Nielsen

20.1 INTRODUCTION

Pandemics and large-scale outbreaks of infectious disease present huge challenges to healthcare systems and in particular to policymakers, public health authorities, clinicians and all healthcare workers. Large numbers of afflicted patients are likely to overwhelm hospital systems, including, importantly, critical care services. The recent COVID-19 pandemic has resulted in an unprecedented number of patients who have required hospital and intensive care unit (ICU) admission, and underscored the relevance and importance of critical care as a discipline. Critical care units are a vital and integral component of pandemic preparedness, providing care to seriously ill patients, many of whom may require organ support. Safe and effective critical care has the potential to improve outcomes, motivate individuals to seek medical attention timeously, and attenuate the devastating sequelae of a severe pandemic. In order to achieve this, suitable planning and preparation are essential. Various excellent publications, guidelines and suggested approaches to ICU pandemic preparedness and organisation have been published in recent years – the additional reading list at the end of this chapter can be consulted for these. This chapter discusses the key principles and strategies that can be used to better prepare critical care services during a pandemic. Many of the lessons learned pertaining to critical care have emanated from recent experiences with the COVID-19 pandemic.

20.2 OBJECTIVES

The objectives of this chapter are:
- To highlight pandemics as inevitable occurrences.
- To underscore advance planning, clear lines of communication, and consistent messaging as essential.
- To discuss why critical care services and staff are an integral and vital component of all pandemic preparation, planning and healthcare delivery.

- To describe the 6 'S's' (Staff, Stuff, Space, Systems, Support, Sustainability) as crucial elements which need to be adequately addressed in pandemic management.
- To emphasise the need to learn from past mistakes in order to optimise for the future.

20.3 HISTORY

More human beings have died from infectious disease than as a consequence of any other entity. The emergence and spread of infectious disease with pandemic potential have occurred regularly throughout history (Humermovic et al, 2019). Conditions such as plague, cholera, influenza, severe acute respiratory syndrome coronavirus (SARS-CoV), Middle East respiratory syndrome coronavirus (MERS-CoV), Ebola virus disease and most recently, coronavirus disease 2019 (COVID-19) have infected vast numbers of individuals and resulted in millions of deaths (Piret and Boivin, 2021; Christian et al, 2007). They have also highlighted the capacity of certain pathogens for rapid transmission and spread as well as the risks posed to healthcare workers. The polio scourge of 1952 marked the start of intensive care medicine and the use of mechanical ventilation outside the operating theatre, a pivotal step that has saved many lives and revolutionised medicine (Lassen, 1953; Reisner-Senelar, 2011; Kelly, 2011).

20.4 TERMINOLOGY

Various terms and definitions are necessary to understand in order to better inform and assist in optimising decisions by those involved in pandemic planning. These include the terms 'outbreak', 'epidemic', 'pandemic', 'critical illness' and 'intensive care unit'.

Outbreaks refer to local increases in disease incidence which may place a significant burden on a healthcare facility or healthcare facilities in a particular region. Epidemics are similar to outbreaks but generally involve larger geographic areas and have a greater potential impact on healthcare services. A pandemic relates to an epidemic that affects multiple areas and regions of the world (Kelly, 2011).

Critical illness is defined as a state of ill health in which vital organ dysfunction is present and where a high risk of imminent death exists. It is the most severe form of acute illness due to any underlying disorder and results in millions of deaths globally annually (Adhikari et al, 2010; Rudd et al, 2020; Razzak et al, 2019). Improving the way healthcare manages critical illness has the potential to save countless lives (Weil and Tang, 2011; Marshall et al, 2017; Schell et al, 2019).

An intensive care unit is an organised system for the provision of care to critically ill patients which provides intensive and specialised medical and nursing care, an enhanced capacity for monitoring, and multiple modalities of physiologic organ support to sustain life during a period of life-threatening organ system insufficiency. Although an ICU may be based in a designated and defined area of a hospital, its activities often extend beyond the walls of the physical space to include the emergency department, hospital ward and follow-up clinic. Various levels of ICU capacity and capability are recognised. These definitions and descriptions can inform healthcare decision-makers in planning and measuring capacity and provide clinicians and patients with a benchmark to evaluate the level of resources available for clinical care (Marshall et al, 2017).

An understanding of these terms has important implications for optimal pandemic preparation and planning.

20.5 KEY ELEMENTS INVOLVED IN PLANNING AND PRINCIPLES OF ICU PROCESSES: THE 'S's'

Several key elements are discussed which are relevant to ameliorate surge capacity and address important aspects pertinent to pandemics with respect to critical care service planning. The COVID-19 pandemic, in particular, and many of the important lessons learned from it and other pandemics, epidemics and outbreaks, have helped to inform a better understanding of what is required. These elements are best considered as the 'S's' (see Figure 1).

The 'S's'

- Staff – supply, safety, 'scarce resource'
- Stuff – supply requirements, consumable and equipment availability
- Space – critical care and critical care practice outside of formally designated ICUs
- Systems – organisational aspects, standard of care, triage, ethics
- Support – elements to address burnout
- Sustainability

Figure 20.1 Key components for critical care pandemic planning, preparation and delivery

20.5.1 Staff

In pandemic conditions, all elements of the healthcare system are placed under additional and often overwhelming stress, and this includes healthcare personnel. The demands generated by a sharp rise in patient numbers and additional challenges posed by the pandemic illness place substantive stress on healthcare workers who may already be functioning in less than ideal conditions at baseline.

Several important considerations must be taken into account when appraising the *Staff* element: (1) essential healthcare staffing incorporates far more than nurses and physicians; (2) different considerations apply to the allocation of different types of healthcare staff; (3) healthcare workers (HCWs) are not readily exchangeable and often are not able to move freely across regional or national borders; (4) HCWs are among the individuals at highest risk during pandemic conditions while simultaneously being among the most difficult to replace should they fall ill.

Modern healthcare is far more complex than just the workings of physicians and nurses – a hospital providing critical care services requires the contributions of allied health professionals and other professionals (such as pharmacists, dieticians, physiotherapists, occupational therapists, respiratory therapists, social workers, chaplaincy staff) and infrastructure staff (including physical plant engineers, environmental engineers, medical device maintenance, housekeepers, food services, laundry services, mortuary services and security personnel amongst others). As patient numbers rise rapidly, the additional workload and demands placed on all these roles increase and expanded staffing (and staffing "backup") plans are as essential to hospital functioning as those for physicians or nurses.

When it comes to direct patient care, another set of considerations apply – due to the nature of their work and required 'hands on time', ideal nurse to patient ratios as may be the norm, may no longer be possible. This may be compounded as patient admission numbers rise by insufficient available skilled nurses – simply put, too many patients, not enough nurses. Similar elements pertain to the number of available physicians and critical care trained specialists. This has the potential to impact on the quality and personalisation of care, increase errors, and enhance the risk of staff burnout. Hospital administrators and planners must be cognisant of these hugely relevant facts, and plan accordingly. It is important to recognise that whilst it may be necessary to 'do more with less', it is just as relevant to ensure that 'less is not done for more' (Mer, 2021).

Not all healthcare workers possess the same skill set – specifically, not all physicians or nurses have the skills, experience or psychological makeup to function at a satisfactory level in the critical care setting, especially as mortality rates begin to climb. Critical care specialists in medicine, nursing and allied health professions are trained to deal with emergencies and acutely ill patients and situations, and while other professionals may be redeployed from other locations and pressed into service, they may not function at the same level as those trained formally in critical care. Some may not be able to function in this arena at all. Another challenge is that the healthcare workforce is not a freely mobile one – matters of licensure, credentialing, and even immigration status can limit the movement of healthcare workers from a location under less stress to a location that is in need. As pandemic waves strike regions and nations at differing times, initiatives to facilitate the mobility of the healthcare workforce to areas in crisis are essential in order to reduce the stress on personnel on the ground. In view of many of these elements, as well as experience gleaned from the COVID-19 pandemic, critical care staff have been referred to as a 'scarce resource'.

A final consideration in the *Staff* element is the acknowledgement of the risks that healthcare workers face in pandemic conditions. In every pandemic, among the most vulnerable are front-line HCWs and any death amongst this group may impact adversely on the collective psyche of these professionals, adding an additional set of fears and stressors on a workforce already under duress. Each individual lost to either convalescence or death generates a trickle-down effect on their colleagues – be it additional shifts to be covered or more patients to be seen. Hospitals that cannot adequately protect their staff in pandemic conditions are at progressive risk for collapse due to simple attrition, and administrators must appreciate their staff as the finite, precious resource that they are.

20.5.2   Stuff

This aspect pertains to the supply requirements necessary to deal with a pandemic and relates to both relevant consumables, including pharmaceuticals, as well as to appropriate equipment required to support patients.

If, as Napoleon stated, 'An army travels on its stomach', then a pandemic hospital travels on its PPE (Personal Protective Equipment). Not only is a reliable supply of PPE a prerequisite for healthcare workers to safely perform their daily tasks, but it also is essential for the maintenance of staff morale and of confidence that they are valued and protected. The lack of proper PPE is one of the major factors leading to HCW attrition, due to either potentially preventable infection or due to fear of the same.

It should be noted that not all PPE is the same – depending on the pathogen involved, different types of equipment may be required. For example, an airborne pathogen requires a certain set of protective equipment as compared to a blood-borne one; a droplet-transmitted pathogen requires different precautions than an aerosolised one. Proper PPE planning for future pandemics needs to account for the differing requirements posed by a wide range of potential pathogens, and not only re-prepare based on the last pandemic.

Maintaining a reliable and flexible supply chain of PPE to strained healthcare facilities is thus of tantamount importance – breakdowns in supply can affect HCW morale and availability, but also lead to in-hospital patient-to-patient transmission of infection or to iatrogenic complications such as in-hospital acquired infection. Supply chains must be flexible in order to maintain safe working conditions during surges in patient numbers as well as to meet unexpected increases in demand.

Other *Stuff* to be accounted for in pandemic preparation is dependent on the nature of the infection that results. A pathogen such as SARS-CoV-2 that predominantly causes respiratory failure led to a demand for mechanical ventilators; other pathogens may generate a similar demand in dialysis machines or blood purification technologies; still others in intravenous fluids, antibiotics or immune-system modulating therapies. A fully functioning supply chain should be able to rapidly adapt to the unique medical challenges posed by rampant pathogen spread and be able to ensure an equitable and timely distribution of such life support materials.

20.5.3 Space

Traditionally, the practice of critical care has occurred in a designated and defined space within a hospital. The COVID-19 pandemic has resulted in a global re-imagining of the critical care *Space* – both within and without the traditional ICU setting. Within the ICU, non-traditional spaces (closets, treatment rooms, offices, hallways) have been transformed into patient 'rooms'; room capacities have been expanded beyond previously prescribed limits. Non-ICU wards have been transformed into ICU-like treatment environments following the requisite re-engineering; critical care has even become 'portable', delivered in non-ICU locales until limited ICU space becomes available.

In the most extreme cases, ICU '*Spaces*' have been created even outside of hospital walls – critical care has been provided in tents, in parking garages, and in open spaces. Redefining and re-evaluating critical care services, including where it can be delivered, is part of a flexible response that is required in pandemic circumstances. Rigidly holding onto 'how it's always been done' is not necessarily an applicable or viable option in the context of a pandemic.

20.5.4 Systems

The COVID-19 pandemic has clearly demonstrated that the proper organisation of healthcare *Systems* translates directly into improved healthcare delivery on the front lines. Properly structured organisational responses, particularly those with tiered responses based upon the number and trajectory of hospitalisations, not only improve the efficiency of patient distribution and the maintenance of equitable access to care, but can reduce anxiety and confusion among frontline healthcare workers, who all too often feel in the dark about rapidly changing administrative priorities and decision-making.

Of particular importance in this regard is the need for well-defined, properly structured triage systems for when the demand for care resources, and in particular critical care, outstrips all available supply. In pandemic times, decisions may have to be made as to who receives certain resources and who does not. Resource allocation schema should be laid out in advance, clearly codified and accessible, be made as transparent as feasible, and based upon objective criteria whenever possible. Decisions regarding allocations should include objective, detached administrators. The psychological trauma experienced by physicians forced into making such immediate life-or-death decisions cannot be understated, and all steps to ameliorate and assist in these difficult decisions should be taken.

In a similar vein, close collaborations between physicians and non-physicians are essential in ensuring that a healthcare *System*, whatever the scale, can operate as efficiently as possible during a pandemic. The skills of non-healthcare workers such as administrators, logisticians, ethicists, lawyers, and particularly government liaisons are as important for framing an adaptive response to a pandemic as are those from clinicians. Lines of communication between medical and non-medical professionals working to address the challenges of a pandemic must be open and readily available. Transparency in decision-making processes and clear, consistent messaging is essential. Adaptability, much as it is for healthcare workers on the ground, is absolutely necessary as is the ability to learn from immediate and past mistakes. Critical care never takes place in a vacuum, and a *System* that can be as flexible and inventive as the practitioners operating within it, can save even more lives, albeit under the most challenging of circumstances.

20.5.5   Support

Burnout is a major risk for every person in the healthcare arena, irrespective of role, during a pandemic (Stocchetti et al, 2021; Azoulay et al, 2020; Khasne et al, 2020; Kerlin, 2020). The reasons for this complex burnout and moral distress are wide-ranging, and its presence and downstream effects need to be acknowledged within any institutional plan for pandemic response. Burnout not only directly increases attrition within the already strained healthcare workforce, it also contributes to poor healthcare outcomes and clinical errors (Reader et al, 2008; Garrouste-Orgeas et al, 2016).

The importance of appropriate *Support* for all the members of the critical care team cannot be sufficiently emphasised, and these support mechanisms should be made available both during and after the pandemic response. A wide range of activities and resources should be provided, ranging from small on-the-job 'morale boosts' to professional psychological counselling. It is important to acknowledge that every individual healthcare worker on the pandemic front lines will cope with the stresses in a different manner and that a 'one size fits all' approach to supporting them will never be effectual. Additionally, putting the onus on front line workers to 'practise self-care' is rarely helpful – persons at the limits of their reserves may see this as yet another demand on their time and energy, another task to accomplish, another potential avenue for failure.

Effective institutional *Support* strategies for strained healthcare workers involves tangible steps to make the workday easier, such as limiting paperwork or documentation requirements, resources that are accessible at the workplace or during convenient times, and interventions that actively reach out and attempt to identify struggling individuals rather than empty encouragements of 'self-care'. For many persons, the psychological trauma of delivering critical care during pandemic conditions will not be a short-term struggle, and institutions should make resources for their staff available for months to years after a pandemic resolves.

20.5.6   Sustainability

All of the above need to be *Sustained* during the time of a pandemic, and *Sustainability* beyond pandemics offers the possibility of enhancing and improving healthcare for many citizens. It also ensures delivery of the best possible care for critically ill patients whilst reducing the risk to healthcare workers.

20.6 SPECIAL AND SPECIFIC CONSIDERATIONS

20.6.1   Interaction with Government and Policymakers

There is little that damages the morale of frontline healthcare workers more than the feeling that 'the government', be it local, regional or national, is not supportive of their life-saving efforts or is providing mixed messages to the public.

Consistent, fact-based messaging from political leadership, ideally grounded in data and science, is important not only to make healthcare practitioners feel supported, but also to help the general public make informed choices regarding safety measures and preventative behaviours. Leaders that involve scientists, physicians or public health experts in the crafting of messaging, and who are seen as listening to evidence and reason, immediately gain credibility and respect from the healthcare community. Well-grounded messaging to the public also has the potential to prevent further spread of the pandemic and thus reduce the pressure on the healthcare system overall.

20.6.2   Early Preparation

'Failing to prepare is preparing to fail.' Early preparation cannot be over-emphasised. A tragic reality of the COVID-19 pandemic is that despite early warnings of potential danger and spread at the outset, the majority of the nations of the world were not properly prepared, politically, structurally or medically, for a scourge as persistent, aggressive and easily transmitted as SARS-CoV-2. Some nations such as Taiwan, Singapore and Japan with prior experience from the first SARS epidemic appeared to have prepared more timeously on all levels, with consequent reduced deleterious impact as compared to those who were lesser prepared.

Preparedness on every level, both prompt and efficient, from national to the individual hospital unit, is pivotal in better preparation for inevitable future pandemics (Mer, 2020).

20.6.3 Involvement of Non-ICU Staff

Because there may be a paucity of adequately trained critical care staff in a pandemic, the pool of physicians, nurses and ancillary healthcare staff may by necessity need to be expanded. Creative measures such as novel restructuring of critical care teams may need to be initiated, for instance, critical care trained practitioners supervising small teams of non-critical care trained practitioners rather than practising direct patient care. In such circumstances, standard credentialing, scope-of-practice and medico-legal rules need to be adjusted accordingly, and both the new supervisors and those supervised informed of the new processes and protocols as well as being reassured that their licensure is protected.

Other creative measures to rapidly increase critical care human resource 'capacity' may be required, and include condensed training programmes or online training programmes created by professional societies or other organisations tailored to specific pandemic-induced demands. These initiatives are complex, however, and will involve not only trained critical care clinician-educators, but also professional societies, licensing authorities, and governmental regulatory agencies.

20.6.4 Review of Therapeutic Approach: Protocols

Protocols play an important role in assisting with a standard accepted approach to the management of patients. They may serve as very useful resources in all settings, but particularly where non-critical care trained practitioners are involved in critical care practice, and where critical care is provided outside of traditional critical care settings. Protocols may include sets of instructions, flow charts, checklists and guidance statements. It is essential, however, that these clinical protocols be practical, easy to follow, situation-relevant, and reflect the resources available at the individual facility. They must also be evidence- or best practice-based whenever possible and be properly vetted by practitioners with the relevant expertise and knowledge of local conditions, resources and epidemiology. Furthermore, these protocols must above all be *adaptable* – in pandemics, local conditions may change rapidly, resources may shift, and knowledge regarding the pathogen involved may itself evolve rapidly. Rigid protocols that cannot adapt to changing circumstances or scientific understanding may become more of a hindrance and a source of waste, inefficiency, and sub-optimal care than no protocols at all.

Thus, in the development and adoption of such protocols, there should be planned periodic updates as well as mechanisms for rapidly implementing changes should circumstances demand.

20.6.5   Clinical Trials

Clinical research undertaken during a pandemic has the potential to positively impact on the pandemic course. Current and future pandemics cannot be overcome without scientific knowledge, and credible knowledge cannot be generated without properly conducted clinical trials.

Healthcare facilities and institutions, including critical care units, can contribute significantly to providing valuable information, imparting a better understanding and supplying pertinent details and facts regarding incidence, case presentation, risks, infection and prevention control aspects, resource elements, management aspects and outcome. This information is key to informing clinical, including critical care, as well as broader public health decision-making (Fineberg, 2009). Research performed during a pandemic should conform to the same vigorous scientific and ethical standards expected during non-pandemic times. All conducted research should have the goal of promoting knowledge and enhancing health, be scientifically and methodologically sound, and where benefits to communities and the individuals supersedes any harm. Ethics and study protocols should ideally be expedited by oversight bodies in order for potentially meaningful and relevant research to take place during a pandemic. Appropriate and ethically correct consent procedures must always be adhered to. Similarly, submitted research must be subjected to the same diligent and meticulous review processes that are present in non-pandemic periods (Tong et al, 2020; Yeoh and Shah, 2021).

20.6.6   Team Work and Support (Including Psychological Support)

Communication with staff is a vital and essential component to fostering good teamwork – engaging, polite, constructive and inclusive with all parties and at all times (Mer, 2020). This approach will often address and overcome many significant challenges, including fear, panic and anxiety. Regular staff debriefings or communication sessions are important to provide positive feedback, encouragement and support, and to acknowledge the input from each team member. It is also important that team members are reassured that when resources are stretched, it may not be possible to treat patients to the high standards usually demanded under normal conditions, and that doing everything possible in these circumstances is suitably appropriate. Psychological support for personnel is imperative and must be available for all medical, nursing and allied teams, as the risk of burnout poses a real possibility and staff well-being is crucial for continued efficiency, productivity and effective functionality of critical care units. Elements pertaining to staff burnout have been alluded to previously.

20.6.7   Family Interaction

Pandemics bring with them real challenges in many instances regarding family-patient interactions related to safety concerns. Consequently, direct patient-family interactions are often not feasible. This frequently creates anxiety and loneliness for both the patient and their family. Regardless of the huge demands that may be experienced in an excessively busy ICU, time must be set aside to communicate with families on a regular basis and to keep them suitably updated on their loved one's condition and progress. Telephonic discussion, text messages and video calls are simple ways of achieving this and go a long way to both creating rapport, as well as to ameliorating family concerns and apprehension. These modalities should be considered as a basic minimum in terms of communication and information sharing. In the sad event of a terminal patient, a dignified video call can often assist families in not feeling that their loved one has died alone, and many have expressed that it has helped enormously in finding closure.

20.6.8   Futility

It is important to appreciate that there is a need to determine futility, particularly in the face of limited resources. Appropriate selection of patients to ICU should be based on unit capacity and patient profile. Triage elements have been previously alluded to, and as a general principle, patients should not be admitted to the ICU or submitted to organ support interventions if they are going to die regardless of the efforts on the part of ICU staff. This is not only a futile and unkind step for the patient and their family, but also impacts on wider society, restricting the availability of such services for those who could genuinely benefit. Moreover, the high mortality rates associated with admitted cases where further care is futile may also impact negatively on the morale of ICU personnel. Formalised criteria for ICU admission and the use of life-support therapies, at all times, including during pandemics, assist enormously in determining that only patients who are likely to benefit are included.

20.6.9   Impact on Patients not Affected by Pandemic

It should always be borne in mind that patients not afflicted by the pandemic but who require ICU services should not be forgotten. Where possible, such patients should be afforded ICU care and provisions for this patient cohort should be part of the planning efforts. Failure to do so may have deleterious consequences and result in unnecessary unfavourable patient outcomes. This has been a neglected issue and frequent oversight during pandemics. The impact of not addressing non-pandemic patients' needs may be seen for years to come. The cancellation of routine procedures, the fear of going to hospital and healthcare facilities during a pandemic and possibly contracting disease, loss of patients to follow-up and missing treatments and delayed presentations are all factors that must be considered during pandemics. The COVID-19 pandemic has highlighted and brought all of these aspects to the fore. Psychological issues as a consequence of lockdowns, social isolation, fear and loneliness amongst those not affected are also important additional considerations.

20.6.10   Low-and-Middle Income Countries (LMICs) / Resource-Limited Region Challenges

Healthcare infrastructures vary widely around the world. Fragile healthcare systems exist in many LMICs and in several domains these are severely resource-constrained. Critical care facilities in some regions are grossly lacking, and this may be further compounded by challenges in oxygen supplies, water safety, electricity, trained personnel and staffing, medical equipment, protective equipment, support services and transportation. Notwithstanding these elements, excellent quality care is feasible and possible with adherence to sound practices and basic clinical principles. This approach should always be strived for, even under extremely difficult circumstances, to ensure that patient care and dignity is never compromised.

Telemedicine has a potentially very useful role to play and this benefit can in fact extend to all global regions, whether resource-limited or not.

20.6.11   Follow-Up Clinics

Long-term sequelae in survivors of pandemics are not an infrequent occurrence, and appropriate follow-up services and rehabilitation programmes should be initiated for these patients to allow for further ongoing management, support and care to enhance recovery. Where appropriate, vaccine education and rollout are additional very important aspects to address.

20.7 FUTURE AND CONCLUSION

Pandemics place unprecedented strains on healthcare systems, with resultant increases in morbidity, mortality and human suffering, including amongst HCWs. These events are inevitable, but can also be powerful drivers of technological, structural and care delivery innovations. Critical care is an integral component of all pandemic preparation, planning and healthcare delivery. The COVID-19 pandemic has emphasised and highlighted the relevance, importance and need for critical care services and staff, and that appropriate planning for such services is vital. Reflection and introspection at all organisational levels, and based on cumulative experiences, will assist in further optimising this indispensable service moving forward.

20.8 SELF-ASSESSMENT QUESTIONS

1. Name the six crucial elements when addressing pandemic management.
2. How is critical care defined?

20.9 REFERENCES

Adhikari, N.K., Fowler, R.A., Bhagwanjee, S. and Rubenfeld, G.D. 2010. Critical care and the global burden of critical illness in adults. *Lancet* 376(9749), pp. 1339–1346.

Aziz, S., Arabi, Y.M., Alhazzani, W., Evans, L., Citerio, G., Fischkoff, K., et al. 2020. Managing ICU surge during the COVID-19 crisis: rapid guideline. *Intensive Care Med* 46, pp. 1303–1325.

Azoulay, E., De Waele, J., Ferrer, R., Staudinger, T., Borkowska, M., Povoa, P., et al. 2020. Symptoms of burnout in intensive care unit specialists facing the COVID-19 outbreak. *Ann Intensive Care* 10, p. 110.

Barbash, I.J. and Kahn, J.M. 2021. Fostering Hospital Resilience – Lessons from COVID-19. *JAMA* 326(8), pp. 693–694.

Christian, M., Lapinsky, S.E. and Stewart, T.E. 2007. Critical Care Pandemic Preparedness Primer. *Intensive Care Med* 2007, pp. 999–1010.

Fineberg, H. 2014. Pandemic preparedness and response – lessons from the H1N1 influenza of 2009. *N Engl J Med* 370, pp. 1335–42.

Garrouste-Orgeas, M., Flaatten, H. and Moreno, R. 2016. Understanding medical errors and adverse events in ICU patients. *Intensive Care Med* 42, pp. 107–109.

Goh, K.J., Wong, J., Tien, J.C.C., Ng, S.Y., Wen, S.D., Phua, G.C., et al. 2020. Preparing your intensive care unit for the COVID-19 pandemic: practical considerations and strategies. *Critical Care* 24, p. 215.

Gomersall, C.D., Loo, S., Joynt, G.M. and Taylor, B.L. 2007. Pandemic preparedness. *Curr Opin Crit Care* 13, pp. 742–747.

Griffen, K.M., Karas, M.G., Ivascu, N.S. and Lief, L. 2020. Hospital Preparedness for COVID-19: A Practical Guide from a Critical Care Perspective. *Am J Respir Crit Care Med* 201(11), pp. 1337–1344.

Humermovic, D. Brief History of Pandemics (Pandemics Throughout History). In: D Huremovic (Ed) *Psychiatry of Pandemics.* Springer Nature Switzerland AG 2019, pp. 7–35. doi: https://doi: 10.1007/978-3-030-15346-5.

Kain, T. and Fowler, R. 2019. Preparing intensive care for the next pandemic influenza. *Critical Care* 23, p. 337.

Kelly, H. 2011. The classic definition of a pandemic is not elusive. *Bull World Health Organ* 89, pp. 539–40.

Kerlin, M.P., McPeake, J. and Mikkelson, M.E. 2020. Burnout and Joy in the Profession of Critical Care Medicine. *Crit Care* 24, p. 98.

Khasne, R.W., Dhakulkar, B.S., Mahajan, H.C. and Kulkarni, A.P. 2020. Burnout among Healthcare Workers during COVID-19 Pandemic in India: Results of a Questionnaire. *Indian J Crit Care Med* 28(8), pp. 664–671.

Lassen, H.C. 1953. A preliminary report on the 1952 epidemic of poliomyelitis in Copenhagen with special reference to the treatment of acute respiratory insufficiency. *Lancet* 1(6749), pp. 37–41.

Marshall, J.C., Bosco, L., Adhikari, N.K., Connolly, B., Diaz, J.V., Dorman, T., et al. 2017. What is an intensive care unit? A report of the task force of the World Federation of Societies of Intensive and Critical Care Medicine. *J Crit Care* 37, pp. 270–276.

Maves, R., Downar, J., Dichter, J.R., Hick, J.L., Devereaux, A., Geiling, J.A., et al. 2020. Triage of Scarce Critical Care Resources in COVID-19. An Implementation Guide for Regional Allocation. An Expert Panel Report of the Task Force for Mass Critical Care and the American College of Chest Physicians. *CHEST* 158(1), pp. 212–225.

Mer, M. 2020. Lessons I have learnt from COVID-19. *Wits Journal of Clinical Medicine* 2(3), pp. 217–220.

Mer, M. Personal quotation. From talk delivered at the 3rd World Sepsis Congress held on 21 April 2021 as well as from talk delivered at Critical Care Society of Southern Africa Symposium, 8 May 2021.

Piret, J. and Boivin, G. 2021. Pandemics Throughout History. *Front Microbiol* 11, p. 631736.

Razzak, J., Usmani, M.F. and Bhutta, Z.A. 2019. Global, regional and national burden of emergency medical diseases using specific emergency disease indicators: analysis of the 2015 Global Burden of Disease Study. *BMJ Global Health* 4(2), p. e000733.

Reader, T., Cuthbertson, B.H. and Decruyenaere, J. 2008. Burnout in the ICU: potential consequences for staff and patient well-being. *Intensive Care Med* 34(1), pp. 4–6.

Reisner-Senelar, L. 2011. The birth of intensive care medicine: Bjorn Ibsen's records. *Intensive Care Med* 37(7), pp. 1084–6.

Rudd, K.E., Johnson, S.C., Agesa, K.M., Schackelford, K.A., Tsoi, D., Kievlan, D.R., et al. 2020. Global, regional and national sepsis incidence and mortality, 1990-2017: analysis for the Global Burden of Disease Study. *The Lancet* 395(10219), pp. 200–211.

Schell, C.O., Beane, A., Kayambankadzanya, R.K., Khalid, K., Haniffa, R. and Baker, T. 2019. Global Critical Care: Add Essentials to the Roadmap. *Annals of Global Health* 85(10), p. 97.

Society of Critical Care Medicine. Configuring ICUs in the COVID-19 era. Rapid Resource Center. Available at: https://www.sccm.org.

Sprung, C.L., Zimmerman, J.L., Joynt, G.M., Christian, M., Joynt, G.M., Hick, J.L., et al. 2010. Recommendations for intensive care unit and hospital preparations for an influenza epidemic or mass disaster: summary report of the European Society of Intensive Care Medicine's Task Force for intensive care unit triage during an influenza epidemic or mass disaster. *Intensive Care Med* 36, pp. 428–443.

Stocchetti, N., Segre, G., Zanier, E.R., Zanetti, M., Campi, R., Scarpellini, F., et al. 2021. Burnout in Intensive Care Unit Workers during the Second Wave of the COVID-19 Pandemic: A Single Center Cross-Sectional Italian Study. *Int J Environ Res Public Health* 18, p. 6102.

Thomas, T., Laher, A.E., Mahomed, A., Stacey, S., Motara, F. and Mer, M. 2020. Challenges around COVID-19 at a tertiary-level healthcare facility in South Africa and strategies implemented for improvement. *S Afr Med J* 110(9), p. 964–967.

Tong, A., Elliot, J.H., Azevido, L.C., Baumgart, A., Bersten, A., Cervantes, L., et al. 2020. Core Outcome Set for Trials in People With Coronavirus Disease 2019. *Crit Care Med* 48(11), pp. 1622–1635.

Weil, M.H. and Tang, W. 2011. From intensive care to critical care medicine: a historical perspective. *Am J Respir Crit Care Med* 183(11), pp. 1451–3.

Wunsch, H. 2020. The outbreak that invented intensive care. *Nature.* Doi: 10.1038/d41586-020-01019-Y.

Wurmb, T., Scholtes, K, Kolibay, F., Schorscher, N., Ertl, G., Ernestus, R.I., et al. 2020. Hospital preparedness for mass critical during SARS-CoV-2 pandemic. *Critical Care* 24, p. 386.

Yeoh, K.W. and Shah, K. 2021. Research ethics during a pandemic (COVID-19). *Int Health* 13(4), pp. 374–375.

Additional reading

Aziz, S., Arabi, Y.M., Alhazzani, W., Evans, L., Citerio, G., Fischkoff, K., et al. 2020. Managing ICU surge during the COVID-19 crisis: rapid guideline. *Intensive Care Med* 46, pp. 1303–1325.

Barbash, I.J. and Kahn, J.M. 2021. Fostering Hospital Resilience – Lessons from COVID-19. *JAMA* 326(8), pp. 693–694.

Goh, K.J., Wong, J., Tien, J.C.C., Ng, S.Y., Wen, S.D., Phua, G.C., et al. 2020. Preparing your intensive care unit for the COVID-19 pandemic: practical considerations and strategies. *Critical Care* 24, p. 215

Gomersall, C.D., Loo, S., Joynt, G.M. and Taylor. B.L. 2007. Pandemic preparedness. *Curr Opin Crit Care* 13, pp. 742–747.

Griffen, K.M., Karas, M.G., Ivascu, N.S. and Lief, L. 2020. Hospital preparedness for COVID-19: A practical guide from a critical care perspective. *Am J Respir Crit Care Med* 201(11), pp. 1337–1344.

Kain, T. and Fowler, R. 2019. Preparing intensive care for the next pandemic influenza. *Critical Care* 23, p. 337.

Maves, R., Downar, J., Dichter, J.R., Hick, J.L., Devereaux, A., Geiling, J.A., et al. 2020. Triage of scarce critical care resources in COVID-19. An implementation guide for regional allocation. an expert panel report of the Task Force for Mass Critical Care and the American College of Chest Physicians. *CHEST* 158(1), pp. 212–225.

Society of Critical Care Medicine. Configuring ICUs in the COVID-19 era. Rapid Resource Center. Available at: https://www.sccm.org.

Sprung, C.L., Zimmerman, J.L., Joynt, G.M., Christian, M., Joynt, G.M., Hick, J.L., et al. 2010. Recommendations for intensive care unit and hospital preparations for an influenza epidemic or mass disaster: summary report of the European Society of Intensive Care Medicine's Task Force for intensive care unit triage during an influenza epidemic or mass disaster. *Intensive Care Med* 36, pp. 428–443.

Thomas, T., Laher, A.E., Mahomed, A., Stacey, S., Motara, F. and Mer, M. 2020. Challenges around COVID-19 at a tertiary-level healthcare facility in South Africa and strategies implemented for improvement. *S Afr Med J* 110(9), pp. 964–967.

Wurmb, T., Scholtes, K., Kolibay, F., Schorscher, N., Ertl, G., Ernestus, R.I., et al. 2020. Hospital preparedness for mass critical during SARS-CoV-2 pandemic. *Critical Care* 24, p. 386.

CHAPTER 21

PANDEMICS AND THE MANAGEMENT OF INFECTIOUS DISEASES

Colin Nigel Menezes

21.1 INTRODUCTION

A disease outbreak occurs when the number of cases of a particular disease exceeds what would normally be seen in a particular geographic area. An epidemic is similar to the definition of an outbreak of a disease but is used in the instance where the disease spreads quickly into a larger geographic area. A pandemic, on the other hand, is defined as an epidemic that spreads globally, crossing international borders (Meningitis Research Foundation, 2020).

Infectious diseases are a leading cause of mortality worldwide and this is mainly due to changes in human behaviour, larger cities being on the increase, travel, misuse of antibiotics, and the emergence of new infections. Infectious disease outbreaks are unpredictable and have serious public health and economic consequences, warranting urgent responses as they may end up as epidemics or pandemics (Verikios, 2020).

There have been several new and serious infections throughout the years, such as the Ebola virus, the human immunodeficiency virus (HIV), the severe acute respiratory syndrome (SARS) virus, the Middle East respiratory syndrome (MERS) virus, and multiple influenza virus outbreaks that spread globally causing fear and panic. Trade, livelihoods, and travel are also impacted (World Health Organization, 2018). The coronavirus disease 2019 (COVID-19) pandemic outbreak started in 2019.

Generally, efforts are focused on limiting the direct health impact of pandemics, which can be catastrophic and result in overwhelming already overstretched healthcare systems. However, the indirect impacts of pandemics can be equally catastrophic with disrupted access to health services when strict lockdowns are put in place. Patients with conditions unrelated to the pandemic often find it difficult to access healthcare services. As a result, morbidity and mortality rates of other diseases rise. Several low-income and middle-income countries have high burdens of HIV infection/acquired immunodeficiency syndrome (AIDS), tuberculosis (TB), and malaria. The impact of the disruption of health services on these major health priorities has long-standing consequences (Hogan et al, 2020).

21.2 OBJECTIVES

At the end of the chapter, one should be able to:

- Explain the different concepts of an outbreak, epidemic, and pandemic.
- Briefly describe the dynamics of a pandemic.
- Briefly describe the interventions applied during a pandemic.
- Discuss the impact of the pandemic on other infectious diseases.
- Discuss the management of other infectious diseases in the setting of a pandemic.

21.3 THE DYNAMICS OF PANDEMIC INFECTIOUS DISEASES

According to the World Health Organization (WHO), planning and preparation are vital in mitigating impact. New infections usually start locally and tend to spread rapidly if the transmission is not interrupted. Therefore, it is important to understand their dynamics to prevent the wide-ranging spread and an overwhelmed healthcare system. In addition, contextual dynamics affect the interventions that are applied. Generally, epidemics and pandemics occur in four phases, with the first phase being the emergence of an infection in a community. This might result in an outbreak with localised transmission during which sporadic infections may occur and result in the second phase. In the third phase, this human-to-human transmission may cause a sustained outbreak, threatening to spread further and amplify into an epidemic or pandemic. The fourth phase is when human to human transmission reduces because of acquired population immunity or effective interventions (World Health Organization, 2018).

21.4 INTERVENTIONS IMPLEMENTED DURING A PANDEMIC

The type of interventions are dependent on the dynamics of the pandemic and are implemented in five stages. The first stage is the anticipation of new and re-emerging infections to facilitate faster detection and response. This is followed by the second stage, which includes early detection of the emergence of infections in animal and human populations. The third stage is the containment of the infection at the early stages of transmission and the fourth stage is that of control and mitigation during its amplification. The fifth stage is the elimination of the risk of outbreak or eradication of the infectious disease (World Health Organization, 2018).

Early interventions, awareness, cooperation, and collaboration between communities, national and local governments, agencies, and organisations are critical. Healthcare systems need to be strengthened so that they can overcome the additional and often excessive strain during pandemics. There is a tendency to move resources to the real-time emergency. Healthcare workers, equipment, and drugs are usually relocated to respond to the emergency with devastating effects on basic and essential health services. It is essential that interventions are put in place to prevent deaths not only from the pandemic but from other causes, including infections (World Health Organization, 2018). The key to the risk mitigation decision-making process is that interventions also minimise adverse indirect impacts of other infectious diseases in addition to the pandemic.

21.5 THE MAGNITUDE OF OTHER INFECTIOUS DISEASES

In 2019, the WHO reported that even though the incidence of TB had dropped to around 9% in the past few years, nearly 10 million people were diagnosed with the disease globally, with 1.4 million people dying from this infection. South Africa was listed as one of the top eight countries in the world, accounting for two-thirds of total new infections. Of concern also was that multidrug resistance TB had increased by 10%, with 206 030 people infected (World Health Organization, 2020h).

HIV/AIDS is another major public health concern, with nearly 38 million people living with the disease in 2019. However, the WHO estimated that new HIV infections dropped by 39% and HIV-related deaths by 51%. Nearly 15.3 million lives were saved because of antiretroviral therapy. It has now become a manageable chronic disease. South Africa also has the highest rates of HIV infection worldwide (World Health Organization, 2020c).

There were 228 million cases of malaria, with 405 000 deaths globally reported by the WHO in 2018. Young children were the most affected, with 67% of the deaths in this group (World Health Organization, 2020f).

According to the WHO, the lack of vaccination coverage has remained unchanged worldwide over the past years. In 2019, only about 85% of infants received the full three doses of the diphtheria-tetanus-pertussis vaccine and one dose of the measles vaccine. Similarly, only 86% received the full three doses of the polio vaccine and only 39% received the rotavirus vaccine (World Health Organization, 2020d).

In its 2019 report, the World Bank estimated that antimicrobial resistance (AMR) accounted for 700 000 deaths yearly (The World Bank, 2019). According to the WHO's Global Antimicrobial Resistance and Use Surveillance System (GLASS), the misuse of antibiotics with resultant antimicrobial resistance continues to grow. The rates of resistance to ciprofloxacin, a common antibiotic that is used to treat urinary tract infections and bacterial associated diarrhoea, is concerning – ranging from 8.4–92.9%. The need for the development of antimicrobial stewardship programmes has become ever more important now (World Health Organization, 2020g).

21.6 THE IMPACT OF PANDEMICS ON OTHER INFECTIOUS DISEASES

According to a report from the Centre for Global Development, the West Africa Ebola epidemic in 2014 resulted in the lack of routine care for HIV/AIDS, TB, and malaria, which led to an estimated 10 600 additional deaths in Guinea, Liberia, and Sierra Leone. This death rate nearly equalled the 11 300 deaths directly caused by Ebola in these countries. Facilities closed as a result of understaffing and fear of contracting Ebola played a large role in the lack of access to or avoidance of routine healthcare. The report described a similar situation during the COVID-19 pandemic. India had a significant drop (80%) in daily TB notifications, with nearly 117 million children missing out on their measles vaccination. In Africa, an additional 225 million malaria deaths were reported because of disruptions in the preventative programmes (Krubiner, Keller and Kaufman, 2020).

In countries with a high burden of HIV, TB, or malaria, the health impact of disruptions during the COVID-19 pandemic is estimated to cause additional mortality over a period of five years – due to HIV infection of up to 10%, TB up to 20%, and malaria up to 36% respectively, this compared to if no pandemic occurred (Hogan et al, 2020).

According to the National Institute of Communicable Diseases (NICD) of South Africa, the strict restrictions during the COVID-19 pandemic resulted in an approximately 48% average weekly decrease in TB GeneXpert® testing numbers. A likely reason included limited access to public transport resulting in limited access to healthcare services that were operational during that time. It has been suggested that only those with advanced TB sought care (National Institute for Communicable Diseases, 2020a). While this resulted in a major setback for the TB control programme, the GeneXpert® machines were repurposed for the diagnosis of COVID-19, as the assay was fully automated and provided results rapidly. In addition, laboratory staff was familiar with the GeneXpert® platform, given that the Xpert® MTB/RIF assay serves as the primary diagnostic assay for drug-sensitive and resistant TB (World Health Organization Regional Office for Europe, 2020). This may have also led to a reduction in TB testing capacity.

According to the 2019 Southern African cryptococcal disease treatment guidelines, all HIV-infected patients with a CD4+ T-lymphocyte (CD4) count of less than 200 cells/μL will need to have a reflex serum cryptococcal antigen (CrAg) screening test done (Govender et al, 2019). A decline in CrAg screening was noted during the COVID-19 pandemic compared to screening done during previous years. Lockdown measures might have led to fewer patients seeking HIV care where they would have a CD4 count test done, and screened for a serum CrAg test if required. The decreased availability of public transportation and the perceived risk of COVID-19 exposure at public health facilities may have influenced patients with advanced HIV disease to avoid healthcare settings (Centre for Healthcare-Associated Infections, 2020).

The World Bank reported in 2019 that the AMR death toll could rise to 10 million deaths annually by 2050 and this could also result in increased deaths during pandemics because of secondary bacterial and fungal infections caused by organisms resistant to antibiotics (The World Bank, 2019). This was seen in other influenza pandemics, where almost one in four patients had pneumococcal pneumonia as the most common secondary bacterial infection (MacIntyre et al, 2018). Appropriate use of antimicrobials guides the principles of antimicrobial stewardship (AMS) activities. During the COVID-19 pandemic, the use of antibiotics for patients admitted with COVID-19 was high, with concerns that interruptions in AMS activities could drive an increase in antimicrobial resistance. It has been reported in the literature that prescription rates were as high as 70% (Rawson et al, 2020). WHO's interim guidance on the clinical management of COVID-19 includes antibiotic stewardship principles. It does not recommend antibiotic therapy or prophylaxis for patients with suspected or confirmed mild or moderate COVID-19 unless signs and symptoms of a bacterial infection exist, or where specific conditions exist (World Health Organization, 2020b).

According to the WHO, UNICEF, and Gavi, the Vaccine Alliance – vaccination rates dropped during the COVID 19 pandemic, with millions of children across the world at risk of getting diphtheria, measles, and polio (World Health Organization, 2020a). In a pandemic setting, immunisation programmes are likely to get disrupted due to the reallocation of healthcare workers, the lack of personal protective equipment, the fear of contracting the pandemic infection by both healthcare workers and parents of the children, and the lack of availability of vaccines (Centers for Disease Control and Prevention (CDC), 2020). On the other hand, hand hygiene and social distancing measures implemented to reduce SARS-CoV-2 virus transmission in all probability played a role in reducing influenza virus transmission. Worldwide, influenza rates were reported at lower levels than expected (World Health Organization, 2020e). Despite continued or even increased testing for influenza in South Africa, very few cases of influenza were reported (National Institute for Communicable Diseases, 2020b).

21.7 MANAGEMENT OF INFECTIOUS DISEASES IN A PANDEMIC SETTING

Maintaining continuity of healthcare services during a pandemic while focusing on the pandemic should be given high priority to reduce the broader health impact of the pandemic. The indirect impact of the pandemic might be avoided through the maintenance of health programmes. When planning, issues to be considered include strengthening of health systems, leadership and governance, resource allocation and financing, service delivery, human resources, diagnostics, and delivery of medical supplies (Krubiner, Keller and Kaufman, 2020).

21.7.1 Streamline Clinical Services

As clinical staff will be reallocated to manage an increased number of in-patients, the Infectious Diseases, HIV, and TB clinics should rapidly streamline their services, to allow for patients to be triaged appropriately. Patients who are ill can be triaged at the entrance of the clinic to be screened for respiratory symptoms and tested accordingly. Those who are screened and found to have no symptoms of the pandemic infection but are ill can be referred to a doctor. The stable patients can be seen by a primary healthcare trained nurse, have their routine blood tests done and a repeat script written up without the need for them to see a doctor. If indicated, patients may be given appropriate vaccinations such as the influenza vaccine in the winter period. To further streamline services, blood results can be checked on free clinic days for booked patients.

21.7.2 Diagnosis and Laboratory Preparedness

Respiratory infections such as pulmonary TB and the pandemic COVID-19 infection have a similar clinical presentation which includes fever, cough, or shortness of breath; therefore a similar strategy is required to be applied in these settings. Similar precautions are needed when collecting, transporting, and handling sputum samples. In the setting of TB, sputum collection should be in an open, well-ventilated area away from crowded patient areas, and away from staff (World Health Organization, 2020i).

Every effort must be made to ensure that the laboratory services are running efficiently and that they are not overwhelmed by the testing for the inter-current pandemic. As capacity will be limited, relevant SOPs should be put in place to prioritise testing of samples for the HIV and TB programme, children, and those failing treatment. In addition to the rapid point-of-care tests that are required for the diagnosis of the inter-current pandemic to allow for appropriate patient management, rapid tests for the diagnosis of other infections should also be made readily accessible, to reduce unnecessary or prolonged use of broad-spectrum antimicrobials. Rapid and affordable diagnostic tests must be introduced to differentiate between bacterial and viral respiratory tract infections (Getahun et al, 2020). Expanding testing facilities by using other research site laboratories would assist in reducing the turnaround time of testing. These laboratories should be assessed for accreditation to meet standards to support public hospitals during the pandemic surge. Besides, this would allow laboratories to focus on other important services. Increased vigilance in laboratory surveillance systems would be necessary to detect any increase in infections during and after that pandemic so that appropriate actions can be instituted.

21.7.3   Availability of Medication

Ensuring the continuity of a regular supply of antiretroviral, antituberculosis drugs, antimicrobials and vaccines is critical. There are major concerns for HIV and TB drug resistance due to interruptions in access to treatment, with the adverse implications of these interruptions manifesting in the long run. Disruptions to supply chains from the lockdown will be affected because of the economic situation and travel restrictions (Krubiner, Keller and Kaufman, 2020).

Several countries have started adopting new policies for multi-month prescriptions. These have been implemented across various clinics and hospitals to allow patients to access longer courses of treatment, especially in HIV and TB programmes. The WHO and the President's Emergency Plan For AIDS Relief (PEPFAR) have recommended providing up to a six-month supply of antiretroviral therapy (ARVs). The Global Fund has advised a three to six month supply and has assisted with medications in various countries (Krubiner, Keller and Kaufman, 2020). In South Africa, one-year scripts have been allowed for stable and compliant patients (Medical Brief, 2020). For patients with chronic conditions who remained stable on their medication, the South African National Department of Health's Central Chronic Medicine Dispensing and Distribution (CCMDD) programme commenced with distributing medicine from a central point to different pharmacies, as well as community-based sites that were located in areas close to patients' homes for easy collection, already before the pandemic (Zeeman, 2017).

21.7.4   Antimicrobial Stewardship

Antimicrobial stewardship activities must be integrated into the pandemic response. Training clinicians on distinguishing COVID-19 infection, which does not require antibiotics, from TB, or a superimposed bacterial or fungal infection would reduce the need for unnecessary antibiotics. Emphasising the need for de-escalation of antibiotics, understanding local resistance patterns when prescribing antibiotics, avoiding prolonged stay of in-patients, and implementing strict infection prevention and control measures are important. This could take place through multidisciplinary AMS meetings via limited physical ward rounds or online virtual tools where advice around antimicrobial management and interpretation of microbiology results can occur. It is also important that AMS activities in non-pandemic wards of hospitals continue taking place (Mazdeyasna et al, 2020).

21.7.5 Malaria Programmes

In the setting of malaria, preventative programmes have to be prioritised, providing long-lasting insecticidal nets and prophylactic treatment either as mass distribution or as part of a seasonal programme, and they have to be planned around the lockdown measures (Hogan et al, 2020).

With the recent breakthrough in malaria control, a vaccine has now been added to the armamentarium of the malaria preventative programmes. On 6 October 2021, the WHO announced that as part of its malaria control programme, it will be recommending that the RTS,S/AS01 (RTS,S) malaria vaccine be used for children in sub-Saharan Africa and other regions with moderate-to-high Plasmodium falciparum transmission. This would be in addition to the long-lasting insecticidal nets, indoor spraying of homes, rapid diagnostic tests, and prophylactic treatment. With this malaria vaccination programme, it is hoped that there will be a further reduction in the burden of malaria morbidity and mortality (World Health Organization, 2021).

21.7.6 Vaccination Programmes

Communication is of vital importance in vaccination programmes. Awareness campaigns must also include the precautions taken to prevent transmission of the pandemic infection to alleviate the fears of communities. Communities must be informed in advance about the availability of routine immunisation services and mass campaigns. Such measures are likely to ensure the safety and concerns of both the health workers and parents. This can take place through advocacy meetings and social mobilisation. Apart from the regular training of healthcare workers on the vaccination programmes, plans need to include special training for pandemic settings. Catch-up immunisation programmes need to be planned around the countrywide lockdown levels (Centers for Disease Control and Prevention (CDC), 2020).

21.8 CONCLUSION

Pandemics are a leading cause of mortality worldwide. Moreover, infectious disease outbreaks have serious public health and economic consequences. While efforts are focused on limiting the direct impact of the pandemics, the indirect impacts of pandemics are equally disruptive. As a result, risk mitigation strategies must also focus on both the direct and indirect impacts of the pandemic, especially on priorities such as TB, HIV/AIDs, malaria, AMR, and immunisation against infections, as these are also likely to contribute to significant morbidity and mortality during the pandemic. Whatever policies are put in place, attention to these issues is critical.

21.9 SELF-ASSESSMENT QUESTION

1. What is a pandemic? Why is it important to understand the dynamics of pandemic diseases?

2. Why is it important to manage other infectious diseases during a pandemic?

21.10 REFERENCES

Centre for Healthcare-Associated Infections, A.R. and M.N.I. for C.D. 2020. The Impact of COVID-19 Public Health Measures on Diagnosis of Advanced HIV Disease, Cryptococcal Antigenaemia and Cryptococcal Meningitis in South Africa. Available at: https://www.nicd.ac.za/wp-content/uploads/2020/06/COVID Impact_CryptoScreening_2020-06_15-002.pdf.

Centers for Disease Control and Prevention (CDC). 2020. Operational Considerations for Immunization Services during COVID-19 in Non-US Settings Focusing on Low-Middle Income Countries | CDC. Available at: https://www.cdc.gov/coronavirus/2019-ncov/global-covid-19/maintaining-immunization-services.html.

Getahun, H., Smith, I., Trivedi, K., Paulin, S. and Balkhy, H.H. 2020. Tackling antimicrobial resistance in the COVID-19 pandemic, challenges to tackling antimicrobial resistance. doi: 10.1017/9781108864121.004.

Govender, N.P., et al. 2019. Southern African HIV Clinicians Society guideline for the prevention, diagnosis and management of cryptococcal disease among HIV-infected persons: 2019 update. *Southern African Journal of HIV Medicine* 20(1), pp. 1–16. doi: 10.4102/sajhivmed.v20i1.1030.

Hogan, A.B., et al. 2020. Potential impact of the COVID-19 pandemic on HIV, tuberculosis, and malaria in low-income and middle-income countries: a modelling study. *The Lancet Global Health* 8(9), pp. e1132–e1141.

Krubiner, C., Keller, J.M. and Kaufman, J. 2020. Balancing the COVID-19 Response with Wider Health Needs: Key Decision-Making Considerations for Low- and Middle-Income Countries, Center for Global Development. Available at: Balancing the COVID-19%0AResponse with Wider Health%0ANeeds.

MacIntyre, C.R., Chughtai, A.A., Barnes, M., Ridda, I., Seale, H., Toms, R. and Heywood, A. 2018. The role of pneumonia and secondary bacterial infection in fatal and serious outcomes of pandemic influenza a(H1N1)pdm09. *BMC Infectious Diseases* 18(1), pp. 1–20. doi: 10.1186/s12879-018-3548-0.

Mazdeyasna, H., Nori, P., Patel, P., Doll, M., Godbout, E., Lee, K., Noda, A.J., Bearman, G. and Stevens, M.P. 2020. Antimicrobial Stewardship at the Core of COVID-19 Response Efforts: Implications for Sustaining and Building Programs. *Current Infectious Disease Reports* 22(23), pp. 1–6. doi: 10.1007/s11908-020-00734-x.

Medical Brief. 2020. Act amendment allows extension of expiring prescriptions from 6 to 12 months. Available at: https://www.medicalbrief.co.za/archives/act-amendment-allows-extension-of-expiring-prescriptions-from-6-to-12-months/.

Meningitis Research Foundation. 2020. Outbreak, epidemic, pandemic – what's the difference? Available at: https://www.meningitis.org/blogs/outbreak-epidemic-pandemic-difference.

National Institute for Communicable Diseases. 2020a. Impact of COVID-19 intervention on TB testing in South Africa. Available at: https://www.nicd.ac.za/wp-content/uploads/2020/05/Impact-of-Covid-19-interventions-on-TB-testing-in-South-Africa-10-May-2020.pdf.

National Institute for Communicable Diseases. 2020b. Weekly Respiratory Pathogens Surveillance Report. Available at: https://www.nicd.ac.za/wp-content/uploads/2020/06/Monthly-Pathogens-surveillance-report-week-24-final.pdf.

Rawson, T.M., Moore, L.S.P., Zhu, N. Ranganathan, N., Skolimowska, K., Gilchrist, M., Satta, G., Cooke, G. and Holmes, A. 2020. Bacterial and fungal co-infection in individuals with coronavirus: A rapid review to support COVID-19 antimicrobial prescribing. *Clinical Infectious Diseases*. doi: https://doi.org/10.1093/cid/ciaa530.

The World Bank. 2019. Pulling Together to Beat Superbugs: Knowledge and Implementation Gaps in Addressing Antimicrobial Resistance. Available at: https://www.worldbank.org/en/topic/agriculture/publication/pulling-together-to-beat-superbugs-knowledge-and-implementation-gaps-in-addressing-antimicrobial-resistance#:~:text=Already%2C AMR causes 700%2C000 deaths, million deaths annually by 2050.

Verikios, G. 2020. The dynamic effects of infectious disease outbreaks: The case of pandemic influenza and human coronavirus. *Socio-Economic Planning Sciences*. Elsevier Ltd, 71(March), pp. 1–15. doi: 10.1016/j.seps.2020.100898.

World Health Organization. 2018. Managing epidemics: key facts about major deadly diseases. Available at: https://www.who.int/emergencies/diseases/managing-epidemics/en/.

World Health Organization. 2020a. At least 80 million children under one at risk of diseases such as diphtheria, measles and polio as COVID-19 disrupts routine vaccination efforts, warn Gavi, WHO and UNICEF. Available at: https://www.who.int/news-room/detail/22-05-2020-at-least-80-million-children-under-one-at-risk-of-diseases-such-as-diphtheria-measles-and-polio-as-covid-19-disrupts-routine-vaccination-efforts-warn-gavi-who-and-unicef.

World Health Organization. 2020b. *Clinical management of COVID-19 – interim guidance*. Available at: https://apps.who.int/iris/bitstream/handle/10665/332196/WHO-2019-nCoV-clinical-2020.5-eng.pdf?sequence=1&isAllowed=y.

World Health Organization. 2020c. HIV/AIDS: Key Facts. doi: 10.1007/978-1-137-00443-7_3.

World Health Organization. 2020d. Immunization coverage: Key Facts. Available at: https://www.who.int/news-room/fact-sheets/detail/immunization-coverage.

World Health Organization. 2020e. Influenza update – 378. Available at: https://www.who.int/influenza/surveillance_monitoring/updates/latest_update_GIP_surveillance/en/.

World Health Organization. 2020f. Malaria: Key Facts. Available at: https://www.who.int/news-room/fact-sheets/detail/malaria.

World Health Organization. 2020g. Record number of countries contribute data revealing disturbing rates of antimicrobial resistance. Available at: https://www.who.int/news/item/01-06-2020-record-number-of-countries-contribute-data-revealing-disturbing-rates-of-antimicrobial-resistance.

World Health Organization. 2020h. Tuberculosis: Key facts. Available at: https://www.who.int/news-room/fact-sheets/detail/tuberculosis.

World Health Organization. 2020i. Tuberculosis and COVID-19: Considerations for tuberculosis care, World Health Organization. Available at: https://www.who.int/docs/default-source/documents/tuberculosis/infonote-tb-covid-19.pdf.

World Health Organization Regional Office for Europe. 2020. Rapid communication on the role of the GeneXpert® platform for rapid molecular testing for SARS-CoV-2 in the WHO European Region. Available at: https://www.euro.who.int/__data/assets/pdf_file/0005/436631/Rapid-communication-COVID-19.pdf.

World Health Organization. 2021. WHO recommends groundbreaking malaria vaccine for children at risk. Available at: https://www.who.int/news/item/06-10-2021-who-recommends-groundbreaking-malaria-vaccine-for-children-at-risk.

Zeeman, H. 2017. CCMDD: A vehicle towards universal access to Anti Retrovirals and other chronic medicines in South Africa. Available at: https://www.hst.org.za/hstconference/hstconference2016/Presentations/hst_conf_ccmdd_h_zeeman_28_04_2016.pdf.

CHAPTER 22

PANDEMICS AND PAEDIATRICS

Robin T Saggers

Daynia E Ballot

"There can be no keener revelation of a society's soul than the way in which it treats its children." Nelson Mandela

22.1 INTRODUCTION

In South Africa, children's rights are enshrined in the Constitution (1996) and the Children's Act of 2005 (South Africa, 2005). However, children are a vulnerable and often overlooked group as they are dependent on caregivers to assist with fulfilling their health needs. Their access to healthcare and uptake of interventions is often related to their parents' culture, level of education and economic access. While there are disparities with regards to healthcare amongst different populations, the gaps are exaggerated amongst children.

Fortunately, COVID-19 seems to have 'spared' children. Theories abound as to the reason for this, yet the cause remains unclear. Nevertheless, it seems that children rarely show symptoms of the disease, and thankfully, rarely become ill enough to require hospitalisation. The mortality amongst children worldwide is negligible. However, deaths in children with a Kawasaki disease-like condition, that is linked to COVID-19, have been reported. The Paediatric Inflammatory Multisystem Syndrome (PIMS), also known as Multisystem Inflammatory Syndrome in Children (MIS-C), commonly presents with hypotension and shock and a variety of other signs. Treatment includes using the traditional modalities known to be effective in the management of Kawasaki disease, such as intravenous immunoglobulin.

While the COVID-19 pandemic has proved challenging in resource-rich settings, it is more challenging in resource-limited settings where healthcare systems are already stretched to capacity with little room to expand in order to accept the influx of COVID-19 patients.

Over and above the care of COVID-19 patients, the healthcare system still needs to provide ongoing care to the multitudes of acute and chronic patients with other illnesses accessing the system daily. A good example of this in the paediatric setting is the Extended Programme of Immunisations. Previous outbreaks of widespread, infectious diseases (for example, Ebola in West Africa) have been associated with massive, concomitant increases in mortality from other vaccine-preventable diseases. This highlights the importance of continuing routine public health programmes related to the prevention of disease and chronic care.

Infection prevention and control practices have never been more important – the basic principles of handwashing, sanitising and maintaining physical distance are the best defences against the spread of disease, be it bacterial, fungal, or viral. Yet, these simple common-sense solutions are difficult to implement and enforce, requiring ongoing education and reinforcement amongst the general population and healthcare workers alike.

22.2 OBJECTIVES

The objectives of this chapter are:

- To place children in global health challenges as a vulnerable, often overlooked population, especially in resource-limited settings.
- To describe COVID-19 in paediatrics, specifically:
    a. Neonatal issues, including breastfeeding;
    b. General paediatrics, including severity of disease and high-risk patients; and
    c. Multisystem Inflammatory Syndrome in children.
- To briefly address mental health amongst children, carers, and healthcare workers.
- To highlight issues in preparing for the pandemic.
- To call attention to the importance of advocating for children during a pandemic.

22.3 A VULNERABLE POPULATION

22.3.1 The Child in Global Health Challenge

Children have been increasingly impacted by COVID-19, both directly and indirectly (Ahmed et al, 2020). Children are a vulnerable population, particularly in low-and-middle-income countries (LMICs). Prior to COVID-19, LMICs already had a 66-fold higher under-five pneumonia mortality rate. Risk factors for poor outcomes in pneumonia include severe malnutrition, low immunisation uptake, nutritional anaemia, HIV-exposure or infection, air pollution, poverty, low parental education and limited access to acute healthcare. These risk factors are overwhelmingly more prevalent in LMICs than high-incoming countries (HICs)

(Ahmed et al, 2020). While COVID-19 does not only manifest as pneumonia, the potential impact of COVID-19 is concerning for children in LMICs (Ahmed et al, 2020).

In LMICs, further threats to the well-being of children include widespread parental unemployment, disrupted education, as well as food and housing insecurity. Threats to vital preventative health programmes, particularly immunisations, further exacerbate the vulnerability of children. Other preventative health programmes, such as antenatal care, infant feeding and nutrition programmes, HIV and malaria prevention, are essential in preventing unnecessary morbidity and mortality amongst children (and their carers) (Ahmed et al, 2020).

With the large burden of disease amongst adults, critical healthcare services may be diverted away from mothers and children. Delays in seeking care due to fear or poor access may result in more severe illness. Pandemic response measures may accentuate well-established risk factors for poor paediatric outcomes and expose long-standing system vulnerabilities. Therefore, by simply strengthening existing healthcare programmes and maintaining vital access to care is likely to save more children's lives than procuring more costly interventions like advanced intensive care (Ahmed et al, 2020).

In South Africa, the lockdown strategy and regulations imposed have affected children's access to healthcare and education, and maternal support for hospitalised children. Questions regarding the care of children arise when healthcare providers decide to empty paediatric wards and prevent caregivers from entering hospitals. In many instances, children are more likely to be the victims of measures taken to halt the spread of COVID-19 rather than the disease itself (van Bruwaene et al, 2020).

22.3.2 Early Childhood Development

Children typically obtain their daily physical activity through walking to school, physical education and recess at school, organised sports, games and dance, and spending time in playgrounds and parks. Most sedentary time and sleep occur at home. The COVID-19 pandemic has resulted in many governments implementing school closures and physical distancing measures resulting in children being unable to meet the movement behaviour guidelines. Lockdown strategies have increased the amount of sedentary time children spend at computer or TV screens and decreased physical activity levels with children not being allowed outdoors (Guan et al, 2020).

Children's health may potentially be even more compromised during COVID-19, given the strong associations between health outcomes and movement behaviours. Periods of home confinement could lead to higher risk of Vitamin D deficiency, mental health issues and myopia. There could be potential long-term health implications if the adverse behaviour adaptations, such as less activity become the new normal (Guan et al, 2020).

In addition to the obvious adverse effects on development and learning, many children rely on school for feeding and safety, hence the closing of schools has resulted in some children experiencing anxiety, isolation, and hunger (van Bruwaene et al, 2020).

22.4 NEWBORN ISSUES

Neonates are a group of patients that require special consideration. There are reports of early detection of the virus in neonates. This is likely to be transmission during or soon after birth. The risk of transmission is in the close contact between the COVID-19 positive breastfeeding mother and the neonate. Hence breastfeeding is a contentious issue, with various countries taking different approaches in their guidelines. Breastmilk has been shown to contain viral RNA (Costa et al, 2020; Tam et al, 2020). While it is unknown whether or not it causes infection via that route, breastmilk is considered safe. As such, some countries have adopted a strategy of separating positive mothers from their infants, others not allowing breastmilk feeding, ignoring the inherent pitfalls with regards to maternal-infant bonding and infant nutrition. However, the WHO recommends that mothers with suspected or confirmed COVID-19 should be encouraged to initiate or continue to breastfeed, since the benefits of breastfeeding substantially outweigh the potential risks for transmission (World Health Organization Scientific Brief, 2020).

The WHO also recommends that 'mother and infant should be enabled to remain together while rooming-in throughout the day and night and to practice skin-to-skin contact, including kangaroo mother care, especially immediately after birth and during establishment of breastfeeding, whether they or their infants have suspected or confirmed COVID-19' (World Health Organization Scientific Brief, 2020).

Data remain scarce about the risk of mother-to-foetal transmission of SARS-CoV-2, but the risk of transmission is estimated to be very low (probably under 1%) (Egloff et al, 2020). The virus has been found in placental tissue, but similar to breastmilk, the significance of this finding is as yet unknown (Costa et al, 2020).

22.5 CHARACTERISTICS OF CHILDREN WITH DISEASE

22.5.1 Epidemiology

The initial observational studies from Wuhan province in China, reported that compared to adults, children do not often experience severe disease. The Chinese CDC reported that only 1.3% of the 72 314 patients diagnosed with COVID-19 were younger than 20. In the largest case series from China, paediatric patients less than 19 years old only accounted for 2.0% of confirmed cases (Wu and McGoogan, 2020). Similarly, in Italy, COVID-19 cases in children accounted for 1.2% of cases, and in Korea, 4.8% (Korean Society of Infectious Diseases et al, 2020; Livingston and Bucher, 2020). Regarding transmission, in Guangzhou, China, only 1.3% of children who were in close contact with COVID-19 infected adults tested positive for SARS-CoV-2 (10/745) (Xu et al, 2020).

22.5.2 Severity

Among children treated at Wuhan Children's Hospital, 15.8% were asymptomatic and 19.3% only had an upper respiratory tract infection. The most common symptoms were cough (48.5%) and fever (41.5%) (W. Guan et al, 2020).

In a report of 171 children younger than 16 years hospitalised in Wuhan province, only three were admitted to the ICU, and one of those children died (Guan et al, 2020). The overall disease severity in children was reported to be significantly milder in children than in adults (Guan et al, 2020).

A study across ICUs in North America revealed 48 children had been admitted to 14 PICUs in the USA; 43/48 (83%) had pre-existing underlying medical conditions, 35 (73%) presented with respiratory symptoms and 18 (38%) required invasive ventilation, and 4.2% died. The authors concluded that COVID-19 could occasionally cause severe disease in children, but early hospital outcomes in children are better than in adults (Shekerdemian et al, 2020).

Shekerdemian et al found comorbidities in more than 80% of patients. These included 'medically complex' (40%) – defined as children who had long term dependence on technological support (including tracheostomy) associated with developmental delay and/or genetic anomalies – immune suppression/malignancy (23%), diabetes (8%). Obesity, which is considered an important risk factor for adult patients with COVID-19, was also a comorbidity amongst children (15%). The mortality rate in children was lower than in adults, leading the authors to conclude that children continue to face a far greater risk of critical illness from influenza than from COVID-19, emphasising the importance of routine non-COVID-19 preventative paediatric health maintenance (Shekerdemian et al, 2020).

22.5.3 Paediatric Inflammatory Multisystem Syndrome – Temporally associated with SARS-CoV-2 (PIMS-TS) / Multisystem Inflammatory Syndrome in Children (MIS-C)

The most serious paediatric complication of COVID-19 is a syndrome found amongst children and adolescents that is similar to Kawasaki Disease (KD), a rare vasculitis occurring in children with an unknown aetiology that causes coronary artery aneurysms. The diagnosis of KD is based on the presence of persistent fever, rash, cervical lymphadenopathy, conjunctival injection and changes to the mucosae and extremities (Viner and Whittaker, 2020). Although the cause is unknown, a preceding or active infection has been suspected due to its temporal association with viral epidemics.

In early May 2020, the first reports of a Kawasaki-like disease began to emerge from Bergamo, Italy, at the peak of the pandemic in that country (Verdoni et al, 2020). They reported 10 cases, of which half had features similar to KD. They reported a high proportion of shock (50% required fluid resuscitation and 20% needed inotropic support).

In late April 2020, clinicians in the UK reported a cluster of eight previously healthy children presenting with cardiovascular shock, fever, and hyperinflammation, requiring critical care. They dubbed the syndrome Paediatric Inflammatory Multisystem Syndrome – temporally associated with SARS-CoV-2 (PIMS-TS) (Riphagen et al, 2020). Other case series reported mucocutaneous manifestations, toxic shock syndrome, secondary haemophagocytic lymphohistiocytosis, or macrophage activation syndrome. In the USA, the syndrome was called 'Multisystem Inflammatory Syndrome in Children' (MIS-C) associated with SARS-CoV-2. It is a serious and life-threatening illness in previously healthy children and adolescents with a range of clinical manifestations and absence of pathognomonic findings or diagnostic tests. One hypothesis is that PIMS-TS/MIS-C is a consequence of immune-mediated injury triggered by SARS-CoV-2 infection (Feldstein et al, 2020).

There are slight differences in the case definitions across the world, but the principles of diagnosis and management are similar. The features include a fever > 38.5 degrees Celsius, single or multi-organ dysfunction, clear evidence of inflammation, with no other clear cause. Importantly, SARS-CoV-2 PCR testing may be positive or negative, and serology should be used to aid the diagnosis (World Health Organization, 2020a).

The principles of early general management and investigation include treating the patient as possibly infective for COVID-19, considering sepsis as a possibility, and treating with appropriate empiric antibiotics early, while performing laboratory investigations to assist diagnosis. Monitoring of cardiorespiratory function is important and early referral to an intensive care centre is advised, as well as other special investigations as required (such as ECG and echocardiogram).

Clinical features may include hypotension, tachycardia, confusion, headache, syncope, conjunctivitis, respiratory symptoms, sore throat, mucous membrane changes, lymphadenopathy, neck swelling, abdominal pain, diarrhoea, vomiting, rash, and swollen extremities. Initial targeted therapy should include intravenous immunoglobulins (IVIg), anticoagulation (with aspirin or heparin/LMWH) and steroids. Further treatment may involve repeat doses of the aforementioned and the addition of biological agents (IL-6 inhibitors or IL-1RA) if available (Henderson et al, 2020).

A study across 26 US states reported on 186 patients with MIS-C (Feldstein et al, 2020). The majority of patients (70%) had laboratory-confirmed previous or concurrent SARS-CoV-2 infection. The median age was 8.3 (IQR 3.3 – 12.5) years, 62% (115) were male, and 73% (135) had been previously well. Most patients had gastrointestinal symptoms (92%), cardiovascular involvement (80%), haematologic in 76%, mucocutaneous in 74% and respiratory in 70%. The median duration of hospitalisation was seven days (IQR 4 – 10), 80% received intensive care, 20% required mechanical ventilation, almost half (48%) required vasoactive support, and four patients (2%) died. Coronary artery aneurysms were found in 15 patients (8%). Nearly all patients (92 %) have elevations in at least four of the following inflammatory biomarkers: elevated ESR or CRP, lymphocytopaenia, neutrophilia, elevated ferritin level, hypoalbuminaemia, elevated ALT, anaemia, thrombocytopaenia, and an elevated D-dimer, prolonged INR, or elevated fibrinogen level. The treatment used included the following immunomodulators: IV-Ig in 77%, glucocorticoids in 41%, and IL-6 or IL-1RA inhibitors in 20%. In a small subgroup (14 patients), the median interval between the onset of COVID-19 symptoms and hospitalisation for MIS-C was reported to be 25 days (Feldstein et al, 2020).

Feldstein et al (2020) highlighted the importance of cardiac consideration in these patients: only 5% of children with KD in the USA required vasopressor or inotropic support for cardiovascular shock, compared to 50% of children with MIS-C. Myocardial dysfunction is a prominent extrapulmonary manifestation of COVID-19, highlighting the importance of performing an echocardiogram in all patients presenting with MIS-C. Since MIS-C is an evolving disease, the authors recommend long-term cardiac follow-up of children with MIS-C, according to the KD guidelines.

The full spectrum of MIS-C disease is not yet known and may be difficult to distinguish from typical KD since the conditions may share overlapping clinical features. Patients with MIS-C encompass a broader age range than typical KD, have more prominent gastrointestinal and neurologic symptoms, present more frequently in shock, and are more likely to display cardiac dysfunction (arrhythmias and ventricular dysfunction). At presentation, patients with MIS-C tend to have lower platelet counts, lower absolute lymphocyte counts, and higher CRP levels than patients with KD (Henderson et al, 2020).

Despite this severe inflammatory syndrome in children, children remain minimally affected by SARS-CoV-2 infection overall. Understanding PIMS-TS/MIS-C may provide information about immune responses to SARS-CoV-2 that might have relevance for both adults and children alike (Viner and Whittaker, 2020).

22.5.4 Treatment

Treatment for COVID-19 infection remains supportive in nature. Since there are no proven therapies, it is recommended to restrict any proposed therapies for the treatment of COVID-19 infection to the context of formal clinical trials. Careful consideration should be taken in children especially because of the continued lack of proven efficacy and concern regarding adverse effects in some cases (Shekerdemian et al, 2020).

Since point of care testing is unavailable, it is recommended that hospitalised children who fit local case definitions for COVID-19 be treated as such until proven otherwise (Ong et al, 2020). Given the relatively low rates of critical illness due to COVID-19, the importance of testing, PPE and personnel safety will likely create more impact than sick patients with confirmed infection (Ong et al, 2020).

It is important to bear in mind that the management of COVID-19 has not been studied prospectively. Recommendations are largely based on retrospective studies, this currently being the best evidence available. As is also often the case, much of paediatric care is extrapolated from adult studies. There have been calls to accelerate COVID-19 clinical research in resource-limited settings by forming coalitions and collaborations (COVID-19 Clinical Research Coalition, 2020). Paediatricians should make use of the opportunities afforded by these sorts of collaborations, or form their own local, national and international networks. Establishing communication channels is essential to disseminate information and education for this emerging infection with rapidly generated data. Moreover, it creates a sense of community amongst practitioners (Ong et al, 2020).

22.6   MENTAL HEALTH

The pandemic is a stressful time for citizens and healthcare workers alike. People are anxious about their personal welfare and that of their loved ones. Viral illness and the novelty of this condition invokes additional concern. This sense of isolation and fear is further exacerbated by the lockdown and physical distancing strategies intended to limit the spread of disease. It is essential during these difficult times for politicians to exhibit strong leadership and have clear communication with the public. Healthcare providers must prioritise the mental well-being of their staff (Ong et al, 2020).

Although children are very unlikely to experience severe disease, anxiety and fear are heightened in the paediatric context. The public has responded negatively to the opening of schools. Parents request advice from paediatricians – a number of position statements from paediatric professional organisations have supported the return to school (South African Paediatric Association, 2020; South African Paediatric Association and Paediatrician Management Group, 2020). Children are less at risk of being infected than adults and are unlikely to be the index case in the household (Munro and Faust, 2020). Most children present with mild symptoms. Although severe disease is possible, it is rare and mortality is negligible when compared with other childhood diseases (Dong et al, 2020). For healthcare workers treating paediatric patients, it is important to maintain perspective, as one is more likely to contract the virus from community transmission than from caring for a COVID-19 infected child.

The importance of non-pharmacological measures in preventing the spread of disease needs to be stressed, that is wearing a cloth mask whenever in public, hand hygiene and regular cleaning of commonly used surfaces in the home, school and at work (Blumberg et al, 2020).

22.7   PREPARING FOR THE PANDEMIC

South Africa benefitted from the seasonal lag in respiratory infections, which allowed time for preparation. Furthermore, the hard lockdown period in South Africa limited the number of admissions during the early phase of the pandemic in the country, allowing much needed time to ready facilities. Preparation for the pandemic is key to limiting its negative effects. Preparation should include preparing the facilities to accommodate patients, both those suspected or proven to have COVID-19, and those without. Patient flow needs to be addressed. While it is difficult and costly to address the infrastructure, simple means of identifying additional areas and separating wards goes a long way to limit the spread of infection. In resource-limited settings, where space is also limited, innovative thinking is needed to address issues for maximum benefit (Ong et al, 2020).

In preparation for a pandemic, identifying potential surge capacity in the form of extra beds, staff, and equipment is essential. Identifying staff who may be able to bolster the response may also be necessary at an early stage (Saggers et al, 2020). This may include the reversal of the traditional hierarchy in order to minimise staff exposure, such as which level of staff attends births (World Health Organization, 2020b).

Further preparation includes the procurement of personal protective equipment (PPE). It is imperative that clear guidelines about the use of PPE are established, and training undertaken at all levels. Shortages of certain items are likely to occur. For this reason, supply chains systems must be strengthened to maintain the safety of healthcare professionals. PPE must also be used rationally, with those at highest exposure to infection using the highest level of protection and those at lower risk using what is appropriate for that setting (Ahmed et al, 2020).

22.8   ADVOCATING FOR CHILDREN DURING A PANDEMIC

Healthcare workers, in particular paediatricians, need to be outspoken in upholding the well-being of children during this pandemic. Political and healthcare workers in positions of authority must be encouraged the make rational and realistic decisions. When decisions that do not hold the best interests of children at heart are made, these must be challenged in the form of petitions and position statements from authoritative, professional, and academic bodies (South African Paediatric Association, 2020; South African Paediatric Association and Paediatrician Management Group, 2020).

A national intersectoral approach with balanced strategies to protect children is central to coordinated pandemic response efforts (van Bruwaene et al, 2020). While it is fortunate that COVID-19 has limited direct effects amongst children, it is time to strengthen existing preventative healthcare programmes and improve access to care for the most vulnerable among us. The health of our children needs to be at the heart of the future of South Africa (Siegfried and Mathews, 2020).

22.9   CONCLUSION

Thankfully, the COVID-19 pandemic relatively spares children. The majority of children are asymptomatic or minimally affected by the infection, but a small number of children and adolescents can develop serious or life-threatening complications. On the other hand, almost all children are indirectly affected by the strategies used to limit the spread of the virus, with the most vulnerable invariably being the hardest hit.

Careful thought needs to be put into planning for pandemics to limit the adverse effects that the disease and policies may have on the children in the country. Paediatricians and other healthcare workers must advocate for the protection of children so as to live up to Nelson Mandela's ideal, as set out by the Children's Act of 2005, 'that the child's best interest is of paramount importance' (South Africa, 2005).

22.10 SELF-ASSESSMENT QUESTIONS

1. What is MIS-C?
2. How should babies born to mothers with COVID-19 be managed?

22.11 REFERENCES

Ahmed, S., Mvalo, T., Akech, S., Agweyu, A., Baker, K., Bar-Zeev, N., Campbell, H., Checkley, W., Chisti, M.J., Colbourn, T., Cunningham, S., Duke, T., English, M., Falade, A.G., Fancourt, N.S.S., Ginsburg, A.S., Graham, H.R., Gray, D.M., Gupta, M., Hammitt, L., Hesseling, A.C., Hooli, S., Johnson, A.W.B.R., King, C., Kirby, M.A., Lanata, C.F., Lufesi, N., MacKenzie, G.A., McCracken, J.P., Moschovis, P.P., Nair, H., Oviawe, O., Pomat, W.S., Santosham, M., Seddon, J.A., Thahane, L.K., Wahl, B., van der Zalm, M., Verwey, C., Yoshida, L.M., Zar, H.J., Howie, S.R.C. and McCollum, E.D. 2020. Protecting children in low-income and middle-income countries from COVID-19. *BMJ Global Health* 5, pp. 1–3. doi: https://doi.org/10.1136/bmjgh-2020-002844.

Blumberg, L., Jassat, W., Mendelson, M. and Cohen, C. 2020. The COVID-19 crisis in South Africa: Protecting the vulnerable. *South African Medical Journal* 110, pp. 825–826. doi: https://doi.org/10.7196/SAMJ.2020.v110i9.15116.

Costa, S., Posteraro, B., Marchetti, S., Tamburrini, E., Carducci, B., Lanzone, A., Valentini, P., Buonsenso, D., Sanguinetti, M., Vento, G.and Cattani, P. 2020. Excretion of SARS-CoV-2 in human breast milk. *Clinical Microbiology and Infection* 26, pp. 1430–1432. doi: https://doi.org/10.1016/j.cmi.2020.05.027.

COVID-19 Clinical Research Coalition. 2020. Global coalition to accelerate COVID-19 clinical research in resource-limited settings. *The Lancet* 395, pp. 1322–1325. doi: https://doi.org/10.1016/S0140-6736(20)30798-4.

Dong, Y., Mo, X., Hu, Y., Qi, X., Jiang, F., Jiang, Z., Jiang, Z. and Tong, S. 2020. Epidemiology of COVID-19 among children in China. *Pediatrics* 145, e20200702. doi: https://doi.org/https://doi.org/10.1542/peds.2020-0702.

Egloff, C., Vauloup-Fellous, C., Picone, O., Mandelbrot, L. and Roques, P. 2020. Evidence and possible mechanisms of rare maternal-fetal transmission of SARS-CoV-2. *Journal of Clinical Virology* 128, pp. 1–8. doi: https://doi.org/10.1016/j.jcv.2020.104447.

Feldstein, L.R., Rose, E.B., Horwitz, S.M., Collins, J.P., Newhams, M.M., Son, M.B.F., Newburger, J.W., Kleinman, L.C., Heidemann, S.M., Martin, A.A., Singh, A.R., Li, S., Tarquinio, K.M., Jaggi, P., Oster, M.E., Zackai, S.P., Gillen, J., Ratner, A.J., Walsh, R.F., Fitzgerald, J.C., Keenaghan, M.A., Alharash, H., Doymaz, S., Clouser, K.N., Giuliano, J.S., Gupta, A., Parker, R.M., Maddux, A.B., Havalad, V., Ramsingh, S., Bukulmez, H., Bradford, T.T., Smith, L.S., Tenforde, M.W., Carroll, C.L., Riggs, B.J., Gertz, S.J., Daube, A., Lansell, A., Coronado Munoz, A., Hobbs, C. v., Marohn, K.L., Halasa, N.B., Patel, M.M. and Randolph, A.G. 2020. Multisystem Inflammatory Syndrome in U.S. Children and Adolescents. *New England Journal of Medicine* 383, pp. 334–346. doi: https://doi.org/10.1056/nejmoa2021680.

Guan, H., Okely, A.D., Aguilar-Farias, N., del Pozo Cruz, B., Draper, C.E., el Hamdouchi, A., Florindo, A.A., Jáuregui, A., Katzmarzyk, P.T., Kontsevaya, A., Löf, M., Park, W., Reilly, J.J., Sharma, D., Tremblay, M.S. and Veldman, S.L.C. 2020. Promoting healthy movement behaviours among children during the COVID-19 pandemic. *The Lancet Child and Adolescent Health* 4, pp. 416–418. doi: https://doi.org/10.1016/S2352-4642(20)30131-0.

Guan, W., Ni, Z., Hu, Y., Liang, W., Ou, C., He, J., Liu, L., Shan, H., Lei, C., Hui, D.S.C., Du, B., Li, L., Zeng, G., Yuen, K.Y., Chen, R., Tang, C., Wang, T., Chen, P., Xiang, J., Li, S., Wang, J.L., Liang, Z., Peng, Y., Wei, L., Liu, Y., Hu, Y.H., Peng, P., Wang, J.M., Liu, J., Chen, Z., Li, G., Zheng, Z., Qiu, S., Luo, J., Ye, C., Zhu, S. and Zhong, N. 2020. Clinical characteristics of coronavirus disease 2019 in China. *New England Journal of Medicine* 382, pp. 1708–1720. doi: https://doi.org/10.1056/NEJMoa2002032.

Henderson, L.A., Canna, S.W., Friedman, K.G., Gorelik, M., Lapidus, S.K., Bassiri, H., Behrens, E.M., Ferris, A., Kernan, K.F., Schulert, G.S., Seo, P., F. Son, M.B., Tremoulet, A.H., Yeung, R.S.M., Mudano, A.S., Turner, A.S., Karp, D.R. and Mehta, J.J. 2020. American College of Rheumatology Clinical Guidance for Pediatric Patients with Multisystem Inflammatory Syndrome in Children (MIS-C) Associated with SARS-CoV-2 and Hyperinflammation in COVID-19. Version 1. *Arthritis & Rheumatology* 72, pp. 1791–1805. doi: https://doi.org/10.1002/art.41454.

Korean Society of Infectious Diseases, Korean Society of Pediatric Infectious Diseases, Korean Society of Epidemiology, Korean Society for Antimicrobial Therapy, Korean Society for Healthcare-associated Infection Control and Prevention, Korean Centers for Disease Control and Prevention, 2020. Report on the epidemiological features of coronavirus disease 2019 (COVID-19) outbreak in the Republic of Korea from January 19 to March 2, 2020. *Journal of Korean Medical Science* 35, e112. doi: https://doi.org/10.3346/jkms.2020.35.e112.

Livingston, E. and Bucher, K. 2020. Coronavirus Disease 2019 (COVID-19) in Italy. *JAMA* 323, p. 1335. doi: https://doi.org/10.1001/jama.2020.4344.

Munro, A.P.S. and Faust, S.N. 2020. Children are not COVID-19 super spreaders: Time to go back to school. *Archives of Disease in Childhood* 105, pp. 618–619. doi: http://dx.doi.org/10.1136/archdischild-2020-319474.

Ong, J.S.M., Tosoni, A., Kim, Y.J., Kissoon, N. and Murthy, S. 2020. Coronavirus Disease 2019 in Critically Ill Children: A Narrative Review of the Literature. *Pediatric Critical Care Medicine* 21, pp. 662–666. doi: https://doi.org/10.1097/PCC.0000000000002376.

Riphagen, S., Gomez, X., Gonzalez-Martinez, C., Wilkinson, N. and Theocharis, P. 2020. Hyperinflammatory shock in children during COVID-19 pandemic. *The Lancet* 395, pp. 1607–1608. doi: https://doi.org/10.1016/S0140-6736(20)31094-1.

Saggers, R.T., Ramdin, T.D., Bandini, R.M. and Ballot, D.E. 2020. COVID-19 Preparedness in a Neonatal Unit at a Tertiary Hospital in Johannesburg, South Africa. *Wits Journal of Clinical Medicine* 2(SI), pp. 43–46. doi: http://dx.doi.org/10.18772/26180197.2020.v2nSIa8.

Shekerdemian, L.S., Mahmood, N.R., Wolfe, K.K., Riggs, B.J., Ross, C.E., McKiernan, C.A., Heidemann, S.M., Kleinman, L.C., Sen, A.I., Hall, M.W., Priestley, M.A., McGuire, J.K., Boukas, K., Sharron, M.P. and Burns, J.P. 2020. Characteristics and Outcomes of Children with Coronavirus Disease 2019 (COVID-19) Infection Admitted to US and Canadian Pediatric Intensive Care Units. *JAMA Pediatrics* 174, pp. 868–873. doi: https://doi.org/10.1001/jamapediatrics.2020.1948.

Siegfried, N. and Mathews, C. 2020. COVID-19 and the school response: Looking back to learn what we can do better. *South African Medical Journal* 110, pp. 727–728. Doi: https://doi.org/10.7196/SAMJ.2020.v110i8.14991.

South Africa, 2005. Children's Act No. 38 of 2005.

South Africa, 1996. Constitution of the Republic of South Africa.

South African Paediatric Association. 2020. Prevention of coronavirus infection (Covid-19) in early childhood development (EDC) programmes.

South African Paediatric Association, Paediatrician Management Group, 2020. POSITION STATEMENT: Public School Closure.

Tam, P.C.K., Ly, K.M., Kernich, M.L., Spurrier, N., Lawrence, D., Gordon, D.L. and Tucker, E.C. 2020. Detectable severe acute respiratory syndrome coronavirus 2 (SARS-CoV-2) in human breast milk of a mildly symptomatic patient with coronavirus disease 2019 (COVID-19). *Clinical Infectious Diseases* 72, pp. 128–130. doi: https://doi.org/10.1093/cid/ciaa673.

Van Bruwaene, L., Goga, A. and Green, R.J. 2020. What are we doing to the children of South Africa under the guise of COVID-19 lockdown? *South African Medical Journal* 110, pp. 574–575. https://doi.org/10.7196/SAMJ.2020.v110i7.14932.

Verdoni, L., Mazza, A., Gervasoni, A., Martelli, L., Ruggeri, M., Ciuffreda, M., Bonanomi, E. and D'Antiga, L. 2020. An outbreak of severe Kawasaki-like disease at the Italian epicentre of the SARS-CoV-2 epidemic: an observational cohort study. *The Lancet* 395, pp. 1771–1778. doi: https://doi.org/10.1016/S0140-6736(20)31103-X.

Viner, R.M. and Whittaker, E., 2020. Kawasaki-like disease: emerging complication during the COVID-19 pandemic. *The Lancet* 395, pp. 1741–1743. doi: https://doi.org/10.1016/S0140-6736(20)31129-6.

World Health Organization. 2020a. Multisystem inflammatory syndrome in children and adolescents temporally related to COVID-19: Scientific Brief 15 May 2020. Available at: https://www.who.int/news-room/commentaries/detail/multisystem-inflammatory-syndrome-in-children-and-adolescents-with-covid-19.

World Health Organization. 2020b. Rational use of personal protective equipment for coronavirus disease (COVID-19): interim guidance. World Health Organization, Geneva.

World Health Organization Scientific Brief, 2020. Breastfeeding and COVID-19, pp. 1–3.

Wu, Z. and McGoogan, J.M. 2020. Characteristics of and Important Lessons from the Coronavirus Disease 2019 (COVID-19) Outbreak in China: Summary of a Report of 72314 Cases from the Chinese Center for Disease Control and Prevention. *JAMA* 323, pp. 1239–1242. doi: https://doi.org/10.1001/jama.2020.2648.

Xu, Y., Li, X., Zhu, B., Liang, H., Fang, C., Gong, Y., Guo, Q., Sun, X., Zhao, D., Shen, J., Zhang, H., Liu, H., Xia, H., Tang, J., Zhang, K. and Gong, S. 2020. Characteristics of pediatric SARS-CoV-2 infection and potential evidence for persistent fecal viral shedding. *Nature Medicine* 26, pp. 502–505. doi: https://doi.org/10.1038/s41591-020-0817-4.

PROVISION OF SEXUAL AND REPRODUCTIVE HEALTHCARE SERVICES DURING PANDEMICS

Lawrence Chauke

23.1 INTRODUCTION

Drawing on local and international lessons learnt from the current and previous infectious disease outbreaks and medical ethics, this chapter presents an argument for the preservation and guidance for the provision of sexual and reproductive health services (SRH) during pandemics. Specifically, we argue that SRH must be prioritised during pandemics because women and children constitute vulnerable groups in most societies. This vulnerability is likely to be exacerbated unless strategic and deliberate efforts are put in place to protect them. For the purpose of this discussion, SRH refers to the following services:

- Prenatal and newborn care
- Labour and deliveries
- Family planning and termination of pregnancy (TOP)
- HIV prevention and treatment.

23.2 OBJECTIVES

At the end of this chapter, the reader is expected to achieve the following learning objectives.

- Describe the effects of a pandemic on SRH.
- Justify the prioritisation of SRH during pandemics.
- Apply medical and ethical frameworks to help guide the prioritisation and configuration of SRH during pandemics in order to minimise both the direct and pandemic-related response to SRH.

23.3   PANDEMICS AND SRH

Pandemics have devastating effects on the health of the population. Outbreaks of infectious diseases are unpredictable and when they occur, leave little time for proper planning mainly because the natural history and healthcare impact of the offending organism is initially not fully understood.

Pandemics have both direct and indirect effects on population health (Detailed discussion follows later in the chapter). For now, it is sufficient to mention that direct effects depend on the characteristics (virulence) of the causative agent and the indirect effects are mediated through multiple pathways which include, among others:

- Country's response to pandemics such as lock downs and restriction of movement of people.
- Prioritisation and repurposing of healthcare services and redeployment of healthcare personnel.
- Disruption in supply chain services which has negative impact on the availability of medicines such as antiretroviral (ART), contraceptives as well as other healthcare resources.
- Negative impact on countries' economic and individuals' ability to secure employment. As a result countries struggle to meet their social obligations while the high level of unemployment and entrenchment limit individual's ability to access healthcare services.

Therefore, pandemics, perforce, have an important bearing on SRH because these services cater for a unique population with special needs. First, this is because the majority of women utilising SRH services (maternity services in particular) are generally young and healthy and as a result are often not prioritised during pandemics due to the assumption that their immune status makes them less vulnerable to infections. Secondly, while pregnancy is a physiological state, women continue to die of avoidable pregnancy-related complications, mainly due to the marginalisation of women in society and because women's health issues are not a priority in many countries around the globe. Thirdly, unwanted pregnancy and unsafe abortion, both of which are associated with high maternal mortality, remain major threats during pandemics as well. This is because during lockdowns, women are likely to fall pregnant, experience high levels of physical and sexual abuse in addition to limited access to contraceptive and TOP services (Adelekan et al, 2020). Consequently, women and children who are already disadvantaged under normal circumstances, often bear an additional, disproportionate burden of disease, firstly due to the direct effect of the pandemic and indirectly as a result of the health system response to the infectious outbreak.

While most pregnant women are young and healthy, obstetric practice increasingly sees women with comorbidities often brought on by social deprivation or unhealthy lifestyles. These patients have additional complex clinical needs which require greater attention. Pregnancy related complications are also unpredictable, affect women considered to be low risk and the limited access to healthcare that often accompanies pandemics adds additional vulnerability to this group (Pattinson, 2015).

The above contributes to the high rate of maternal deaths as a result, it does not come as a surprise that maternal deaths remain a top priority on the global health agenda. It would be a travesty of justice if SRH services fall through the cracks or are relegated to the sidewalk during pandemics (Jolivet et al, 2018). The death of a mother is a violation of women's rights which has disastrous long-term social, economic and psychological consequences for the surviving children and affected families (Table 23.1). Neglecting SRH services during pandemics would make it impossible for countries to meet the United Nation' Sustainable Development Goals (SDGs), particularly SDG 3 which, among others requires countries by 2030 (United Nation, 2015) to:

- Reduce maternal mortality to less than 70 per 100 000 livebirths.
- End preventable deaths of new-borns and children under 5 years of age.
- End the epidemics of AIDS, tuberculosis, malaria, neglected tropical diseases, combat hepatitis, water-borne diseases, and other communicable diseases.
- Ensure universal access to sexual and reproductive healthcare services, including family planning, access to information and education, and the integration of reproductive health into national strategies and programmes.

The above factors are perhaps compelling reasons for the prioritisation of SRH services even in times of crisis (Molla et al, 2015; Reed et al, 2000).

Table 23.1 Negative effects of the death of a mother

• Loss of a maternal caregiver disrupts family life, results in broken families and orphaned children.
• Surviving children experience adverse health and social outcomes, among those, premature death, poor school outcomes, child abuse and neglect as well as behavioural problems such as illicit drug abuse and sexual inhibition.
• Financial and economic burden on extended family members have to take additional responsibilities of looking after orphaned children.

23.4 EFFECT OF PANDEMICS ON MATERNAL HEALTH AND RELATED HEALTHCARE SERVICES

Previous pandemics have highlighted the need to prioritise and preserve SRH services. As discussed in the previous section, the effect of pandemics on SRH services are both direct and indirect (direct effect of infectious agent and indirectly (country, public and health system responses to the pandemic).

23.4.1 Direct Effects

Pregnant women are at increased risk of viral and bacterial infections and, when they are infected, have more severe illnesses particularly respiratory infections as a result of physiological adaptations which occur during pregnancy:

- Immune: The altered cellular immunity associated with pregnancy renders women more susceptible to infections (Jamieson et al, 2006).
- CNS: Increase in CSF pressure.
- Cardiovascular Systems: There is an increase in cardiac output (CO), stroke volume(SV), heart rate (HR) as well as hypertrophy of the left ventricle.
- Respiratory system: Increase in minute volume (MV), decrease in functional residual capacity (FRC), increase in partial pressure of oxygen (PaO2) and decrease in partial pressure of carbon dioxide (PaCO2).
- Endocrine: Thyroid hyperplasia, transient hypothyroidism and insulin resistance (increases the risk of glucose hyperglycemia).

These changes are thought to be responsible for the increase in both the incidence and severity of hypoxia when pregnant women present with respiratory diseases.

During the 1918 and 2009 influenza and H1N1 outbreaks, pregnant women were more likely to present with severe disease, require ICU admission and had a higher risk of dying compared to the general population (Kourtis et al, 2015; Kuehn, 2009; Saleeby et al, 2010). In a Swedish study, Colins et al (2020) reported that pregnant women (including those that were in the immediate postpartum period) with COVID-19 were more likely to be admitted to ICU compared to non-pregnant infected women.

However, the reported obstetric effects of pandemics vary, calling for more vigilance when managing pregnant women during infectious outbreaks:

- Infuenza (1918), Severe Acute Respiratory Sydrome, SARS (2002-2003), Middle East Respiratory Syndrome or MERS (2012) were associated with an increase in severity of respiratory disease, ICU admission, maternal death, spontaneous miscarriages, congenital anomalies such as hydrocephalus, neural tube defects, cleft lip and palate, congenital heart disease, intrauterine growth restriction (IUGR), preterm births and neonatal ICU (NICU) admission (Korutis et al, 2015).

- Ebola: Similarly, the Ebola pandemic was associated with a higher incidence of miscarriage, stillbirth, maternal morbidity and mortality (Bebell et al, 2017).
- Zika: The Zika virus has been associated with an increase in foetal anomalies, in particular, microcephally while the effect on pregnant women of this usually mild and self-limiting infection was similar to that of the general population (Lin et al, 2017).
- COVID 19: Evidence linking COVID-19 with increased maternal morbidity and mortality without increase in congenital anomalies, is starting to emerge (Basu et al, 2021; Silveira Campos and Peixoto Caldas, 2020; Westgren et al, 2021).

23.4.2 Indirect Effects

The indirect effects are two-fold:

23.4.2.1 Public health response to pandemics

The emergence of a pandemic triggers a public health response that is directed at containing the spread of infection, minimise the detrimental effects of the outbreak on the health of the population and reduce pressure on the healthcare system. Common country-level interventions include:

- Lockdowns to reduce movement of people and person-to-person contact thereby minimising the spread of the infection;
- Prioritisation of specific healthcare services by shifting healthcare resources to pandemic-related healthcare needs; and
- Suspension of some of the health services in order to free up resources in order to manage the outbreak.

Evidence from the 2013–2016 Ebola epidemic in Guinea, Liberia and Sierra Leone has conclusively demonstrated that infection containment measures had a negative effect on services and reproductive healthcare services. These countries experienced a decrease in antenatal clinic attendance and of deliveries in healthcare facilities during the duration of the outbreak (Delamou et al, 2017; Sochas, 2017). This resulted in an increase in the number of maternal deaths, completely reversing the gains made prior to the start of the epidemic. Similarly researchers have been trying to draw the world's attention to the observed increase in maternal mortality associated with COVID-19 (Amorim et al, 2020; Basu et al, 2021; Takemoto et al, 2020). The 2017–2019 Saving Mothers' Report in South Africa included a section on COVID-19 and maternal deaths (NCCEMD, 2021).

This report found an increase in maternal mortality which peaked around June, one month before the peak was observed in the general population (NCCEMD, 2021). This finding suggests that pregnant women suffer disproportionately from the COVID-19 pandemic yet little attention is being paid to this vulnerable group in the world's response to the pandemic.

During a pandemic, healthcare services are configured to respond to the unfolding crisis. This usually requires prioritisation of hospital beds and staff to deal with pandemic-related healthcare needs. Routine services and operations are either temporarily suspended or adjusted, to free resources for the outbreak.

Restrictions on movement also have a negative impact on women and pregnant women's ability to access transport and healthcare services resulting in failure to access help timeously in times of need. These are among the known driving factors of maternal mortality, particularly in low- and middle-income countries (Dahab and Sakellariou, 2020). A South African study on the early effects of COVID-19 on the utilisation of family planning and the termination of pregnancy reported a marked decline in the use of these services compared to a similar period prior to the pandemic (Adelekan et al, 2020). The authors ascribed their findings to the effect of the country's lockdown.

23.4.2.2 Women's response to a pandemic

A pandemic causes psychological distress and uncertainties, and pregnant women are not exempted. Lockdowns also result in economic hardship, which further exacerbates an already difficult situation. Women therefore delay seeking help because of the fear of contracting an infection while in hospital. There is also a reduced availability of health services and difficulties in accessing transport due to a lack of funds and/or limited availability of transport services.

23.5 SUMMARY OF THE EFFECTS OF PANDEMICS OF SRH SERVICES

In summary, infectious outbreaks have the potential to exacerbate negative health outcomes in vulnerable groups, such as women and children. The negative outcomes are mediated via multiple mechanisms such as a lockdown, fear of contracting infection, limited availability of healthcare services and difficulty in accessing transport (either due to economic reasons or reduced availability). Furthermore, a pandemic generates emotional distress particularly in pregnant women, who worry about their own health and that of the unborn child. These and other factors contribute to adverse pregnancy outcomes, in particular, increases in maternal and perinatal mortality (Jones et al, 2016). The death of a woman is a violation of women's rights and a social disaster that has far-reaching consequences for the surviving children and affected families. The above highlights the need to prioritise SRH services during pandemics.

23.6 MANAGEMENT OF SRH AND RELATED HEALTHCARE SERVICES DURING A PANDEMIC

23.6.1 Health Systems' Response to Pandemics

Three main issues underpin health system response to pandemics:

- Healthcare services prioritisation;
- Infection control; and
- Promotion of mental wellbeing for patients, families, communities and the healthcare workforce (Figure 23.1).

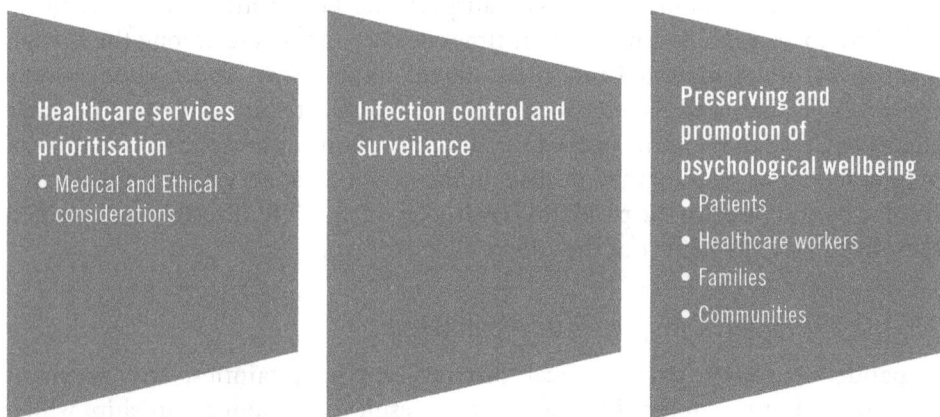

Healthcare services prioritisation
- Medical and Ethical considerations

Infection control and surveilance

Preserving and promotion of psychological wellbeing
- Patients
- Healthcare workers
- Families
- Communities

Figure 23.1 Pandemic response framework

23.6.2 Operational Guidance and Ethical Principles

Prioritisation of healthcare services during a crisis is complex and must be based on sound medical and ethical principles.

23.6.2.1 Operational guidance

The World Health Organization (WHO, 2020) developed a set of general guidelines to assist countries and concerned parties in managing healthcare services during outbreaks (Table 23.2).

Table 23.2 Guidance for the management of healthcare services during infectious outbreaks

Strategy	Action
1. *Governance and coordination mechanisms*	• Establish mechanisms and protocols to guide the governance and coordination of healthcare services • Establish triggers for the reallocation of routine healthcare capacity towards essential services in a phased manner • Embark on ongoing monitoring of the delivery of essential health services in order to identify ongoing gaps and respond accordingly
2. *Identification of context-relevant essential services*	Prioritise: • SRH services • STIs and HIV prevention • Services aimed at prevention of communicable diseases (e.g., vaccination) • Medication supply for chronic diseases • Management of time sensitive conditions (e.g., some cancers) and emergencies • Radiology, laboratory and blood bank services • Critical care services and other critical care therapies
3. *Optimisation service delivery platforms*	• Compile a list of country's essential services • Compile a list of routine and elective services that can be delayed or redirected to non-affected areas • Establish a strategy and protocol for reduction (and re-introduction) of healthcare services when conditions permit) in a progressive manner
4. *Establishment of effective patient flow protocol encompassing screening, triage, and referral between and across different all levels of care*	• Map and designate functions to existing healthcare facilities • Designate 24hrs acute care to some of the hospitals, taking into consideration competing needs and contextual capacity • Redirect chronic care to community-based and other facilities that have been identified for this purpose • Set up outreach mechanisms to maintain delivery of essential services

➡

Strategy	Action
5. *Redistribution and repurposing of health workforce*	• Implement screening protocol at care sites (e.g., universal screening) • Establish a triage system based on disease acuity • Establish isolation areas for infected patients • Establish care referral pathways and protocols for different categories of patients (e.g., isolation, hospital care, ICU care, etc.)
6. *Establishment of mechanisms to ensure continued availability of essential medications, equipment and supplies*	• Conduct needs and skills assessment for different clinical areas • Distribute healthcare workers according to their skills level • Upskill healthcare workforce (task shifting) where possible to respond to contextual needs • Establish on the job training programmes focusing on diagnosis, triage, clinical management of the infection, including infection prevention and control measures

(Adapted from WHO, 2020)

23.6.3 Ethical Principles

Three ethical principles are relevant for the provision of SRH services during pandemics and therefore worthy of discussion. The reader is referred to WHO (2016) for detailed discussion.

23.6.3.1 Justice

In the context of competing needs and inadequate resources, the first principle is that of justice. How do decision-makers ensure fairness in the allocation of scarce resources during an outbreak? Equity, utility and procedural justice are some of the main pillars that form the principle of justice. Equity is concerned with making sure that people with similar needs and similar circumstances, are treated the same, in order to avoid unfair discrimination. Assuming all things are equal, equity requires that special attention is provided to marginalised and vulnerable groups. This principle paid valid argument to prioritise SRH services during pandemics and natural disasters. Utility, on the other hand, focuses on maximising the benefit and cost-efficiency of an intervention. It is about choosing the option that is likely to provide maximum impact at the lowest cost. Utility and equity are however not necessarily mutually exclusive because utility should also consider the need of the vulnerable and the marginalised. Balancing the need for cost-effectiveness with inclusiveness and equitable distribution of resources when allocating resources is of paramount importance.

The focus of procedural justice is on fairness and transparency of the decision-making process. This is made possible by making sure that all relevant and key stakeholders are given an opportunity to contribute to the decisions that are made. Extensive engagement with stakeholders ensures accountability and shared decision-making in terms of healthcare service design, prioritisation and oversight.

23.6.3.2 Beneficence

The second principle, beneficence, states that an action is justified by its outcome. In healthcare, the expected outcome is either a reduction/removal of pain/suffering. Healthcare workers have an ethical obligation to always act in the best interests of patients and the communities they service.

23.6.3.3 Respect for persons

The third principle is respect for persons. This principle states that an individual has a right to make decisions about his/her own health and related matters (autonomy). This right must be respected at all times.

23.6.3.4 Reciprocity

Fourth, the principle of reciprocity requires that those who contribute to a cause should have proportional return for their contribution. This argument has been used to prioritise health workers in terms of allocating scarce resources, such as ICU beds, based on the risk they face when treating patients. The challenge is on who should be given priority between clinical and non-clinical staff, all of whom complement each other in the provision of healthcare services in a situation where the two compete for the same resource. An argument can also be made that health workers have an ethical obligation and a social contract to provide frontline healthcare services without expecting special treatment or favours. This line of thought is supported by the fact that medical practice is a risky business and by choosing the profession, health workers accept the risk, irrespective of whether it is done explicitly or implicitly. Additionally, health workers have committed to act in the best interest of the patient (Voo and Capps, 2010). In this setting, the ethical principle of reciprocity could be satisfied by prioritising health workers in terms of access to personal protective equipment (PPE), ensuring that health workers have access to social and mental support services, creating an enabling and safe working environment and not necessarily giving them unfair advantages over patients with similar competing needs (WHO, 2016).

23.6.3.5 Solidarity

The fifth principle, solidarity is when communities and members of society stand together to fight a common threat. In a pandemic, solidarity requires that everyone does their part, in order to reduce the spread and impact of infection. This could be in the form of pooling limited resources, adhering to social distancing and supporting those who are infected and affected by the pandemic. Solidarity also requires the inclusion of the marginalised and vulnerable members of society in healthcare interventions and planning.

23.6.4 Implications for SRH services

Both the WHO Guidance on Management of Healthcare Services (WHO, 2020) and the Ethical Framework (WHO, 2016) guidance on management of healthcare services during outbreaks are important and useful tools to consider when managing outbreaks and pandemics with special focus on prioritising SRH services. What is the relevance of the above in terms of prioritising SRH? SRH services serve vulnerable groups and as a result, should be prioritised during infectious outbreaks and natural disaster. By doing so, society would be demonstrating its commitment (solidarity) to safeguard the right to dignity of its marginalise and vulnerable members. Prioritisation of SRH services should be deliberate, guided by ethical principles of justice, beneficence, solidary and autonomy by not taking away services earmarked for women and instead making them widely available and accessible so that women can make their own choices regarding their utilisation. In doing so, health workers should always prioritise the vulnerable groups despite scarce resources while adhering to stringent infection prevention and control measures to minimise getting infected.

23.7 HOW SHOULD SRH SERVICES BE CONFIGURED DURING OUTBREAKS AND NATURAL DISASTERS?

The answer to the above will depend on what is known about the offending organism and also contextual factors. Table 23.3 and 23.4 are examples of service configurations for maternity and reproductive services, respectively.

Table 23.3 Maternity services

---

1. *Antenatal care*

   - Treat antenatal clinics as medium risk and use risk-appropriate personal protective equipment (PPE) based on the infectious agent

   - Do not interrupt antenatal care schedules for high-risk pregnancy

   - Use virtual platform for some of the consultation if feasible and safe to do

   - Tailor antenatal care according to the need. The following antenatal schedules are suggested (some can be replaced or supplemented with virtual antenatal care where available:

     - Booking for pregnancy confirmation and to rule out abnormal pregnancy

     - Aneuploidy screening visit at 11–13 weeks and 6 days if missed, 16 weeks

     - Foetal anomaly scan and general check-up at 18–22 weeks

     - Foetal growth and maternal check-up: 26, 30–32, 36, 38, 40 weeks

     - Assessment for postdates and induction: 41 weeks

2. *Foetal Medicine services*

   - Continue to provide foetal scan but under stringent infection prevention and control measures

   - Consult existing professional guidelines on invasive testing. When not available, benefits should be weighed against the risks and discussed with the woman

3. *Labour ward and deliveries*

   - Manage labour ward high-risk area (maximum PPE recommended)

   - Avoid invasive procedure unless unavoidable

   - Maintain routine and safe labour practices

   - Implement strict infection prevention and control measures

   - Develop visiting policy based on expert advice and what is known about the infectious agent

   - Women should have access to support during labour if safe to do so

   - Allow mothers to stay with their new-born children and to breastfeed

3. *Caesarean sections*

   - Implement routine laboratory-based screening/testing of the infectious agent for all elective caesarean sections

   - Develop theatre protocols to minimise risk of infections between staff and staff and patients

   - Set aside dedicated theatre(s) for the management of positive cases or if not possible, strict risk reduction theatre management protocol

4. *Antenatal, post-delivery and high care wards*

   - Separate negative and positive antenatal and postpartum women

   - Identify an area that can be used to managed suspected cases/persons under investigation (PUIs)

Table 23.4 Reproductive services

1. *Family planning*
   - Continue to provide a range of contraceptive services to allow women to make choices
   - Family planning should provide closer to communities where practical possible
   - Promote self-care if safe to do so (self-administration of injectable contraceptives supported by virtual consultations)
   - Ensure a continued supply of all forms of contraceptive through strengthening of supply chain management
   - Promote use of reversible long-acting (Intrauterine contraceptive devices, IUCD or implants) as well as non-reversible method of family planning (male and female sterilisation)
2. *Termination of pregnancy (TOP) services*
   - Continue to provide both first and second trimester TOP in places where it is legal to do so
   - Use medical methods where possible and if acceptable to women seeking TOP services
   - Use virtual consultation platform to support TOP services

23.8 PSYCHOLOGICAL SUPPORT

An infectious outbreak causes excessive psychological distress to patients, health workers and the general population. Outbreaks destabilise social support structures and generate fear because of the loss of significant family members, colleagues and friends, lockdowns and the need to adhere to social distancing. The fear of infecting a family member is a special concern more especially among healthcare workers. This is in addition to the sense of vulnerability that is common during a pandemic.

All pandemic and disaster response plans should include detailed programmes on psychological support for patients, healthcare workers, families and communities. Part of the strategy would be to place psychological support teams in communities and at different levels of care. Healthcare workers with basic training in mental health can provide these services at a primary healthcare level and refer complex cases to the next level of care. All admitting healthcare facilities should have a mental health unit as part of their pandemic response plan. Similarly, health workers should have regular debriefings as well as mental health support as part of the employee wellness program.

23.9   VACCINATION

To date, vaccination remains the most effective public health strategy against infectious diseases and outbreaks. The importance of vaccination for at-risk groups and the general population, including non-pregnant women, is without dispute, however vaccination of pregnant women in the context of new pandemics will always be marred by controversies, partly because of the initial lack of evidence regarding safety of vaccination in pregnant women, including concerns regarding the effects of vaccines on the developing foetus. Drawing from available evidence, expert opinion and position statements from professional bodies worldwide, the following points are made (ACOG, 2021; Moodley et al, 2021; Poliquin et al, 2021; RCOG, 2021; SASOG, 2021):

- Pregnant women constitute a vulnerable group partly because of the physiological changes that occur during pregnancy.
- Drawing from the experience gained from previous and the current COVID-19 pandemic, pregnant women are more likely to experience severe forms of infection, related respiratory illness, require ICU care and also likely to die from the infection.
- Application of the risk-benefit framework provides a compelling argument to offer pregnant women vaccinations unless contraindicated on medical ground.
- In doing so, women should be counselled about the benefits, risks and uncertainties and be given enough information to enable them to make informed decisions (informed consent).
- Based on the above, COVID- 19 vaccines can be given to pregnant women in the absence of medical contraindications from 14 weeks to prevent excess COVID-19 related maternal deaths.

23.10 CONCLUSION

The threat of future pandemics is real. There is a need to build resilient health systems which can weather the storms. It is equally important to ensure that SRH services are included in pandemic management strategies, in particular, the provision of contraceptive and termination of pregnancy services as well as the continuity of antenatal and maternity care. Protection of healthcare workers should occupy centre stage in pandemic response plans as a large number of infected health workers will result in the collapse of the health system. This is possible through provision of adequate PPE, strict infection control practices and early vaccinations.

23.11 SELF-ASSESSMENT QUESTIONS

1. Which of the following is true regarding the increase in susceptibility of pregnant women to respiratory infections?
    A. Respiratory adaptation that occurs during pregnancy.
    B. Placenta acts as a reservoir for microorganism.
    C. Decrease in cellular immunity and respiratory adaptation that occurs in pregnancy.
    D. Decrease in cellular immunity that occurs during pregnancy.

2. With regard to vaccination, which of the following statement is true?
    A. Vaccination is always contraindicated in pregnancy.
    B. Pregnant women must sign a legal waiver should they request vaccination because of the medicolegal risks.
    C. Benefits must be weighed against the risk and women counselled accordingly.
    D. All known vaccines are teratogenic to the developing foetus.

23.12 REFERENCE

ACOG. 2020. Vaccinating pregnant and lactating women against Covid-19. Available at: https://www.acog.org/clinical/clinical-guidance/practice-advisory/articles/2020/12/vaccinating-pregnant-and-lactating-patients-against-covid-19#:~:text=ACOG%20recommends%20COVID-19%20vaccines,otherwise%20meet%20criteria%20for%20vaccination.

Adelekan, T., Mihretu, B., Mapanga, W., Nqeketo, S., Chauke, L., Dwane, Z. and Baldwin-Ragaven, L. 2020. Early Effects of the COVID-19 Pandemic on Family Planning Utilisation and Termination of Pregnancy Services in Gauteng, South Africa: March–April 2020. *Wits Journal of Clinical Medicine* 2(2), pp. 145–152. doi: https://doi.org/10.18772/26180197.2020v2n217.

Amorim, M.M.R., Soligo Takemoto, M.L. and Da Fonseca, E.B. 2020. Maternal deaths with coronavirus disease 2019: a different outcome from low- to middle-resource countries? *American Journal of Obstetrics and Gynecology* 223(2), pp. 298–299. doi.

Basu, J.K., Chauke, L. and Magoro, T. 2021. Maternal mortality from COVID 19 among South African pregnant women. *The Journal of Maternal-Fetal & Neonatal Medicine*, pp.1–3. doi: https://doi.org/10.1080/14767058.2021.1902501.

Bebell, L.M., Oduyebo, T. and Riley, L.E. 2017. Ebola virus disease and pregnancy: A review of the current knowledge of Ebola virus pathogenesis, maternal, and neonatal outcomes. *Birth Defects Research* 109(5), pp. 353–362. Available at: https://www.ncbi.nlm.nih.gov/pmc/articles/PMC5407292/.

Carlo, W.A. and Travers, C.P. 2016. Maternal and neonatal mortality: time to act. *Jornal de Pediatria* 92(6), pp. 543–545. doi: https://doi.org/10.1016/j.jped.2016.08.001.

Collin, J., Byström, E., Carnahan, A. and Ahrne, M. 2020. Pregnant and postpartum women with SARS-CoV-2 infection in intensive care in Sweden. *Acta Obstetricia et Gynecologica Scandinavica* 99(7), pp. 819–822. doi: https://doi.org/10.1111/aogs.13901.

Dahab, R. and Sakellariou, D. 2020. Barriers to Accessing Maternal Care in Low Income Countries in Africa: A Systematic Review. *International Journal of Environmental Research and Public Health* 17(12), p. 4292. doi: https://doi.org/10.3390/ijerph17124292.

Delamou, A., Ayadi, A., Sidibe, S., Delvaux, T., Camara, B.S., Sandouno, S.D., Beavogui, A.H., Rutherford, G.W., Okumura, J., Zhang, W.H. and De Brouwere, V. 2017. Effect of Ebola virus disease on maternal and child health services in Guinea: a retrospective observational cohort study. *The Lancet. Global health* 5(4), pp. e448–e457. doi: https://doi.org/10.1016/S2214-109X(17)30078-5.

Huntley, B.J.F., Huntley, E.S., Di Mascio, D., Chen, T., Berghella, V. and Chauhan, S.P. 2020. Rates of Maternal and Perinatal Mortality and Vertical Transmission in Pregnancies Complicated by Severe Acute Respiratory Syndrome Coronavirus 2 (SARS-Co-V-2) Infection. *Obstetrics & Gynecology* 136(2), pp. 303–312. doi.

Hussein J. 2020. COVID-19: What implications for sexual and reproductive health and rights globally? *Sexual and reproductive health matters* 28(1), p. 1746065. doi: https://doi.org/10.1080/26410397.2020.1746065.

Jamieson, D.J., Theiler, R.N. and Rasmussen, S.A. 2006. Emerging infections and pregnancy. *Emerging infectious diseases* 12(11), pp. 1638–1643. doi: https://doi.org/10.3201/eid1211.060152.

Jolivet, R.R., Moran, A.C., O'Connor, M., Chou, D., Bhardwaj, N., Newby, H., Requejo, J., Schaaf, M., Say, L. and Langer, A. 2018. Ending preventable maternal mortality: phase II of a multi-step process to develop a monitoring framework, 2016–2030. *BMC Pregnancy and Childbirth* 18(1). doi: https://dx.doi.org/10.1186%2Fs12884-018-1763-8.

Jones, S.A., Gopalakrishnan, S., Ameh, C.A., White, S. and Van den Broek, N.R. 2016. 'Women and babies are dying but not of Ebola': the effect of the Ebola virus epidemic on the availability, uptake and outcomes of maternal and newborn health services in Sierra Leone. *BMJ global health* 1(3), p. e000065. doi: https://doi.org/10.1136/bmjgh-2016-000065.

Kourtis, A.P., Read, J.S. and Jamieson, D.J. 2015. Pregnancy and Infection. *Obstetric Anesthesia Digest* 35(2), pp. 67–68. doi: https://doi.org/10/1097/01.aoa.0000463812.15481.00.

Kuehn, B.M. 2009. Pregnancy and H1N1 Flu. *JAMA* 301(24), p. 2542. doi: https://doi.org/0.1001/jama.2009.858.

Lin, H., Tambyah, P., Yong, E., Biswas, A. and Chan, S. 2017. A review of Zika virus infections in pregnancy and implications for antenatal care in Singapore. *Singapore Medical Journal* 58(4), pp. 171–178. doi: https://doi.org/10.11622/smedj.2017026.

McDougall, L., Sharma, A., Franz-Vasdeki, J., Beattie, A.E., Touré, K., Afsana, K., Boldosser-Boesch, A., Dare, L., Draganus, F., Eardley, K., Ruiz, C.G., Gronseth, L., Iversen, K., Kuruvilla, S., Marshall, A., McCallon, B. and Papp, S. 2015. Prioritising women's, children's, and adolescents' health in the post-2015 world. *BMJ*, 351(S1), pp. 60–70. Available at: https://www.bmj.com/content/bmj/351/bmj.h4327.full.pdf.

Molla, M., Mitiku, I., Worku, A. and Yamin, A.E. 2015. Impacts of maternal mortality on living children and families: A qualitative study from Butajira, Ethiopia. *Reproductive Health* 12(S1). Available at: https://www.ncbi.nlm.nih.gov/pmc/articles/PMC4423766/.

Moodley, J., Ngene, N. C., Khaliq, O. P. and Hunter, M. 2021. An imperative to offer pregnant and lactating women access to the COVID-19 vaccination roll-out programme. *South African Medical Journal* 111(6), pp. 567–569. Available at: http://www.samj.org.za/index.php/samj/article/view/13271.

NCCEMD. 2021. Saving Mothers and Babies 2017–2019: Executive Summary plus the Final Report on the use of maternal and reproductive health services and maternal and perinatal deaths in South Africa. Pretoria: National Department of Health, South Africa.

Pattinson, R.C. 2015. Safety versus accessibility in maternal and perinatal care. *South African Medical Journal* 105(4), pp. 261-265. doi: https:/::/doi.org/10.7196/samj.9182.

RCOG. 2021. Covid-19 vaccines, pregnancy and breastfeeding. Available at: https://www.rcog.org.uk/en/guidelines-research-services/coronavirus-covid-19-pregnancy-and-women-health/covid-19-vaccines-and-pregnancy/covid-19-vaccines-pregnancy - breastfeeding/#: ~:text=You%20should%20not%20stop%20breastfeeding,19%20vaccines%20will%20affect%20fertility.

Poliquin, V., Castillo, E., Boucoiran, I., Wng, J., Watson, H., Yudin, M., Money, D., Van Schalkwyk, J. and Elwood, C. 2021. SOGC statement on Covid-19 vaccination in pregnancy. Available at: Pdf.

Reed, H.E., Koblinsky, M.A., Mosley, W.H. and National Research Council (Estats Units D'amèrica), Committee On Population. 2000. *The Consequences of maternal morbidity and maternal mortality: report of a workshop*. Washington, Dc: National Academy Press.

Renfrew, M.J., Cheyne, H., Craig, J., Duff, E., Dykes, F., Hunter, B., Lavender, T., Page, L., Ross-Davie, M., Spiby, H. and Downe, S. 2020. Sustaining quality midwifery care in a pandemic and beyond. *Midwifery* 88, p. 102759. doi: https://doi.org/10.1016/j.midw.2020.102759. Estimates of the Potential Impact of the COVID-19 Pandemic on Sexual and Reproductive Health In Low- and Middle-Income Countries.

Riley, T., Elizabeth Sully, E. , Zara Ahmed , Z and Biddlecom A. (2020). International Perspectives on Sexual and Reproductive Health, pp74-76. https://www.guttmacher.org/sites/default/files/article_files/4607320.pdf.

Royal College of Obstetricians and Gynaecologists (2021). *COVID-19 vaccines, pregnancy and breastfeeding*. Available from: https://www.rcog.org.uk/en/guidelines-research-services/coronavirus-covid-19-pregnancy-and-womens-health/covid-19-vaccines-and-pregnancy/covid-19-vaccines-pregnancy-and-breastfeeding/.

Saleeby, E., Chapman, J., Morse, J.E. and Bryant, A. 2010. H1N1 Influenza in Pregnancy: Cause for Concern. *Obstetrics & Gynecology* 115(1), pp.185–186. Available at: https://pubmed.ncbi.nlm.nih.gov/19888049/.

SASOG. 2021. Covid-19 vaccination advice for pregnant and breastfeeding women. Available at: https://sasog.co.za/wp-content/uploads/2021/02/covid-19-vaccination-advice-pamphlet-28-Jan.pdf.

Sochas, L., Channon, A.A. and Nam, S. 2017. Counting indirect crisis-related deaths in the context of a low-resilience health system: the case of maternal and neonatal health during the Ebola epidemic in Sierra Leone. *Health Policy and Planning* 32(suppl_3), pp. iii32–iii39. Available at: https://academic.oup.com/heapol/article/32/suppl_3/iii32/4621472.

Takemoto, M.L.S., De O Menezes, M., Andreucci, C.B., Nakamura-Pereira, M., Amorim, M.M.R., Katz, L. and Knobel, R. 2020. The tragedy of COVID-19 in Brazil: 124 maternal deaths and counting. *International Journal of Gynecology & Obstetrics* 151(1), pp. 154–156. doi: https://doi.org/10.1002/ijgo.13300.

United Nations. 2015. Transforming governance for the 2030 agenda for sustainable development. Available at: https://sustainabledevelopment.un.org/post2015/trasnformingourworld/publiation.

United Nations (2021). COVID-19 pandemic has amplified the risks of vulnerable children to trafficking and sexual exploitation, Special Rapporteur on the sale of children tells Human Rights Council. https://www.ohchr.org/EN/HRBodies/HRC/Pages/NewsDetail.aspx?NewsID=26825&LangID=E.

Voo, T.C. and Capps, B. 2010. Influenza and the duties of healthcare professionals. *Singapore Med J* 51(4), pp. 275–281. Available at: http://www.smj.org/sites/default/files/5104ra1.pdf.

Westgren, M., Pettersson, K., Hagberg, H. and Acharya, G. 2021a. Severe morbidity and mortality associated with COVID-19: The Risk Should not be Downplayed. *Obstetric Anesthesia Digest* 41(2), pp. 58–59. doi: https://doi.org/10.1097/01.aoa.0000744020.14892.8e.

WHO. 2020. COVID-19: Operational guidance for maintaining essential health services during an outbreak, Interim guidance. Available at: https://apps.who.int/iris/bitstream/handle/10665/331561/WHO-2019-nCoV-essential_health_services-2020.1-eng.pdf?sequence=1&isAllowed=y.

WHO. 2016. *Guidance for Managing Ethical Issues in Infectious Disease Outbreaks.* Geneva, Switzerland, World Health Organization. Available at: https://apps.who.int/iris/handle/10665/250580.

CHAPTER 24

PANDEMICS AND THE SURGICAL DISCIPLINES

Prof Martin D Smith

Rachel Moore

24.1 INTRODUCTION: GLOBAL SURGERY

Access to safe and affordable surgical care is recognised as an 'indivisible part' of improving global healthcare (Debas et al., 2015). Historical misperceptions of the contribution of surgical care in achieving Universal Health Coverage (UHC) and the Sustainable Development Goals (SDG) has meant that not enough focus has been placed on the role of surgery. The appreciation of the role of surgery in global health and managing the unmet need for surgery has resulted from the development of a now widely recognised field of study, Global Surgery. Surgical providers have embraced this rapidly advancing field, which has resulted in a better understanding of how surgical systems can have a positive impact on UHC. Since 2015 a number of seminal publications and resolutions have highlighted the need to integrate surgical care into the Primary Health Care agenda. These include the Lancet Commission on Global Surgery (LCOGS) 2015 (Meara et al, 2015), the World Health Organisation (WHO) resolution 68.15 (WHO, 2014), and World Bank Disease Control Priorities 2015 (Debas et al, 2015). A wide range of role players, including policy makers, non-governmental players, and academics, have recognised that a systems approach to improving surgical care is required.

As stated by the South African Deputy Minister of Health in his keynote address at the National Forum for Global Surgery in 2015: '*This objective cannot be fully achieved without recognising the importance of the universal access to safe and affordable surgical and anaesthetic care. Hence it is imperative that improving access to surgery and anaesthetic care should be part of the global health agenda*' (Rayne et al, 2017). In most low- and middle-income countries (LMICs), progress in advancing this agenda is gaining traction and, in some of these countries, National Surgical, Obstetric and Anaesthesia Plans (NSOAPs) have been or are being developed. These initiatives are led by the health departments to drive the integration of surgical care into national health policies. To facilitate a more complete understanding of the current impact of the COVID-19 pandemic on surgical care, a more in-depth review of the pre-COVID-19 access to surgical care in South Africa is required.

Surgical care can cure or alleviate up to one-third of the global burden of disease. Robust surgical services have been recognised as an important component of health system strengthening and of achieving universal health coverage in South Africa. Access to safe, high-quality surgical care, when needed, especially for essential and emergency surgical conditions, has been inequitable even before the onset of the COVID-19 pandemic (Reddy et al, 2019). There are a number of metrics that reflect this inequity in access to surgical care as well as the extent of the unmet need in South Africa. Time to hospital care is one such metric (Meara et al, 2015), but while in South Africa, more than 96% of the population lives within two hours of a government hospital (Juran et al, 2018), the surgical services and the quality of surgical care available at these facilities is variable and lags behind global standards (Bishop et al, 2019). The global unmet need for surgical procedures was estimated at 143 million procedures annually (Meara et al, 2015). We do not know the extent of this gap in South Africa.

With the global burden of disease shifting towards non-communicable diseases (NCD), oncology services will need to be expanded to meet the growing need. An estimated 14.1 million new cancer cases occurred worldwide in 2012 (Torre et al, 2012), with more than 8 million of these occurring in LMICs. In addition, cancer cases in LMICs are projected to increase from 15% of the world's cancer burden in 1970 to an estimated 70% in 2030 (Economist Intelligence Unit, 2009).

The surgical workforce is a critical component of a functional healthcare system, and has also been studied in South Africa. Significant disparities were demonstrated in the number and distribution of general surgeons. There were 1.78 specialist general surgeons per 100 000 population, of which 0.69 specialist general surgeons per 100 000 population were working in the public sector. There were 2.90 non-specialist (medical officers) surgeons per 100 000 population. There were six specialist general surgeons per 100 000 insured population working in the private sector, which is comparable with the United States (Dell and Kahn, 2018). Surgical services, which include operative treatment of elective and emergency conditions, are hospital-based and often include the need for care in an Intensive Care Unit (ICU) or High Care Unit (HCU), especially post-operatively. South Africa has only 2.8 hospital beds per 1 000 persons and 0.8–0.9 ICU beds per 1 000 persons, compared to the United States which has 2.3–3.2 ICU beds per 1 000 persons (Dell et al, 2018).

24.2 OBJECTIVES

The objectives of this chapter are to:

- Contextualise surgery within a pandemic.
- Contextualise the pandemic within the concepts of Global Surgery and access to surgical care.
- Highlight human factor issues including risk stratification of patients and procedures; safety of healthcare professionals.
- Delivery of surgical services against the background of resource constraints and healthcare systems in the setting of a pandemic.
- Raises questions about the ethical delivery of surgical care during a pandemic.

24.3 SURGICAL SERVICES DURING COVID-19 PANDEMIC

Since early 2020, with the focus of health systems on managing the COVID-19 pandemic, the gains made in advocating for a Global Surgery approach have been under threat. Understandably, managing this infectious disease has had to become the central focus and mobilising health resources to combat the pandemic has been essential. As we move beyond the peak of the pandemic, the focus is shifting and the need for strategies to manage the 'reopening' of surgical care is required. The challenges faced before the COVID-19 pandemic have been exacerbated and the gaps in access to surgical care will have to be addressed. The pathological consequences of the novel coronavirus SARS-CoV-2 do not seem to need a surgical solution in itself, yet the pandemic has had a significant impact on surgical care. As of May 2020, almost 30 million elective procedures have been cancelled globally due to the pandemic. Many cancellations have been for benign conditions; however over 80% of cancer operations have been postponed, as well as a quarter of elective Caesarean sections (COVIDSurg Collaborative, 2020a). The collateral damage of reduction of surgical care worldwide will be great and will be felt for a significant time period.

The impact on surgical care has first been as a consequence of the necessary resource reallocation, including surgical workforce and hospital beds, and secondarily due to the impact that the virus has on patients undergoing surgical care, which has been shown to be associated with an increased morbidity and mortality when surgery is performed on infected patients (COVIDSurg Collaborative, 2020b). The third component is the need to ensure the safety of the health care professionals involved in the operations. Adequate personal protective equipment (PPE) and additional perioperative safety procedures are essential to prevent infections in the workplace (Brindle and Gawande, 2020).

The national response in South Africa to the pandemic through a number of phases of 'lockdown' has resulted in the delayed presentation of patients to healthcare facilities. Patients presenting with surgical problems are often sicker with more advanced diseases. This may be somewhat expressed in the rising 'unexpected deaths' reported during this time. In July 2020, there were 59% more deaths from natural causes than would have been expected based on historical data (South African Medical Research Council, 2020). In a survey conducted by the Association of Surgeons of South Africa (ASSA) (Chu et al, 2020), some participants noted that even though access to emergency surgical care was still available at their hospitals, fewer patients with emergency conditions were presenting than expected. This same reduction in health-seeking behaviour has been reported worldwide for non-surgical emergency conditions such as heart attacks and strokes (Krumholz, 2020).

Decisions regarding delaying of procedures have often been based on opinion or guidelines that are not based on good evidence and hence, through the best intentions, it is possible that many patients (particularly those with cancer) have had a delay in treatment with the consequent increase in disease stage (Spolverato, 2020). Several studies have supported the mandatory postponement of elective surgery (Aminian et al, 2020). For patients with cancer, case-by-case evaluation should be performed and surgery may be warranted, especially among patients in whom a delay would lead to negative long-term outcomes (e.g. those scheduled for diagnostic or therapeutic procedures) (Brindle and Gawande, 2020). In contrast, some have argued that among confirmed COVID-19 patients, only emergency and not elective surgery should be performed (Spolverato et al, 2020). The restrictions imposed during lockdown, including the impact of the ban on alcohol sales (and hence consumption) and curfews, have reduced the burden of the trauma epidemic well known to South Africans. Motor vehicle and pedestrian-vehicle accidents have reduced significantly and the pattern of interpersonal violence may have changed as well. What is not disputed is that the volume of trauma cases seen in emergency departments has decreased and thus facilitated the necessary shift in resources to the management of the COVID-19 pandemic. A two-month ban on alcohol sales has seen potentially 50 000 fewer trauma patients presenting at public hospitals (South African Medical Research Council, 2020).

The 'collateral damage' of hospital COVID 19 preparedness on non-COVID-19 activities has been noted by several authors, including the loss of elective operations and outpatient care. Pre-COVID-19 surgical services in the public and rural private sectors were already limited, and these increased barriers will lead to an increase in morbidity and mortality (Chu et al, 2020).

Accepting that some surgery is required and must be performed, a better categorisation of the need for care is required. The separation into only emergency and elective surgery are not adequate to allocate the scarce resources available for surgical care during the pandemic. The concept of an emergency procedure which, if delayed, will have significant consequences for the patient in the short term, is easily understood. The definition of elective surgery as procedures that have at best a quality of life impact (such as uncomplicated hernia or hip replacements) is also easily understood. Elective procedures, from a practical point of view, could be classified into two broad categories: essential and non-essential or discretionary. The latter alludes to purely elective procedures that are not time-sensitive from a surgical and/or medical perspective. The precise definition of essential surgery is still not well defined but broadly refers to operations that will prolong life; improve the quality of that life; and, if delayed, have a significant negative impact on the patient's outcomes. In the essential group are mostly NCDs such as cancer or vascular occlusions, with the impact of delaying or cancelling care being significant. As NCDs become a greater proportion of our burden of disease as a middle income country (MIC), and given the range of constraints imposed by the pandemic on resources, we as surgical care providers have a greater responsibility to ensure that we remain advocates for our patients and ensure that their needs are not ignored in the urgent preparations for the surges associated with COVID-19. Failure to operate on patients requiring essential surgery may also have a negative financial impact on patients, their families and their communities. While this may be a secondary consequence, it should still be factored into decision-making.

Key to determining what is essential surgery is the need to have significant physician discretion in determining the appropriate care for the individual patient and their disease process. When faced with external forces requiring difficult clinical decisions regarding delaying or cancelling operations, it is imperative that the treating physician retains some autonomy. There is a greater demand on the physician to advocate for the patient, yet broad guidelines are imperative to guide the decision-making process. A survey by ASSA showed that in the majority of hospitals (59 (69.4%)), surgeons were involved in the decision to de-escalate surgical services. At some facilities, surgeons are members of multidisciplinary committees to determine the urgency of specific procedures. In 77 (92.1%) hospitals, surgeons were involved in determining if an operation was considered urgent enough to be performed (Chu et al, 2020).

To implement essential surgery, it is imperative that this concept be understood and included in the development of guidelines. The evidence supporting surgical decision-making is often lacking due to the challenges faced in developing high-level evidence in surgery in general. This body of work is growing but the tenets of evidence-based medicine, which includes both best evidence and experience, must be followed and allow for the appropriate physician discretion. As such, in planning limited surgical services during the pandemic, the term essential surgery becomes more appropriate and relevant.

Decisions around the allocation of healthcare resources during a pandemic are complex and a multitude of factors need to be considered, including the burden of the disease, the availability of PPE, and the overall resources of the hospital to treat surgical and non-surgical conditions. As surgical care is 're-opened' and yet still limited by a number of issues, in particular the huge backlog that will aggravate the already significant unmet need for surgical care, there is a greater need to understand the consequences of prioritisation of surgical care. We have recently developed a tool that can be used as a calculator to more objectively determine the potential impact of operating on a patient who has COVID-19 infection or has the potential to contract the virus during their in-hospital stay.

Table 24.1 Factors to consider when scheduling surgery during the COVID-19 pandemic

1.	Safe re-introduction of surgery in the presence of community transmission of COVID-19 requires assessment of individual patient risk as well as health facility readiness.
2.	Surgery with co-existing COVID-19 infection poses an increased risk of morbidity and mortality and should be avoided for non-emergency surgery.
3.	Pre-operative COVID-19 testing should ideally be performed on all patients scheduled for non-emergency surgery and surgery postponed if positive (for at least 14 days after last day of symptoms or from test if asymptomatic).
4.	Where testing is not available or turnaround time is prohibitively long, patients with COVID-19 symptoms should be postponed for at least 14 days.
5.	For patients recovered from COVID-19 (> 14 days after last day of symptoms or from test if asymptomatic), assessment for COVID-19 sequelae is part of the risk evaluation. Routine repeat PCR testing is not recommended.
6.	Risk of concimitant and nonsocomial COVID infection should be discussed as part of the consent process.

Table 24.2 Risk scoring calculator

PART 1: Individual Patient Risk Score:

a) Patient Factors: Total ____ /30

		1	3	5	10
1	Age	<40	41-60	61-70	>70
2	Diabetes	None	Yes, well controlled	Poorly controlled	
3	BMI	<30	31-40	>40	
4	ASA Category	1-2 (Well/Mild systemic disease)	3 (Severe systemic disease)	4 (Systemic disease - threat to life)	
5	Functional capacity (Metabolic equivalents)	Engages in strenuous sporting activity (METS 10)	Climbs 2 flights of stairs/can jog (METS 4-9)	Walks on flat, light housework (METS <4)	

b) Disease Factors: Total ____ /30

		1	5	10
1	Non operative Mx	Not available	Available, poorer outcome	Available, similar outcome
2	2-week delay (impact on outcome)	Significant	Moderate	Minimal
3	3-month delay (impact on outcome)	Significant	Moderately	Minimal

c) Procedure Factors: Total: ____ /20

		1	3	5
1	Operating Time	< 60 mins	61 – 180mins	>180mins
2	Expected Post op care	General Ward	High Care Unit	Planned ICU post op
3	Type of Anaesthetic	Local/Regional	Possible GA	Planned GA
4	Ext length of Stay	<24 hrs	1 – 3 days	>4 days

Total Score a + b+ c = _____   (12-80) Patient Score to be plotted here   - with Pandemic Score Guidance

12	Proceed		⟷ Team Review ⟷		Postpone	80

PART 2: Facility Readiness – Pandemic Score
To be calculated weekly or monthly by designated hospital team

		1	3	5
1	Community COVID-19 numbers	Decreasing over 2/52	Plateau over 2/52	Increasing over 2/52
2	COVID Test Turn-around time	<48 hours	2 – 3 days	>3 days
3	Reallocation of Hospital Beds and Staff for COVID	Minimal/no reallocation	Significant reallocation	Majority of beds/staff reallocated
4	PPE	Adequate supplies	Rationed	Limited or uncertain availability

Pandemic Score: ____ /20

Guide for Pandemic Score (PS) Adjustment

PS Score 4-9

12	20	30	40	50	60	70	80

PS Score 10 - 15

12	20	30	40	50	60	70	80

PS Score >15

12	20	30	40	50	60	70	80

This guide is a working document from the NDOH Technical Working Group on COVID-19 and Surgery and is in the process of validation.
Clinical judgement and informed consent remain critical to the decision to proceed with surgery during the COVID-19 Pandemic. V² 26 August 2020

The literature is awash with case studies and guidelines indicating how this prioritising may occur. However, the evidence on which much of this is based is missing. The likelihood of this evidence emerging in the near future is limited. A recent search of the surgical literature reported that there were 59 COVID-19 original articles (8%). The great majority of articles were opinion articles (83.4%). Almost 40% of COVID-19 articles were published in the top 10 surgical journals (Slim et al, 2020). There have however been some useful observational studies such as the CovidSurg study published in *The Lancet* journal, which concluded that operating on patients with COVID-19 infection has up to a five-fold higher mortality rate. This study is based on multi-centre data, with some centres having enrolled as few as five patients. In this series, 75% of the procedures were classified as urgent and as such it is difficult to extrapolate this data to essential surgery.

The analysis was well done but the numbers were too small to make any firm conclusions (COVIDSurg Collaborative, 2020b), yet this is the best evidence we have. A study from Iran reported only four patients with a worse perioperative outcome (Aminian et al, 2020). As such, we do accept that unless required to save a life, surgery in COVID-19 positive patients should be delayed, with the major source of morbidity being pulmonary. However, we do not as yet know exactly how long we should delay surgery and under what circumstances the delay may be shortened or lengthened. Delaying surgery in patients who have had a severe physiological response has been recommended. The emerging evidence supporting a thrombotic component and the role of anticoagulants in improving survival has been valuable but has not answered the fundamental questions about the duration of the delay. The role of inflammatory mediators to mitigate the inflammatory response in the perioperative period is also unknown and thus, a risk-benefit ratio is very difficult to understand.

24.4 THE FUTURE

The current trend of COVID-19 indicates that this pandemic may continue longer than initially expected. Recently, the WHO has suggested that this virus may become just another endemic virus in our communities, similar to HIV, and it may never go away (Ghai, 2020). In the unfortunate but increasingly likely event of COVID-19 becoming endemic, will our current strategies remain relevant? The extent to which the 'epidemic' will then impact on surgical services remains unclear, but the current approach of postponing all elective surgery will have significant negative consequences for many individuals and will not be feasible.

As we begin to formalise the approach to surgical care, we need to bear in mind a number of key ethical questions. How does this affect long-term outcomes and does the short-term benefit outweigh the long-term risk? Is it possible to safely deliver the accepted standard of care in surgery? Based on the current evidence, when alternatives are available, what is the ethical justification for performing a substitute procedure? During the pandemic, how do we ethically offer the standard of care or alternatives? In answering these questions during a time of ethical upheaval, it is essential to use an ethical framework to guide decision-making. This allows a structured method of resolving conflicting moral duties. One such framework, initially proposed by Beauchamp and Childress in 1979, has formed the basis of healthcare ethics; with the four principles of patient care being beneficence, non-maleficence, respect for autonomy, and justice (Beauchamp and Childress, 1979). Even if the level of available evidence is poor and we do not have good guidelines to determine the best procedure or approach to the individual patient's needs, we can, at the very least, meet the obligations of beneficence and non-maleficence through only performing essential operations. The real impact of the pandemic on the unmet need is impossible to determine, making a utilitarian argument difficult to defend (Maclead et al, 2020).

During a global pandemic, most healthcare institutions will reach a point at which the department or discipline managing infected patients will become overwhelmed due to the magnitude of the case volume. When this stage is reached, it is imperative that other departments are actively involved in supporting the care of patients infected by the organism responsible for the pandemic (Wira et al, 2020). Without this support, patient care will be compromised; healthcare workers will experience high rates of burnout; and the healthcare systems both within the institution and within the community will be at risk of collapse. Despite the non-surgical nature of pandemics, specialist surgeons and surgical trainees have an important role to play in this situation. Although their focus is on surgical pathologies, they are first doctors and then specialists and as such, their responsibility is to the community as a whole. Surgeons also have a very good understanding of the importance of robust systems and thus have a critical role to play in the development of systems and pathways to strengthen care delivery.

Deployment of surgical staff to support the care of infected patients outside of the surgical areas is dependent on the ability of surgical departments to rationalise their services and restructure accordingly. It is advisable to formulate a plan for this restructuring early in the pandemic, i.e. before it is necessary, however the rapidly changing nature of a pandemic makes it difficult to formulate a detailed plan in advance. To illustrate this process, we now describe the approach taken by the Department of Surgery (DoS) at Chris Hani Baragwanath Academic Hospital (CHBAH) in response to the COVID-19 pandemic.

The DoS was able to support the initial hospital response to the pandemic without changing the existing departmental structure. However when the COVID-19 caseload increased exponentially at the beginning of July 2020, a rapid restructuring was necessary to allow deployment of surgical teams into the COVID-19 wards. In preparation for this, the DoS reviewed the literature and experiences of the global surgical community. From the start, the leadership of the DoS agreed that three principles were paramount when making changes:

1) frontline services (Trauma and Acute Care Surgery (ACS)) must be maintained;

2) the subspecialty units' core business must be protected; and

3) the interdepartmental COVID-19 staffing response should be collaborative, structured in teams and overseen by a central logistics group comprised of representatives from all clinical departments.

The restructuring of the DoS involved the following changes:

- decreasing the overall number of staff in the subspecialty units at all levels;

- leaving most senior registrars in their allocated subspecialty units to protect their training as far as possible (ensuring senior registrar exposure to their allocated subspecialty rotation);

- reducing the number of junior registrars, medical officers and interns in the subspecialty units to the minimum numbers necessary to maintain the core functions;
- redistributing the junior staff who were formerly in subspecialty units to either join the frontline service units (Trauma and ACS); or to be deployed to work in the COVID-19 areas of the hospital;
- forming consultant-led teams of surgical staff to deploy to the COVID-19 areas;
- allocating consultants from subspecialty units to support the ACS Unit (ACSU); and
- added support for the Trauma Unit once the lockdown level 4 and 5 restrictions on the sale of alcohol were lifted. The Trauma Unit at CHBAH is an internationally recognised training centre for surgical trainees and specialists, and under normal circumstances, service provision is supported by a significant number of clinicians from across the world. Travel and lockdown restrictions during the pandemic completely removed this cadre of healthcare professional from the Trauma Unit. Following the lifting of lockdown level 4 and 5 restrictions on the sale of alcohol, the burden of trauma patients presenting to CHBAH increased dramatically and thus the Trauma Unit required additional support from the DoS as a whole.

The already established ACSU was central to the success and relative ease of the rapid response of the DoS to the needs created by the COVID-19 pandemic. This Unit was launched in September 2018, but due to staffing constraints had not been able to function as a fully standalone unit in managing emergency general surgery patients and a complex system of support and calls was developed based on the previous Unit system of emergency calls. However, since its inception, much time and effort had been focused on developing and implementing sustainable systems in the Unit to maximise efficiency. Thus when the need for departmental restructuring arose, the ACSU provided a stable structure as the foundation for integration into the overall response. The effects of the precipitous increase of the COVID-19 caseload in the hospital in July 2020 was first experienced in the frontline spaces, with the very real potential for services to be overwhelmed and deteriorate into chaos. The surgical frontline services of the Trauma Emergency Unit and Surgical Emergency Unit (delivered by the Trauma Unit and ACSU, respectively) had pre-existing robust systems in place which allowed delivery of quality care to continue with only minor disruptions. The structured systems approach is intuitive to surgical thinking and thus experienced surgeons are a valuable part of a collective response to a pandemic.

The approach was premised on the understanding that this was a dynamic process and once implemented, the system must be flexible and accommodate either an increase or a decrease in the pandemic burden. This was an important undertaking in the process of achieving buy-in from all staff members of the DoS. Formal recognition was also given to the fact that change is generally uncomfortable, but especially so in the high-pressure setting of a global pandemic. Formal meetings with each group of junior doctors were held to discuss concerns and challenges, and a consultant working in the COVID-19 stream was designated as the contact person for on the ground issues. The group of senior surgeons that formulated the initial response plan remained the coordinators of the department's COVID-19 response and thus the initial point of contact for any issues or queries arising from this response. Outside the department, a senior DoS clinician along with a senior clinician from the Department of Internal Medicine coordinated the central staffing logistics group. This group met regularly using an online platform to keep all clinical departments updated as to the situation and needs in the COVID-19 areas, as well as to address issues as they arose. Restructuring of the bed allocation was also required to embrace the principle that all COVID-9 positive and persons under investigation (PUI's) would be managed in a geographically centralised area. As such, the DoS allowed the Department of Internal medicine to house and manage their non- COVID-19 patients in surgical wards. This process allowed the development of defined COVID-19 and non- COVID-19 areas within the hospital.

The positive impact of the support of the DoS for the COVID-19 wards was almost immediately recognised. Patient care improved; morale of colleagues in the Department of Internal Medicine improved due to the interdepartmental collaborative approach; after-hours cover of the COVID-19 wards was extended; and efficiency of the functioning of the COVID-19 wards improved.

The responsiveness of this group and the demonstration of concerns being addressed and changes being made as necessary were major factors in the relatively smooth establishment and functioning of the new system. From the beginning, it was recognised that stress and anxiety levels were high in most clinicians and, instead of being taken for granted, needed to be intentionally acknowledged. It was agreed that it was important that all members of the department should be allowed to continue taking planned leave and that there should be no restrictions on leave outside of usual departmental policy. Psychological support for healthcare professionals was also made available in the hospital.

There are multiple learning points that can be taken from this approach, but a few must be highlighted:

1) When a rapid response is necessary, canvassing opinions from all members of a large department before formulating a plan is neither practical nor possible. The process described above allows for input from all staff without sacrificing speed or responsiveness.

2) It is important for the human resource response from departments or disciplines outside those managing infected patients to be integrated into the overall pandemic response. The 'working together' ethos allows more functionality than a 'filling gaps' course of action.

3) Deploying teams rather than individuals reinforce an integrated response. The sense of cohesiveness within the department is improved and avoids the sense of being completely isolated from the home department or discipline.

4) Regular intentional communication is essential in sustaining a prolonged coordinated crisis response, both within the surgical department and between departments or disciplines.

5) Responsiveness to a rapidly changing situation and acknowledgement of stress and anxiety levels are key factors in securing buy-in for change from clinicians.

As the COVID-19 pandemic spread across the world, most countries took the decision to cancel all elective surgery (COVIDSurg Collaborative, 2020a). Initially, non-emergency surgeries were significantly curtailed during Level 5 lockdown, mostly due to COVID-19 infection-related staffing constraints, but as theatre capacity increased, it became clear that a systematic approach to allocation of list space was necessary. Two interventions were put in place in our hospital, which we strongly recommend and are applicable to all surgical settings.

The first was a so-called Theatre Vetting Committee. This group was made up of senior clinicians representing surgical and anaesthetic departments, the head theatre nurse, and a senior hospital manager. Their role was to review all elective surgeries booked to determine appropriateness of booking, and to allocate list space to ensure prioritisation as well as equity amongst various surgical departments. This committee met at the end of every day to review elective surgical lists booked for the following day.

The second intervention was the introduction of a COVID-19 Surgery Prioritisation Calculator developed by a technical working group established by the National Department of Health in South Africa (see above). This score guides the prioritisation of surgical operations, taking into account individual patient risk (patient, disease and procedure factors) and facility readiness (COVID-19 cases in the community, testing time, level of bed reallocation for COVID-19 patients, personal protective equipment (PPE) availability). The combination of the vetting committee and the prioritisation score allowed essential elective surgery to go ahead in an orderly fashion by using a logical, pragmatic and transparent process.

The timing of the reintroduction of non-essential surgery cannot be uniformly predicted as it is dependent on multiple variables which will differ both within and between countries. The surge capacity of a healthcare institution is influenced by its ability to create extra physical space to house patients, to procure sufficient equipment and consumables to meet the increased demand, to increase human resources across all areas of the hospital, and to adapt its management structure in response to the increased load on the facility (Felland et al, 2008). Once the surge of a pandemic has passed and surgical staff have returned to their home department, a structured approach to the resumption of non-essential surgery must be adopted. It is estimated that over 28 million surgeries would be cancelled due to the COVID-19 pandemic, with the vast majority of these being for benign diseases. In South Africa, this translates to at least 150 000 procedures that will need to be accommodated (Biccard, 2020).

A pivotal component of a healthcare institution's response to a pandemic is the ability to carry out accurate testing with a turnaround time of less than 24 hours. This is obviously important to facilitate management of symptomatic patients in appropriate areas in a hospital, but is equally important for asymptomatic patients requiring surgery (Van Waart et al, 2020). The operating theatre becomes a high-risk environment in a pandemic due to healthcare professionals working in close proximity to the patient and to each other in a confined space for prolonged time periods. Pandemics are caused by highly contagious agents thus it is imperative to mitigate the risk of transmission in the working environment and so protect healthcare professionals. Therefore patients booked for non-emergency essential surgery should have a recent negative test result (taken less than 48 hours prior to surgery) before undergoing surgery. In the initial phase of the COVID-19 pandemic, a polymerase chain reaction (PCR) of a nasopharyngeal swab was the mainstay of diagnosis. Computed tomography of the chest has high sensitivity in diagnosing COVID-19 and can be used as the primary diagnostic modality. However in the South African public health sector and in most LMICs, this is not a feasible option due to resource constraints in the healthcare system.

Although a lower priority in the initial response to a pandemic, the impact of a pandemic on the academic aspect of surgery and the surgical training of both undergraduate and postgraduate trainees has to be taken into account (Dedilia et al, 2020). The immediate and most obvious effect on registrar training was the reduction in operative case numbers in subspecialty units due to the cancellation of elective surgery. The negative effect of this in our setting was mitigated by the presence of a dedicated ACSU, which allowed redistribution of registrars from subspecialty units to the ACSU, which allowed greater exposure to 'true General Surgery' in a structured and consultant supervised fashion. Over the last two decades, the focus of postgraduate surgical training internationally has shifted away from traditional General Surgery towards subspecialty training. The cost of this in our local context was the perception amongst trainees that the management of patients presenting with general surgical pathologies was of lesser importance than of those presenting with subspecialty pathologies and should be assigned to junior trainees. It has been recognised worldwide that this is not true, as evidenced by the drive to create dedicated ACS services to give specialised surgical care to this unique group of patients with time-sensitive disease processes (Hameed et al, 2010). The COVID-19 pandemic highlighted this concept and emphasised the important role of the ACSU in registrar training.

Undergraduate training in the surgical disciplines was also affected by the COVID-19 pandemic. After a lengthy absence from the clinical setting, medical students in our institution returned to surgical units but a different approach to training had to be taken. The focus was on more comprehensive integration of students into surgical units than previously, with students learning in a service delivery model with informal 'on the job' teaching largely replacing formal tutorials and lectures. This addressed both academic and practical learning needs, ensured continuation of surgical services, and established physical safety of students and clinicians by doing away with the need to meet in large groups.

24.5 CONCLUSION

The nature of a pandemic is that it exposes and highlights pre-existing fault lines in healthcare systems, which may be addressed to some degree by the pandemic response. Unfortunately, this is not the case with regard to rescheduling surgeries cancelled as the initial pandemic response correctly focuses on increasing the surge capacity of healthcare systems. In South Africa and other LMICs, the challenge of rescheduling surgeries will be added to the pre-existing challenge of sub-optimally resourced surgical services, which translates to a significant unmet need in surgical care. Healthcare systems that were already pressurised before the COVID-19 pandemic will require considerable focus and ingenuity to address the backlog of delayed surgical operations.

24.6 SELF-ASSESSMENT QUESTIONS

1. What principles regarding Global Surgery are relevant to a pandemic response?

2. What are priorities to be considered when rationalising surgical services during a pandemic?

24.7 REFERENCES

Ai, T., Yang, Z., Hou, H., et al. 2020. Correlation of Chest CT and RT-PCR Testing for Coronavirus Disease 2019 (COVID-19) in China: A Report of 1014 Cases. *Radiology* 296(2), pp. E32-E40. doi: 10.1148/radiol.2020200642.

Aminian, A., Safari, S., Razeghian-Jahromi, A., Ghorbani, M. and Delaney, C.P. 2020. COVID-19 Outbreak and Surgical Practice: Unexpected Fatality in Perioperative Period. *Ann Surg* 272(1), pp. e27–e29. doi: 10.1097/sla.0000000000003925.

Beauchamp, T. and Childress, J. 1979. *Principles of biomedical ethics.* 1 ed. New York: Oxford University Press; 5 ed, 2001.

Biccard, B.C.L. Over 70% of surgeries in SA will be cancelled or postponed due to Covid-19 – how will we catch up? Available at: https://www.dailymaverick.co.za/article/2020-05-31-over-70-of-surgeries-in-sa-will-be-cancelled-or-postponed-due-to-covid-19-how-will-we-catch-up/.

Bishop, D., Dyer, R.A., Maswime, S., et al. 2019. Maternal and neonatal outcomes after caesarean delivery in the African Surgical Outcomes Study: a 7-day prospective observational cohort study. *The Lancet Global health* 7(4), pp. e513–e522. doi: 10.1016/s2214-109x(19)30036-1.

Brindle, E.M. and Gawande, A. 2020. Managing COVID-19 in Surgical Systems. *Ann Surg* 272(1), pp. e1–e2. doi: 10.1097/sla.0000000000003923.

Chu, K.M., Smith, M., Steyn, E., Goldberg, P., Bougard, H. and Buccimazza, I. 2020. Changes in surgical practice in 85 South African hospitals during COVID-19 hard lockdown. Vol 1102020.

COVIDSurg Collaborative. 2020a. Elective surgery cancellations due to the COVID-19 pandemic: global predictive modelling to inform surgical recovery plans. *BJS (British Journal of Surgery).* doi: 10.1002/bjs.11746.

COVIDSurg Collaborative. 2020b. Mortality and pulmonary complications in patients undergoing surgery with perioperative SARS-CoV-2 infection: an international cohort study. *The Lancet* 396(10243), pp. 27–38. doi: https://doi.org/10.1016/S0140-6736(20)31182-X.

Debas, H.T., Donkor, P., Gawande, A., Jamison, D.T., Kruk, M.E. and Mock, C.N. (Eds). 2015. *Essential Surgery: Disease Control Priorities, Third Edition (Volume 1).* Washington (DC): The International Bank for Reconstruction and Development / The World Bank.

Dedeilia, A., Sotiropoulos, M.G., Hanrahan, J.G., Janga, D., Dedeilias, P. and Sideris, M. 2020. Medical and Surgical Education Challenges and Innovations in the COVID-19 Era: A Systematic Review. *In vivo (Athens, Greece)* 34(3 Suppl), pp. 1603–1611. doi: 10.21873/invivo.11950.

Dell, A. and Kahn, D. 2018. Where are general surgeons located in South Africa? *South African Journal of Surgery* 56, pp. 12–20. Available at: http://www.scielo.org.za/scielo.php?script=sci_arttext&pid=S0038-23612018000100003&nrm=iso.

Dell, A., Kahn, D. and Klopper, J. 2018. Surgical resources in South Africa: an analysis of the inequalities between the public and private sector. *South African Journal of Surgery* 56, pp. 16–20. Available at: http://www.scielo.org.za/scielo.php?script=sci_arttext&pid=S0038-23612018000200006&nrm=iso.

Economist Intelligence Unit. Breakaway: The global burden of cancer – challenges and opportunities. 2009. Available at: http://graphics.eiu.com/upload/eb/EIU_LIVESTRONG_Global_Cancer_Burden.pdf..

Felland, L.E., Katz, A., Liebhaber, A. and Cohen, G.R. 2008. Developing health system surge capacity: community efforts in jeopardy. *Research brief* 2008(5), pp. 1–8.

Ghai, S. 2020. Will the guidelines and recommendations for surgery during COVID-19 pandemic still be valid if it becomes endemic? *Int J Surg* 79, pp. 250–251. doi: 10.1016/j.ijsu.2020.06.011.

Hameed, S.M., Brenneman, F.D., Ball, C.G., et al. 2010. General surgery 2.0: the emergence of acute care surgery in Canada. *Canadian journal of surgery Journal canadien de chirurgie* 53(2), pp. 79–83.

Juran, S., Broer, P.N., Klug, S.J., et al. 2018. Geospatial mapping of access to timely essential surgery in sub-Saharan Africa. *BMJ Global Health* 3(4), p. e000875. doi: 10.1136/bmjgh-2018-000875.

Krumholz, H.M. Where Have All the Heart Attacks Gone? 2020. *New York Times.* Available at: https://www.nytimes.com/2020/04/06/well/live/coronavirus-doctors-hospitals-emergency-care-heart-attack-stroke.html.

Macleod, J., Mezher, S. and Hasan, R. 2020. Surgery during COVID-19 crisis conditions: can we protect our ethical integrity against the odds? *Journal of Medical Ethics* 46(8), pp. 505–507. doi: 10.1136/medethics-2020-106446.

Meara, J.G., Leather, A.J., Hagander, L., et al. 2015. Global Surgery 2030: evidence and solutions for achieving health, welfare, and economic development. *Lancet* 386(9993), pp. 569–624. doi: 10.1016/s0140-6736(15)60160-x.

National Cancer Registry. Full Report. 2009. Available at: https://www.nicd.ac.za/centres/national-cancer-registry/.

Rayne, S., Burger, S., Straten, S.V., Biccard, B., Phaahla, M.J. and Smith, M. 2017. Setting the research and implementation agenda for equitable access to surgical care in South Africa. *BMJ Global Health* 2(2), p. e000170. doi: 10.1136/bmjgh-2016-000170.

Reddy, C.L., Makasa, E.M., Biccard, B, et al. 2019. Surgery as a component of universal healthcare: Where is South Africa? *South African Medical Journal* 109(9). Available at: http://www.samj.org.za/index.php/samj/article/view/12697.

Slim, K., Mattevi, C., Badon, F., Lecomte, C. and Selvy, M. 2020. The wave of "opinion articles" in the coverage of COVID-19 in surgical literature. *Langenbeck's Archives of Surgery* 405(6), pp. 877–878. doi: 10.1007/s00423-020-01932-w.

South African Medical Research Council. 2020. A 'relentless increase' in excess deaths from natural causes. Available at: https://www.medicalbrief.co.za/ archives/a-relentless-increase-in-excess-deaths-from-natural-causes-samrc/.

South African Medical Research Council. 2020. MRC modelling shows alcohol ban will cut trauma patients by 50,000. Available at: https://www.medicalbrief. co.za/archives/mrc-modelling-shows-alcohol-ban-will-cut-trauma-patients-by-50000/#:~:text=MRC%20modelling%20shows%20alcohol%20ban%20will%20cut%20trauma%20patients%20by%2050%2C000,-July%2015th%2C%20 2020&text=The%20MRC's%20modelling%20found%20the,and%20save%20 the%20government%20R1.

Spolverato, G., Capelli, G., Restivo, A., et al. 2020. The management of surgical patients during the coronavirus disease 2019 (COVID-19) pandemic. *Surgery* 168(1), pp. 4–10. doi: 10.1016/j.surg.2020.04.036.

Torre, L.A., Bray, F., Siegel, R.L., Ferlay, J., Lortet-Tieulent, J. and Jemal, A. 2012. Global cancer statistics. *CA Cancer J Clin* 65(2), pp. 87–108. doi: 10.3322/ caac.21262.

Van Waart, J., Matley, P. and Brand, M. 2020. Federation of Surgeons of South Africa consensus document for the resumption of elective surgery after level 5 COVID-19 "lockdown" period in South Africa. *South African Journal of Surgery* 58, pp. 61–63. Available at: http://www.scielo.org.za/scielo.php?script=sci_arttext&pid=S0038-23612020000200005&nrm=iso.

Wira, C.R., Goyal, M., Southerland, A.M., et al. 2020. Pandemic Guidance for Stroke Centers Aiding COVID-19 Treatment Teams. *Stroke* 51(8), pp. 2587–2592. doi: 10.1161/strokeaha.120.030749.

World Health Organization. 2014. Strengthening emergency and essential surgical care and anaesthesia as a component of universal health coverage. Report by the Secretariat. Available at: https://apps.who.int/gb/ebwha/pdf_files/EB135/B135 _3-en.pdf.

CHAPTER 25

SELF-ASSESSMENT QUESTIONS AND ANSWERS

The objective of this chapter is to allow the reader, the educator and the student to check his/her response to the short answer questions at the end of each of the previous 24 chapters in this book. Short answers have been provided as guidance. These can be used in assessments and can be expanded upon.

CHAPTER 1

1. What are some of the twenty-first-century risks for epidemics and pandemics?

Risks include trade, urbanisation and environmental degradation, and climate change.

2. Discuss some considerations for pandemic preparedness programmes for Africa.

Developing and improving health systems and the social determinants of health, should also target the informal sector if lives and livelihoods are to be saved. Social protection programs need to be expanded, access to health services ensured, and efforts towards achieving universal health coverage must be accelerated.

CHAPTER 2

1. Discuss the role of the Global Alliance for Vaccines and Immunisation with reference to its resource allocation and pricing of vaccines.

It primarily partners with and subsidises firms such as Pfizer, Johnson & Johnson, and GlaxoSmithKline (GSK). These firms have been known to charge premiums of up to 180% for their vaccines.

2. Discuss some of the country level deficiencies which contributed to the spread of COVID-19 globally.

Deficiencies in international surveillance and diagnostics capabilities contributed to the rapid global spread of COVID-19. Many countries lacked the infrastructure for both surveillance and testing capacities necessary to identify and prevent widespread outbreaks. Other causes include neglectful leadership and supply chain deficiencies and technical limitations on appropriate diagnostics, both in quality and efficacy.

CHAPTER 3

1. What are the benchmarks in the framework based on African indigenous values that guide prioritisation of COVID-19 vaccines?

Affirming the humanity of others, survival of communities, social solidarity, and meaningful community engagement.

2. Discuss some of the challenges to professionalism in healthcare during pandemics.

Fear, misinformation and a detachment from one's calling challenge professionalism even more strongly during pandemics. Further compounding the challenge is that even a caring response may not always translate into pragmatic ends.

CHAPTER 4

1. Discuss the legal protection of workers during pandemics.

The law in most countries usually protects workers who have a constitutional and statutory right to a working environment that is not harmful and which threatens their health and safety. Mandatory vaccination for South African health care workers, as happened in Italy would pass constitutional muster as a reasonable and justifiable limitation on the right to freedom and security of the person. The reason for this is that such limitation would be regarded as rational and proportional considering the significance of the reason for the limitation, which is public health. Since health care workers are most likely more exposed to potential COVID-19 infection, it would be in both their interests, as well as those of other patients, to require that they are vaccinated.

2. Why is consent not a legal requirement for autopsies during pandemics?

In South Africa deceased persons are not protected by the Constitution and only partially protected by the common-law crime of interfering with a corpse and statute law governing the removal of tissue (National Health Act, 2003). Hence, consent and the need for consent to autopsies may be dispensed with altogether under the common-law doctrine of 'necessity' (Neethling et al, 2001) during pandemics.

CHAPTER 5

1. What are the specific ethical principles requiring special attention during pandemics?

Scientific Validity and Social Value; Distributive Justice: Equitable Distribution of Risks and Benefits; Emergency Use of Investigational Interventions; Safety and Risks; Informed Consent; Building Trust: Community Consultation and Engagement; Research Ethics Review and Oversight.

2. Name the four principles of the SAN Code of Research Ethics.

Respect, honesty, fairness and care.

CHAPTER 6

1. What does the public think of the news media's reporting on COVID-19?

Although surveys show that the public mostly feels that journalists have done a relatively good job of informing them about COVID-19, the results are contradictory. One poll, conducted in the United States, found that 70% of respondents believed that the news media either did 'a very or somewhat well' job of covering the new coronavirus. But at the same time, about four-in-ten also said the journalists had greatly exaggerated the risks associated with SARS-CoV-2 (Pew Research Centre, 2020). Similarly, a poll that was run in the United Kingdom showed 56% of people there believed news coverage had enhanced their understanding of COVID-19, but simultaneously more than a third said news coverage made the crisis worse (Nielsen, Kalogeropoulos and Fletcher, 2020). In both studies, political affiliations strongly influenced respondents' opinion of the news media's performance: participants who supported conservative parties were far more likely than those who identified with progressive parties to say that the news media performed badly.

2. Has the news media helped scientists to identify gaps in pandemic responses?

In the Bay area in the United States, journalists noticed that sports teams, such as basketball teams, were having in-door practises after larger gatherings in enclosed areas had been restricted. They asked scientists and policymakers in the area to comment on the issue (on whether smaller groups such as sports teams also faced a high infection risk), which brought the matter to their attention. As a result, restrictions were put on sports practises. 'These issues came from journalists identifying the problems, asking the academics to comment on them — the relationship between scientists and journalists has to be hand in glove' (Swartzberg, 2020).

CHAPTER 7

1. What role does leadership play in the achievement of dynamic capabilities in the public health system?

The dynamic capabilities approach emphasises continuous organisational learning as an approach for public sector organisations facing complexity. It requires that leaders are highly skilled, understand the relevant public sector organisation's public value mission and can set up processes of continuous strategy development and implementation at all management levels. Poor leaders centralise processes and decisions, stifle spaces for innovation and penalise experimentation. Such organisations are therefore unable to learn and adapt when facing complexity.

2. What features of the dynamic capabilities approach generate continuous improvement in public sector organisations?

Public health organisations, including departments, regulators and health services, face extreme complexity and contexts of continuous and rapid change. They therefore need to be able to continuously adapt. This requires the institutionalisation of processes of innovation, learning and feedback, which entails decentralisation of decision-making together with processes that enhance rather than diminish trust. Experimentation requires space to try and fail without penalties. With discretion comes the risk of a deviation from mission. Well-designed corporate governance approaches are therefore essential to avoiding capture, selecting highly skilled senior executives and keeping management on mission and avoiding corruption.

CHAPTER 8

1. What advances to PPE are needed to enhance effectiveness?

There has been much uncertainty on the types of PPE items (especially masks) needed or worn by HCPs, essential workers or communities. Further progress is needed to address mainly the confounding variables to enhance PPE effectiveness. This includes testing alternative PPE interventions that includes variation in PPE types or fits, measuring compliance and hand hygiene, assessing contamination levels, the duration and intensity of exposure variability among patients and HCPs as well as susceptibility on dispersing infectious particles post-recovery. In addition, addressing the confounding variables in PPE testing interventions is also crucial in terms of more robust study designs to avoid bias, account for confounders, measure modes of transmission, increasing study power and measure infection accurately to ensure the role of PPE is optimised during pandemics.

2. What are the key areas of PPE research that should be strengthened?

A more integrated and longitudinal approach to PPE research is needed (even between pandemics) which addresses the continuum from the basic sciences to policy research that translates into making improvements. This approach will ensure that new concepts derived from the basic sciences are explored while also making the result translatable to real-world settings. Active collaboration is needed among scientists and clinicians involved in PPE research to build new PPE concepts via the basic sciences (i.e. design, quality, reusability, repurposing and safety), proof of concept via the clinical sciences (i.e. efficacy and effectiveness testing) and standard of practice via policy and regulatory sciences (i.e. to derive new models for disease reduction in populations).

CHAPTER 9

1. Why is it important to address the SDH?

The SDH are the conditions in which people are born, grow, live, work and age, which in turn are shaped by the distribution of money, power and resources at global, national and local levels. The SDH are responsible for these health inequities, which are unfair and avoidable.

2. What action is needed to address the SDH and health inequities during pandemics?

Government has an important stewardship role in maximising the public good. Pandemics provide the opportunity to introduce legislation to redress the historical fault-lines in society. Examples of laws are those that prioritise early childhood development, education, protect the natural environment, mitigate climate change, and achieve equitable health systems.

3. What are the priority research areas on SDH and health equity?

Research is needed to analyse the impact of the different SDH (e.g. socioeconomic position, structural factors, such as climate change, environmental threats, impact of colonialism and racism, etc.) on the health status of populations. There is also the need for research on the specific policy actions to improve health status and to reduce inequities.

CHAPTER 10

1. What are some of the psychological effects that are experienced within populations during pandemics?

Increased levels of bodily and health awareness, help-seeking behaviours, anxiety and depression, compassion fatigue, burnout, substance abuse, interpersonal violence, and stigmatisation.

2. What are some of the interventions and strategies that can be employed to mitigate the psychological sequelae of pandemics for populations?

Developing an awareness of the differential vulnerabilities across populations; developing appropriate psychosocial referral networks; upskilling practitioners in appropriate therapeutic modalities; building social cohesion through community interventions to offset the effects of stigmatisation; providing sound and timely information through communication strategies to dispel myths and reduce anxiety and uncertainty; ramping up health and mental health systems to avoid burnout and compassion fatigue; and implementing policy measures proactively to ensure adequate funding/resourcing of appropriate psychosocial and health services.

CHAPTER 11

1. How was the South African government's economic response during the COVID-19 pandemic different to that of developed countries globally?

Unlike most developed countries whose macroeconomic response to COVID-19 was to follow expansionary fiscal and monetary policy, South Africa adopted a programme of austerity, which limited the government's ability to implement counter-cyclical measures to boost the level of economic activity and protect households and economic infrastructure. Though some stimulus measures were followed, these were much too limited for an effective response to the deleterious effects of the pandemic on the economy.

2. What are the two serious failures of not integrating health considerations with economic imperatives, in particular, during a pandemic?

From the perspective of South Africa's experience, the lack of integration has caused permanent scarring of the economy, with a significant increase in unemployment and an undermining of key parts of the economic infrastructure in the long term. Moreover, health challenges themselves are further accentuated.

CHAPTER 12

1. What are the three types of knowledge indicated by Kereluik et al (2015) that were embedded in the Lived 21st Century Learning Framework: Learning Through a Pandemic?

Foundational, meta and humanistic knowledge

2. What pragmatic approach to assessment emerged during the pandemic?

Programmatic assessment

CHAPTER 13

1. Define eHealth and list the six broad areas in which it can be used to address the impacts of epidemics and pandemics.

eHealth is the use of information and communication technologies for health, and it can address epidemics and pandemics by impacting policy, process, and practice in information, clinical, administrative, research, education and surveillance areas.

2. The COVID-19 pandemic has led to an unparalleled increase in the practice of telemedicine – medical service provided remotely using information and communication technologies (ICT). What are some of the reasons for this?

Necessity: the need to overcome problems related to the protection of patients and providers from infection while providing services (triage, diagnosis and management, follow-up).

Relaxation of existing legal, regulatory, and ethical guidelines and requirements permitting broader use of telemedicine.

New approaches to remuneration for telemedicine.

The ubiquity of relatively simple and low-cost ICT solutions.

CHAPTER 14

1. What are some of the comorbidities included in the Gauteng Department's datasets?

The data sets from the GDoH contain comorbidities as an index of vulnerability that covers comorbidities relevant to COVID-19. These include diabetes, hypertension, emphysema, bronchitis, asthma, pneumonia, heart disease, stroke, HIV/AIDS and tuberculosis.

2. Why is the Google Mobility Report useful?

The Google Mobility Report data is useful to understand the geo-spatial movement of people during the pandemic. Movement trends of people over time and over different categories of places are tracked. The report contains three location categories namely: retail, recreation, groceries, pharmacies, parks, transit stations, workplaces, and residential. These indicators provide a valuable resource for understanding how people interact with different types of locations. All of the Google Mobility indicators have the same overall trend with minor differences except for the residential, which has an almost opposite behaviour due to the increased numbers of people staying in their homes as a result of the pandemic.

CHAPTER 15

1. Which technologies for COVID-19 vaccines were unproven before 2020?

The two technologies are the use of ribonucleic acid (RNA) and non-replication viral vectors for vaccine development. No vaccine licensed before 2020 used any of these technologies. COVID-19 RNA vaccines use genetic instructions, in the form of RNA for a coronavirus protein that prompts an immune response. A non-replicating viral vector COVID-19 vaccine uses a chemically weakened virus (such as the adenovirus) which is genetically engineered to produce coronavirus proteins in the body.

2. What is vaccine hesitancy, and how might it affect containment of spread of the virus for COVID-19?

Vaccine hesitancy refers to the reluctance to accept vaccines, despite the availability of vaccination services. Vaccine hesitancy poses significant risks not only for the hesitant people but also the wider community, as it makes communities unable to reach thresholds of coverage necessary for containment of spread of the virus.

CHAPTER 16

1. How has the COVID-19 pandemic been handled in sub-Saharan Africa?

Despite the health systems being underprepared for the COVID-19 pandemic, most countries directed efforts and resources towards controlling the spread of the virus. This is observed by the formation of task forces and the imposing of country lockdown measures as earlier discussed. All these have been done in the effort to prevent virus transmission.

In South Africa, however, there are suggestions that measures were put in place a little too late and would have been tailor-made to fit the country's economy. This is evidenced in the increase in the unemployment rate and this might have led to higher morbidity from ailments other than COVID. Additionally, there is a notion that the lockdown measures were negligible as the second wave had more impact in terms of the number of new cases and COVID related mortality.

2. What is the way forward for COVID-19 management in sub-Saharan Africa?

Currently, most countries have relaxed on the country lockdown measures mostly to recover from the declined economies. The focus has now diverted to prevention by reaching out to as many people of the population with the COVID-19 vaccines while reinforcing all other known public health interventions such face masks, social distancing, avoiding massive gatherings, etc. The effort to vaccinate a larger part of the population is to allow for heard immunity to take effect and ultimately reduce continued spread of the virus in the population.

CHAPTER 17

1. List the key technical requirements for a successful hospital surveillance system to monitor the COVID-19 pandemic in South Africa

The South African response to COVID-19 required rapid and decisive action towards an innovative, creative, flexible, secure and user-friendly hospital surveillance system with real-time data availability to monitor the epidemic and guide interventions.

2. Describe some key outcomes of the DATCOV hospital surveillance system during the COVID-19 pandemic in South Africa.

The data has been used to inform hospital resource needs and to identify hospitals with higher case fatality rates which require additional support. DATCOV provided insight during the second wave of COVID-19 when the new variant 501Y. V2 predominated, with high volumes of admissions and an increased in-hospital mortality rate. Through DATCOV, risk factors for morbidity and mortality were identified, including an increased risk for COVID-19 mortality if HIV co-infected. Such information is critical for guiding the prevention of COVID-19 in vulnerable groups and for appropriate clinical monitoring of infected persons for interventions, including vaccine prioritisation. Analysis of COVID-19 in special groups such as children, pregnant women and people living in care homes has informed guidelines and best practices for prevention, early alerts and care. Data has been used for reproductive rate modelling and also to describe 'Long COVID' sequelae.

CHAPTER 18

1. What are the common neuropsychiatric manifestations of COVID-19?

- Delirium, mood, anxiety, psychotic disorders in children and adults
- Neurocognitive impairment is increasingly being recognised
- Causes range from direct pathophysiological mechanisms to contextual and psychosocial reactions to the infection as well as socioeconomic impact.

2. What important public mental health solutions can one consider when managing pandemics?

- Telemedicine, adapting medical education/curriculae, psychosocial support for frontline healthcare workers;
- A consideration for adaptation of therapeutic modalities to suit specific needs at the time is important; and
- The use of technology.

CHAPTER 19

1. In what ways does a COVID-19 pandemic directly and indirectly affect access to primary healthcare services?

COVID-19 can directly infect staff members and patient alike. Patients may not easily assess normal chronic services, as they battle with COVID-19 (and are at greater risk of poorer prognosis with comorbidities). Facilities may even close, due to lack of staff and/or cleaning/fumigation (often not evidenced-based). Lockdown levels impact public transport to access the PHC facility. COVID-19 results in a weaker economy resulting in less disposable income for over-the-counter medications and/or medical aid cover. The anxiety around COVID-19 may reduce clinic visits. For groups who are marginalised already (e.g. migrants, disabled), these factors accentuate the existing difficulties accessing care.

2. Explain what is meant by the phrases 'agility of response' and 'continuity of care' with respect to the value that a field hospital may provide to a COVID-19 referral hospital

'Agility' with which clinicians may respond to patients' clinical progression (improvement/deterioration) with up/down referral accordingly. The approach favours the lower-acuity patient, and/or patients with more certain prognosis (e.g. step-down vs PUIs), where there is less risk of deterioration. It is of greater assistance if it is geographically close to parent/referring facilities.

The critical resources by which to manage to ensure 'continuity of care' is time and bed space. It operates as an auxiliary service receiving down-referred patients, whether or not operating separately to a parent. This provides capacity to continue lower-acuity care under less time pressures, by transfer from regional/tertiary COVID wards. It may also facilitate on-referral from PHC to secondary/tertiary, through temporary admission, in select circumstances.

CHAPTER 20

1. Name the six crucial elements when addressing pandemic management.

Staff, stuff, space, systems, support and sustainability.

2. How is critical care defined?

Critical care is a state of ill health in which vital organ dysfunction is present and where a high risk of imminent death exists. It is the most severe form of acute illness due to any underlying disorder and results in millions of deaths globally annually.

CHAPTER 21

1. What is a pandemic? Why is it important to understand the dynamics of pandemic diseases?

A pandemic is defined as an outbreak that spreads quickly into larger geographic areas crossing international borders.

Planning and preparation are important in risk mitigation as new infections tend to spread rapidly. Understanding the dynamics of the pandemic affects what interventions are applied. Transmission can be interrupted in any of the four phases of the pandemic – measures must be put in place to control the pandemic in the initial stages of the outbreak when there is localised transmission, rather than waiting for it to amplify into an epidemic or pandemic.

Early interventions are important as healthcare systems come under great strain during a full-blown pandemic as resources are moved to the management of the real-time emergency. Healthcare workers, equipment, and drugs are relocated to respond to the emergency and this affects basic and essential health services.

2. Why is it important to manage other infectious diseases during a pandemic?

Many countries, especially low-income and middle-income countries, have made substantial progress in reducing their burden of TB, HIV/AIDs, malaria, antimicrobial resistance, and improving their immunisation programmes against major childhood infections. Rates of these issues are extremely high and put a major strain on the already overwhelmed healthcare system. Interruptions in their control programmes during a pandemic could result in major setbacks, compounding the direct impact of the pandemic.

When planning, the risk mitigation process needs to look at the strengthening of health systems, service delivery, human resources, diagnostics, and delivery of medical supplies not only for the pandemic infection but also to minimise adverse indirect impacts on these infectious disease issues in addition to the pandemic.

CHAPTER 22

1. What is MIS-C?

The most serious paediatric complication of COVID-19. It is a syndrome similar to Kawasaki Disease, a rare vasculitis occurring in children with an unknown aetiology, that causes coronary artery aneurysms.

2. How should babies born to mothers with COVID-19 be managed?

Babies should remain with their mothers, and breastfeeding should be encouraged.

CHAPTER 23

1. Which of the following is true regarding the increase in susceptibility of pregnant women to respiratory infections?

   A. Respiratory adaptation that occurs during pregnancy

   B. Placenta acts as a reservoir for microorganism

   C. Decrease in cellular immunity and respiratory adaptation that occurs in pregnancy

   D. Decrease in cellular immunity that occurs during pregnancy

ANSWER: D

2. **With regard to vaccination, which of the following statements is true?**

   A. Vaccination is always contraindicated in pregnancy
   B. Pregnant women must sign a legal waiver should they request vaccination because of the medicolegal risks
   C. Benefits must be weighed against the risk and women counselled accordingly
   D. All known vaccines are teratogenic to the developing foetus

ANSWER: C

CHAPTER 24

1. **What principles regarding Global Surgery are relevant to a pandemic response?**

   • Surgical care can alleviate up to 1/3 of the global burden of disease, thus access to safe and affordable surgical care should be maintained.
   • Robust surgical services are an important component of health systems that are necessary to achieve universal health coverage by allowing access to safe, high-quality surgical care.

2. **What priorities are to be considered when rationalising surgical services during a pandemic?**

   • Concept of essential surgery rather than emergency vs elective categorisation.
   • Impact of cancelled surgeries once full surgical services are 'reopened'.
   • Physical safety of healthcare workers.
   • Awareness of burnout and mental health repercussions in healthcare workers.

INDEX

Page references in italics refer to tables, graphs and figures.

www.ingramcontent.com/pod-product-compliance
Lightning Source LLC
Chambersburg PA
CBHW061738210326
41599CB00034B/6724